Dr. Peter Scardino's
PROSTATE
BOOK

AVERY

a member of Penguin Group (USA) Inc.

New York

Dr. Peter Scardino's
PROSTATE BOOK

The Complete Guide to Overcoming

Prostate Cancer, Prostatitis, and BPH

2ND EDITION

PETER T. SCARDINO, M.D.,

and

JUDITH KELMAN

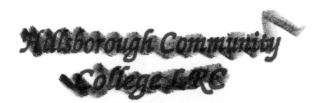

Published by the Penguin Group

Penguin Group (USA) Inc., 375 Hudson Street, New York, New York 10014, USA • Penguin Group (Canada), 90 Eglinton Avenue East, Suite 700, Toronto, Ontario M4P 2Y3, Canada (a division of Pearson Penguin Canada Inc.) • Penguin Books Ltd, 80 Strand, London WC2R 0RL, England • Penguin Ireland, 25 St Stephen's Green, Dublin 2, Ireland (a division of Penguin Books Ltd) • Penguin Group (Australia), 250 Camberwell Road, Camberwell, Victoria 3124, Australia (a division of Pearson Australia Group Pty Ltd) • Penguin Books India Pvt Ltd, 11 Community Centre, Panchsheel Park, New Delhi—110 017, India • Penguin Group (NZ), 67 Apollo Drive, Rosedale, North Shore 0632, New Zealand (a division of Pearson New Zealand Ltd) • Penguin Books (South Africa) (Pty) Ltd, 24 Sturdee Avenue, Rosebank, Johannesburg 2196, South Africa

Penguin Books Ltd, Registered Offices: 80 Strand, London WC2R 0RL, England

Most Avery books are available at special quantity discounts for bulk purchase for sales promotions, premiums, fund-raising, and educational needs. Special books or book excerpts also can be created to fit specific needs. For details, write Penguin Group (USA) Inc. Special Markets, 375 Hudson Street, New York, NY 10014.

Library of Congress Cataloging-in-Publication Data

Scardino, Peter T.
[Prostate book]
Dr. Peter Scardino's prostate book : the complete guide to overcoming prostate cancer, prostatitis, and BPH / Peter T. Scardino and Judith Kelman.—2nd ed.
p.   cm.
Includes bibliographical references and index.
ISBN 978-1-58333-393-8 (alk. paper)
1. Prostate—Popular works.   I. Kelman, Judith.   II. Title.   III. Title: Prostate book.
RC899.S28   2010   2010012311
616.99'463—dc22

Printed in the United States of America
5   7   9   10   8   6

Book design by Meighan Cavanaugh

Neither the publisher nor the authors are engaged in rendering professional advice or services to the individual reader. The ideas, procedures, and suggestions contained in this book are not intended as a substitute for consulting with your physician. All matters regarding your health require medical supervision. Neither the authors nor the publisher shall be liable or responsible for any loss or damage allegedly arising from any information or suggestion in this book.

While the authors have made every effort to provide accurate telephone numbers and Internet addresses at the time of publication, neither the publisher nor the authors assume any responsibility for errors, or for changes that occur after publication. Further, the publisher does not have any control over and does not assume any responsibility for author or third-party websites or their content.

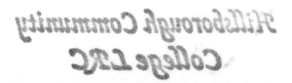

To the new generation: Cecilia, Lillian, Caroline, Ryan, Gus, Lucy, John, and Caroline. May cancer become a distant memory within your lifetime.

To all the dedicated, talented, caring professionals at Memorial Sloan-Kettering Cancer Center, an extraordinary institution devoted to finding the cause of and cure for cancer. We are fortunate to work in an environment where the only limitation to the good we can do is our own energy and imagination.

To all the patients and their families whose courage has been a constant source of wonder and whose insightful questions inspired this book.

And to Uri Herscher and Bill Tully, who helped us make our collaboration permanent and official.

ACKNOWLEDGMENTS

This book is not intended to offer one doctor's point of view. To provide comprehensive, up-to-date information, we sought the help of top medical experts, scientists working in cutting-edge research, nurses, and many patients and their loved ones who have experienced these problems themselves. The authors wish to thank the following for their thoughtful, generous input.

Memorial Sloan-Kettering Cancer Center urologists Drs. James Eastham, Bertrand Guillonneau, Vincent Laudone, Karim Touijer, Brett Carver, and Jonathan Coleman provided countless insights from their vast experience in caring for patients with prostate cancer.

Dr. Howard Scher leads the team of superb medical oncologists who have pioneered the treatment of prostate cancer with new hormones and other drugs. He and Dr. Michael Morris provided valuable perspectives on advanced prostate cancer.

Drs. Zvi Fuks and Michael Zelefsky, pioneers in the development of modern radiation oncology, offered many helpful suggestions about radiation therapy and its complications.

Dr. Victor Reuter contributed his insights as one of the world's leading experts in genitourinary cancers. Dr. Hedvig Hricak, an outstanding radiologist who virtually invented MRI of the prostate, added greatly to our understanding of modern medical imaging and its applications to prostate cancer.

Dr. Hans Lilja, who discovered "free" PSA, and Dr. Andrew Vickers, a brilliant statistician, have greatly expanded our understanding of the relationship between PSA and diseases of the prostate. Dr. Michael Kattan, a wizard of medical informatics, offered many insights on decision-making and those invaluable predictive tools: nomograms.

Research in prostate cancer has made enormous strides in the past five years, in no small part as a result of the contributions of Drs. Charles Sawyers, James

Allison, and Neal Rosen. Their work has heavily influenced our understanding of prostate cancer and its treatment.

Dr. Andrew Roth shared with us his insights into the emotional and psychiatric problems of prostate cancer patients and their partners. Gastroenterologist Dr. Moshe Shike provided valuable advice about the treatment of intestinal complications of radiation therapy for prostate cancer. Dr. Jaspreet Sandhu helped us better understand the diagnosis and treatment of urinary problems, and Dr. John Mulhall, who has written his own book on the sexual complications of prostate diseases, generously shared his expertise. Dr. Barrie Cassileth, a leading thinker in alternative and complementary medicine with an exhaustive up-to-date website about herbs, botanicals, and other products, offered the latest scientifically grounded information.

We are especially grateful to Mary Schoen, N.P., an extraordinary nurse practitioner, who understands so well the long-term burden of prostate cancer and its treatment. Christine DePierro and Alison Costalos, brilliant nurse practitioners, shared countless important observations and practical suggestions. We are also grateful to Dr. E. Darracott Vaughan of Weill Cornell Medical College of Cornell University for his wise counsel and his insights about BPH. Thanks to Dr. Anthony Schaeffer of Northwestern University, one of the country's leading experts on prostatitis, for offering his up-to-date views on a difficult field. Many of the staff at Memorial Sloan-Kettering Cancer Center (MSKCC) provided valuable assistance. Special thanks to Lavanya Reddy and Michael McGregor for their editorial and organizational skills; to Ignacia Ruiz-Garcia, a deft scheduler who helped us find the time; and to Jean Jordan, for her administrative support. Thanks also to Larissa Regala, Elizabeth Manzolillo, and many others.

We are indebted to Sandy Warner, Jim Robinson, Dick Beattie, Paul Marks, Bob Wittes, and Harold Varmus. Without them the Prostate Cancer Program at Memorial Sloan-Kettering Cancer Center would not exist. Heartfelt thanks to Sidney Kimmel, Michael Milken, Joe Allbritton, Uri Herscher and the Skirball Foundation, the Leon Lowenstein Foundation, the Rona Jaffe Foundation, David Storrs, Grant Gregory, and many others who have so generously supported the program, including special friends: Tina and Bill Greenberg, Marc and Mady Simon, Patricia and Tom Shiah, and Patricia and Jose Kuri. Kudos to Anne McSweeney for her magic touch in the development arena. Above all, we are grateful to David H. Koch, a giant in the world of philanthropy, who is uncommonly generous with his time and with his treasure. His personal involvement has catalyzed research in prostate cancer all over the country.

Thanks also to Virgil Simons, Steve Gragg, Ken Borow, Salvatore and Connie Natale, David Elsasser, Richard Barlow, Gregg Wiita, both Ed Grossmans, Steve Joseph, Jamie Janoff, Randolph Duke, Mel Lerman, and Karl Seib for all the thoughtful discussions and valuable input. Frank Forney produced the detailed illustrations throughout.

It's been a privilege to work with top-notch literary agent Peter Lampack, and with all the good people in the Penguin Group, especially Miriam Rich, Megan Newman, and Marilyn Ducksworth.

FOREWORD TO THE SECOND EDITION

When I mentioned that I was working on a new edition of this book, friends and patients were surprised. The last one came out only five years ago. Has that much changed in the field? Are there important new studies? Has the management and understanding of these diseases really progressed enough to warrant a new book?

From inside the field, down in the trenches, the need for a major update was clear. For those of us working in the office with patients, attending research meetings with scientists, going to medical conferences with other physicians, and teaching students and fellows, this has been an exciting time. New studies roll out almost weekly that profoundly challenge our old assumptions about prostate diseases or promise breakthroughs in prevention, detection, and treatment. Many major advances, fascinating new possibilities, and tantalizing missteps that have yielded important insights are detailed in these pages.

Here are some highlights: Research has revolutionized our understanding of the molecular changes that drive the development and growth of prostate cancer and enable it to become resistant to hormone therapy. In 2004, Charles Sawyers discovered the key to "hormone resistance." He found that prostate cancer was able to flourish in the absence of androgens (male hormones) because of the action of the androgen receptor. When this internal amplifier that spurs cell activity is turned up in advanced prostate cancer, cancer cells do not need male hormones to thrive. Armed with this knowledge, Sawyers went on to develop a more powerful antiandrogen to block the androgen receptor. Called MDV3100, this new pill is in the final stages of testing for FDA approval. An even stronger antiandrogen is at an earlier stage in the pipeline. In 2005, Arul Chinnayian discovered an unusual "fusion" gene that stimulates cell growth in response to androgens. Such fusions had rarely been found in any of the common cancers, such as breast or lung, and new drugs are being developed to target this mutant gene.

For decades, researchers have sought a way to prevent prostate cancer, and most clues pointed to diet. In large, government-sponsored trials of dietary supplements, vitamin E and selenium—the prime candidates—proved disappointing. The good news: finasteride (Proscar), a well-known drug that has been used to shrink the prostate, proved highly effective in reducing the risk of developing prostate cancer., and its cousin dutasteride (Avodart) works as well.

"Active surveillance" is gaining popularity as more men and more doctors recognize that small, early cancers found in men of any age can be closely watched, with regular checkups and occasional biopsies, with little risk that the cancer will spread before there are clear signs that the time to begin active treatment has come.

Robotic surgery burst onto the scene amid great marketing fanfare claiming that the side effects of surgery would disappear with the use of the da Vinci robot. Unfortunately, studies found that robotic prostatectomy is no safer than the open operation, and the long-term results no better, leaving little to justify the increased costs of the robotic operation. Similarly, proton beam radiation has been touted as highly curative with virtually no side effects. Careful comparisons with high-dose, image-guided radiation have yet to show any real benefit of this expensive new technology.

For advanced prostate cancer that has spread to bones or other organs, the treatment possibilities are multiplying. New antiandrogens are most promising, and fifty to one hundred new drugs for prostate cancer are currently being studied in the laboratory or early clinical trials. One of the most astonishing is a drug that had been sitting on the shelf for years, which was capable of completely shutting down the body's ability to synthesize male hormones. Abiraterone, recently acquired by Johnson & Johnson for nearly $1 billion, has proven remarkably effective against "hormone resistant" prostate cancer, even though it works by blocking the production of male hormones. Vaccines and antibodies that enhance the immune system are in the final stages of testing. And metastases in bone are being eliminated with a single dose of radiation.

The best news of all: The death rate from prostate cancer continues to fall nationwide. Mortality from this disease in the United States has declined more than 40 percent since 1993, much faster than in Great Britain or Scandinavia, reaching levels not seen since the early 1970s. If the tools of modern medical science can help us to better understand the threat posed by each man's cancer, we may soon be able to determine with greater certainty which cancers can be safely monitored, without unnecessary therapy and its side effects, and which need to be treated immediately. Also, now that we know that many prostate cancers can be prevented with a simple medication, the risk of getting this cancer may steadily fall over the next generation and become one fewer worry for our grandchildren.

CONTENTS

Part Three

■

PROSTATE CANCER

INTRODUCTION

In 1971, the U.S. government declared war on cancer, and for men with prostate cancer, there is excellent news from the front! The risk of dying of prostate cancer in this country has fallen more than 40 percent in the past fifteen years, thanks largely to early detection and effective treatment with surgery or radiation therapy. Modern techniques have lowered the risk of troubling side effects from these treatments, improving quality as well as length of life. Chemotherapy has proven effective and prolongs life in men with advanced prostate cancer. We now understand how some prostate cancers become resistant to hormone treatment, and this knowledge opens the door to rapid development of powerful new hormones, which are remarkably effective against cancers previously thought to be impervious to hormonal manipulation. More than fifty new drugs are in the development pipeline, targeting the key molecular and genetic changes that have been identified in prostate cancer over the past decade. Perhaps most exciting is the fact that we've discovered prostate cancer can be prevented with a simple pill!

Decades of intense research efforts are also paying off in the diagnosis and treatment of other prostate diseases. New medical therapies for benign prostate hyperplasia (prostate enlargement, BPH) shrink the gland and reduce the need for surgery. The scientific study of prostatitis (inflammation or infection in the gland) is finally offering clues to the causes and treatment of this perplexing disease.

Still, despite all the progress we've made, men facing these diseases continue to grapple with troubling questions. Should you have your PSA tested, or could testing lead to unnecessary treatment of an innocent cancer? Should you take medication to prevent prostate cancer? If you have prostate cancer, how dangerous is it? Do you need to be treated now, or can you wait and monitor the disease, hoping the cancer will not progress, avoiding the troublesome side effects of treatment? Is there a way to slow the growth of prostate cancer? If you need treatment, is surgery or radiation the better choice? What about robotic surgery instead of the traditional open procedure? If you opt for radiation, should you have seed implants, external beam therapy, proton beam therapy, or a combination of these treatments? Do you need hormone therapy, and if so, which drugs should you take, and when should you start? What about alternative and complementary medicine? Should you consider experimental therapies or a clinical trial? The vast array of diagnostic tests and treatment alternatives leaves many men frustrated and confused.

If you have urinary problems because of an enlarged prostate, should you take medicine or have surgery? If medicine is the answer, is one drug enough, or do you need two? If surgery is the best option for you, should the tissue be removed by laser? Is hyperthermia (heating the prostate) as effective as TURP (removal of excess tissue through a scope)? Which treatment is safer? Which is more likely to solve the problem permanently? Should you start taking a powerful antibiotic if your PSA rises even though you feel fine, or is there a better approach? Prostate diseases are highly variable and enormously complex. Until trouble strikes, most men know little about their prostate gland. Knowledge in the field is constantly evolving. Persistent myths and misconceptions abound, not only among the general public but among doctors as well. To find the right answers, you may have to navigate some very tricky terrain, including a minefield of marketing-inspired "evidence" and baseless advice on the Internet.

Over the years, I've met with thousands of men in my office face-to-face and tried to arm them with sound, up-to-date, comprehensive, and comprehensible information about their medical issues and options. In these pages, I hope to make the same information available to all men confronting serious prostate problems and to their loved ones. Understanding what you're up against and how to respond can make all the difference. As baseball great Joe Torre said of his own experience with prostate cancer, "When you get the information, the fear just sort of melts away."

To equip you with the knowledge you'll need to make wise choices, this book is organized into three parts. Part One deals with the normal prostate, where it is located, what it does, and how it relates to urinary, bowel, and sexual function. Since many prostate problems are closely associated with aging, we'll go on to explore what typically happens to sexual and urinary function as men age and what you can do to increase your odds of aging successfully. Part Two focuses on prostate problems other than cancer—prostatitis and BPH—that cause so much grief for so many men. We'll look at strategies for dealing with these strikingly common prostate ailments, and we'll also examine how these conditions can confound our ability to diagnose prostate cancer and how they might affect your treatment options if you develop a malignancy in the gland. Part Three takes an in-depth look at prostate cancer: what it is, how it develops and progresses, and what can be done about it. I'll introduce you to state-of-the-art predictive tools called nomograms that have helped many patients and physicians to make sound treatment choices. In these pages, you'll find the facts you need to resolve the major issues: Is treatment necessary now? If so, which approach makes the most sense? Which is more important—the type or the quality of treatment? How can you ensure that you'll get the best available care and the best possible outcome?

Being diagnosed with a prostate disease is no picnic. But today we have the necessary information and tools to provide real options and enable men to make informed decisions. Not long ago, things looked very different indeed.

I first heard about prostate cancer as a teenager, when one of my father's close friends, I'll call him Dan O'Conner, developed the disease. Mr. O'Conner was a strapping, vibrant man in his fifties, a highly successful businessman with an amazing intellect and a terrific sense of humor. He was always great fun to be around, always armed with a fascinating story—someone who seemed to me larger than life.

My father was both Mr. O'Conner's friend and his urologist. I'll never forget the day Dad came home from the office in an uncharacteristically somber mood. When I asked what was wrong, he told me that he had just had to tell a dear friend that he had prostate cancer. Mr. O'Conner was an extrovert in the best sense of the word, always open about the critical events of his life. His daughter was in my high school class, and she had her father's honesty and directness, so her dad's illness was no secret.

Several weeks later, my father operated to remove Mr. O'Conner's prostate gland. To my young mind, that surely meant that he would be fine, back to his old self again as soon as the effects of the surgery wore off. For a while this proved true, but some years later the cancer recurred. While it responded initially to further treatment, over the next few years his condition deteriorated. Even though Mr. O'Conner remained outwardly cheerful, it was clear that he was sinking. He was weakened by bone pain and the narcotic medication needed to control it. He had difficulty walking. I could tell from the bleak look on my father's face when it was Mr. O'Conner on the phone, asking for advice about another in the endless string of medical crises. Back in those days, there was little my dad could do beyond being there for his friend, listening with empathy and trying to keep him as comfortable as possible.

When Mr. O'Conner died, my friends and family went to his funeral. By then I was in my last year of medical school at Duke. I had begun to learn about cancer in general, but the medical school curriculum in those days included almost nothing about prostate cancer. During the funeral service and for weeks afterward, I kept thinking that there had to be a better way to battle this disease. My father's outlook was not encouraging. Though prostate cancer was far more common than most people realized, medical science had made little progress toward detecting it early or figuring out better ways to treat it and save men's lives.

As I went through my own specialty training at the Massachusetts General Hospital, the National Cancer Institute, and UCLA, I became increasingly determined to focus on prostate cancer: to understand it better and to try to develop or apply new treatments. Like my father, my professors unanimously discouraged that choice. Prostate cancer was far too complex, they argued. The disease typically grew and spread so slowly that confirming whether a particular treatment worked or not took longer than the duration of most doctors' careers! Inexplicably, some men with this disease lived for decades without treatment, yet most cancers had already spread to distant sites (metastasized), as Dan O'Conner's had, by the time they were detected. While hormone therapy brought dramatic relief of painful metastases to bone, the remission typically lasted for only a few years and the cancer always recurred. Treating advanced prostate cancer with the chemotherapy that was then available was like rearranging the deck chairs on the *Titanic,* for all the difference it made.

Fortunately, my dad and my teachers were wrong. The slowly expanding research in prostate cancer in the 1970s began to pay off in the 1980s, and the outlook for men with prostate cancer improved dramatically. By the late 1980s, a simple blood test for prostate-specific antigen (PSA), a protein made in the prostate that leaks into the blood when the prostate is disrupted by disease, revolutionized the diagnosis of prostate cancer. For the first time, most prostate cancers could be detected at an early, curable stage. Using ultrasound imaging, we could see the internal structure and measure the size of the prostate, but a major breakthrough came with the development of ultrasound-guided needle biopsy of the prostate. A biopsy of the gland became a fairly safe, simple office procedure— last year over a million were performed in the United States—so doctors could easily diagnose whether a patient had cancer. Refinements in testing and imaging have enabled us to monitor, rather than treat, men with early, favorable cancers that pose no immediate risk to life and health. For those with more serious cancers, advances in surgery have placed the radical prostatectomy (complete removal of the prostate) on firm anatomical ground, improving the chances for cure and reducing the onerous side effects. Both brachytherapy (seed implants) and external beam radiation therapy have been refined to increase the dose of radiation that can be delivered precisely to the prostate to maximize the chance of curing the cancer, while minimizing damage to surrounding structures and decreasing the risk of urinary, sexual, and bowel complications. Drugs to promote penile erections or to relax an irritated bladder, and devices and procedures to control urinary incontinence, give us highly effective means to deal with the side effects of treatment that sometimes occur.

Nevertheless, many doctors continue to have an incomplete understanding of prostate diseases, and even seasoned experts can disagree. When Ralph S., a 62-year-old financial planner, learned that he had prostate cancer, he used his well-honed research skills to track down top-notch professionals to consult. The first urologist he saw recommended surgery as the best way to get rid of the cancer. Ralph expected a second opinion to confirm this, but the next urologist was firmly in favor of seed implants. After all, he said, seeds were much less invasive and would require little lost time from work. Hoping to break the tie, Ralph went to see yet another specialist, this time a medical oncologist, who disagreed with the first two doctors and weighed in strongly on the side of external beam radiation. Ralph's reward, for all his scrupulous efforts, was utter confusion. How could three capable doctors with fine reputations have such strikingly different ideas about what he should do? Were they analyzing and interpreting the data differently? Or were there simply three equally effective alternatives from which he could choose? How on earth was he supposed to make such a daunting decision when, weeks before, he barely knew where his prostate was?

To make a wise choice, you need to understand exactly what you're up against, the risks and benefits of each treatment alternative, and—perhaps most critically—yourself. It's crucial to assess your personal values and concerns. What are the key issues driving your decision? Might some unrealistic expectations or unnecessary concerns be standing in your way?

Take the case of Frank R. When I saw him recently, he was in a panic over the news that his prostate biopsy was positive for cancer. His uncle had suffered with unspecified "prostate troubles" when Frank was a child, with memorably disastrous consequences. Now, Frank was convinced that he would wind up as his uncle had: in diapers, sexually disabled, isolated, lonely, and depressed. He told me he thought his wisest course would be to forget about treatment and retire immediately, so that he could spend what little good time he had left with his wife, children, and friends.

Frank's diagnostic results painted a completely different picture. He was 69 years old, and his biopsy had turned up only one minuscule area of low-risk cancer. In my mind, the central question was whether Frank needed treatment at all. Given the typical slow course of such an early cancer, a reasonable alternative was to monitor him closely, postponing treatment unless and until there were warning signs that the cancer was beginning to grow. There was a good chance that he would live out the rest of his natural life with no problems from his prostate cancer whatsoever.

Frank's situation is far from unique. With prostate cancer, the gulf between reality and expectation can be enormous. Finding accurate, reliable information to narrow that breach is not easy. Advice from other men who have experienced prostate cancer may be misleading, outmoded, or entirely irrelevant to you. If you seek enlightenment from the Internet, you'll find plenty of wishful thinking, blind supposition, and raw bias overwhelming the sound, scientific advice. To make wise choices and cope well with this disease, you have to understand exactly what you're up against. To that end, this book reflects the generous input of leading specialists working to conquer prostate diseases, including medical oncologists, radiation oncologists, radiologists, pathologists, research scientists, biostatisticians, nurses, and mental health practitioners, as well as other urologists from around the country who specialize in prostate cancer, infections in the gland, BPH, infertility, erectile dysfunction, and incontinence. In addition, many of our patients and their partners have graciously contributed their valuable insights, illustrative anecdotes, and practical advice.

As you read, keep in mind that you can and will get through this. Millions of men have weathered serious problems with their prostates successfully. Today, most patients are spared the urinary problems and sexual decline that were once seen as virtually inevitable. Given good modern care, they are able to put the disease behind them and get on with their lives.

Getting the word out is crucial. Ironically, though most men have scant knowledge about their prostates, nearly everyone has heard that prostate diseases and their treatments can impair or alter a man's most intimate personal functions. Preferring not to think about such things, some young, healthy men at high risk for prostate cancer avoid screening for the disease, even though regular testing would virtually guarantee that any cancer they developed would be discovered at an early, curable stage. Out of fear of side effects, some men forgo lifesaving treatment for serious cancers, even though the side effects of modern treatment are not inevitable, are often temporary, and are almost always correctable when they occur. Some men refuse treatment even though the disease itself, if left to progress, can cause serious side effects.

Thankfully, many prominent men have come forward in recent years to discuss their experiences with prostate diseases frankly and to encourage others to become more vigilant, better informed, and more proactive about their own health. Leading political figures Rudolph Giuliani, Colin Powell, Senators Christopher Dodd, Bob Dole, and John Kerry; Nelson Mandela; Intel CEO Andy Grove; baseball legend Joe Torre; Archbishop Desmond Tutu; leading educator Cornel West; and entertainment greats Jerry Lewis, Mandy Patinkin, and Harry Belafonte represent the new forthright face and increasingly optimistic voice of male prostate health. Their message and examples are clear, inspiring, and true: Prostate diseases can be confronted, treated, and overcome.

The American public supports prostate cancer research generously, with more than $200 million in federal funds channeled through the National Cancer Institute and the Department of Defense. Through the Herculean efforts of Michael Milken and his dedicated colleagues at the Prostate Cancer Foundation, private research funding has supplemented public funds and helped us make great strides toward understanding this disease. This organization, with Milken at the helm, has also worked tirelessly and effectively to promote public awareness.

I'm grateful to these remarkable individuals and to all the men with prostate cancer I've been privileged to know over the years, especially my family friend Dan O'Conner. Witnessing his struggle against this disease all those years ago gave me the will to join in the fight against prostate cancer. I know Dan would be delighted by how things have changed for men with this disease and what huge strides we've made toward winning the battle.

Dr. Peter T. Scardino

Part One

THE PROSTATE
AND THE
NORMAL MALE

1

The Prostate

READ THIS CHAPTER TO LEARN:

- Where does the prostate lie, how is it constructed, and what does it do?
- What can go wrong with this troublemaking gland?
- Why do these problems develop so frequently?
- Are prostate diseases inherited?

What is the prostate? Where is it? What does it do? Can you live without it? Or perhaps more to the point if you're plagued by prostate problems: Is there any way that you and this gland can peacefully coexist?

Few men are able to answer any, let alone all, of these fundamental questions. Until trouble strikes, the prevailing attitude holds that this small, obscure gland is probably best ignored. If you're a typical man, you were aware that you have a prostate; you knew that it could cause all manner of unpleasantness; and, quite frankly, you preferred not to think about it.

But now you have no choice. If you or someone you love has been diagnosed with prostate cancer or another serious prostate disease, you need to understand precisely what you're up against in order to determine the best course of action.

WHAT IS THE PROSTATE?

The **prostate** is a gland, the term used to describe fluid-producing organs. Salivary glands, predictably, manufacture saliva, which aids in digestion. Sweat glands secrete sweat to regulate body temperature. Mammary glands in the female breast produce milk. The prostate churns out part of the seminal fluid, which protects and nourishes sperm as they navigate the female reproductive tract.

Terminology related to the prostate and its function can seem deliberately geared to maximize confusion. In a prime example, the plum-shaped prostate "gland" is made up of many fluid-producing sacs that are also called "glands" (just as many hairs on a person's head are collectively referred to as "hair"). Another name for these microscopic glands, though it may not strike you as particularly user-friendly, is **acini**.

In addition to abundant microscopic glands, the prostate contains a network of internal piping (**ducts**) and supporting muscle and fibrous cells (**stroma**). When ejaculation occurs, the muscular stroma contracts like a pumping fist, deploying the seminal fluid out through the penis, along with the sperm it is charged to preserve and defend.

NOTE: People writing about the prostate commonly describe the gland as resembling a walnut. While the general size and shape are somewhat similar, the analogy evokes a hard shell and dry, solid contents, which in no way resemble the healthy human prostate. A small plum, with its spongy, fluid-filled interior and soft skin, is far closer to the way a typical prostate appears after puberty. With the **benign enlargement (BPH)** or prostate cancer that so often accompanies advancing age, a larger and sometimes more irregular plum would serve as a reasonable surrogate image.

WHAT DOES THE PROSTATE DO?

In young boys, the prostate gland is minuscule. It lies dormant until puberty, when, stimulated by a surge of male **hormones**, the gland grows and begins its lifelong task of churning out seminal fluid (**semen**). The seminal vesicles (attached just above the prostate) and Cowper's glands (along the urethra just below the prostate) also add to the seminal fluid that is released during ejaculation. Within the prostate, fluid manufacturing occurs in the **epithelial cells** that line the microscopic glands and ducts.

Seminal fluid contains a complex stew of proteins and minerals specially designed to preserve and protect sperm as they make their way along the female reproductive tract. A critical component, contributed by the prostate, is a protein called **prostate-specific antigen (PSA)**. While finding a high level of PSA on the blood screening test for prostate cancer can be a harbinger of trouble, PSA in the seminal fluid is perfectly normal. In fact, PSA plays the essential role of liquefying coagulated semen so the sperm are free to journey toward an egg.

WHERE IS THE PROSTATE LOCATED?

Deep in the pelvis, below the urinary bladder, the prostate encircles the **urethra**, the conduit that allows both urine and semen to pass through the penis to the outside. The prostate lies directly behind the pubic bone and in front of the rectum, which is why the rear surface of the gland can be felt by a doctor during a **DRE**.

In the 1966 sci-fi film classic *Fantastic Voyage,* an intrepid rescue team is drastically miniaturized and deployed through the circulatory system of a brilliant government scientist to track down and eradicate a life-threatening blood clot in an artery. Had Command Central sent these germ-sized heroes southward to tackle a troubling condition in Professor Benes's prostate gland instead, getting there would have been the least of their troubles. The crew's greater challenge by far would have been

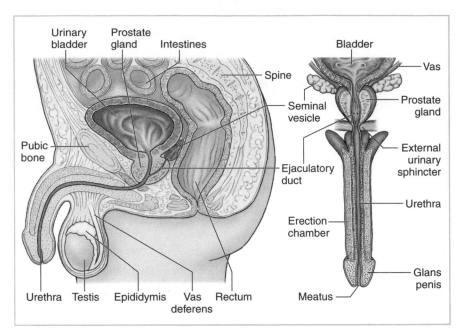

The prostate and neighboring organs. Cutaway views from the side (in left-hand drawing) and from the front (in right-hand drawing).

finding a way to treat Benes's prostate problem without damaging his urinary, bowel, or sexual functions.

While some major organs—such as the kidneys, liver, and lungs—live in relative isolation akin to a private home on a quiet suburban street, the prostate sits smack at the hub of a frenzied anatomical intersection. Here, structures responsible for sexual, urinary, and bowel function operate in perilously close proximity to one another. Like an accident at the frantic juncture of a major highway, a minor glitch in any one of these structures can precipitate a chain of destructive events. One driver stops short, and the trailing vehicles pile up in a mile-long fender bender. One lane is consumed by construction, and smoothly flowing traffic slows to a frustrating trickle. The prostate enlarges with benign **BPH**, becomes inflamed (**prostatitis**), or develops a malignant tumor (**prostate cancer**), and suddenly a man collides head-on with the frightening specters of erectile dysfunction, urinary incontinence, or bowel problems—whether from the disease itself or from the treatment.

Mere millimeters separate the rear of the prostate from the rectal wall, so the rectum lies directly in the line of fire of a radiation beam targeted at a cancerous prostate. Running in the neurovascular bundle just beside the prostate and rectum are the exquisitely delicate **cavernous (erectile) nerves**, which control penile erections. These nerves can be easily damaged by imprecise attempts to treat prostate cancer, whether with surgery, radiation, heating (**high-intensity focused ultrasound, HIFU**) or freezing (**cryotherapy**). Since the urethra runs from the bladder directly through the prostate, BPH or a large cancer can slow the urinary stream and eventually block its flow completely. In front of the prostate looms the pubic bone, which can add to the challenge faced by a surgeon trying to remove the gland, by a radiation therapist doing seed implants, or during cryotherapy.

The bladder and delicate **ureters** (tubes that channel urine from the kidneys to the bladder) perch directly above the prostate, and the penis extends out from below. These organs can be injured if treatment for prostate cancer is not targeted with scrupulous care. For example, if the bladder, urethra, or ureters are hit by damaging rays during radiation therapy, **inflammation** or bleeding (**radiation cystitis**) can result. Radiation damage to erection chambers within the penis or the erectile nerves could result in severely impaired erections. The **bladder neck,** which contains the muscular trapdoor known as the **internal urinary sphincter**, connects to the top—confusingly called the base—of the gland. At their juncture the two organs are enmeshed like zipper teeth and are virtually indistinguishable. Unless the bladder neck is adequately removed during surgery for prostate cancer, the malignant cells left at the edge could grow back. When we perform a radical prostatectomy to cure cancer, the **external urinary sphincter** takes over the job of holding back urine, so this muscular structure must be carefully preserved to avoid urinary incontinence.

The prostate is so closely intertwined with adjacent structures that the inflammation of prostatitis readily causes rectal and perineal pain, lower abdominal aches, burning at the tip of the penis, and the need to urinate frequently.

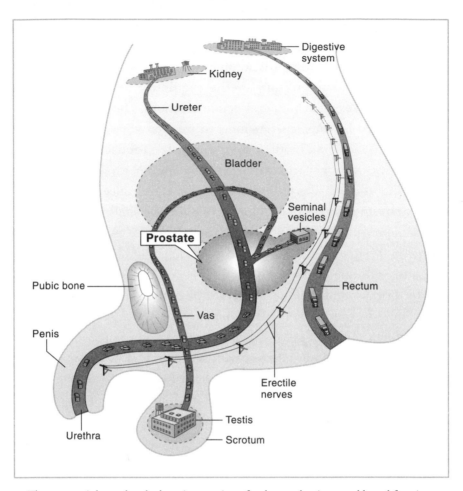

The prostate is located at the busy intersection of male sexual, urinary, and bowel functions.

HOW WAS THE PROSTATE DISCOVERED?

Considering the prostate's remote location and obscure function, it is not surprising that scholars who worked to map human anatomy centuries ago were late to recognize the gland's very existence. In fact, we are still struggling to divine some of its mysterious secrets and fully understand its strikingly eccentric ways.

Though references to urological diseases—most notably, bladder and kidney stones—date back to an ancient Egyptian papyrus written in 1550 BC, the prostate was first described by an Italian physician, Niccolo Massa, nearly 3,000 years later in Renaissance Venice. The gland's given name, *prostate*, derives from a Greek term meaning "to set before," a reference to the prostate's position in relation to the bladder. The word *prostitute* derives from similar Greek roots, meaning "to place before" or "to offer." Given the gland's persistent obscurity, its name is commonly confused with the similar-sounding *prostrate*, which refers to a posture of submission or humility, lying flat with one's face to the ground.

In sixteenth-century Europe, a French military surgeon named Ambroise Paré frequently took embalmed cadavers home to study and practice new medical techniques. Though his family might not have appreciated such unorthodox houseguests, medical science—and urology in particular—owe Paré a considerable debt. He was the first to recognize that the prostate gland is a distinct organ, separate from the bladder. He detailed the gland's intimate relationship to the **seminal vesicles** and **ejaculatory ducts** and explained how it operates during ejaculation. His work added immeasurably to our understanding of how the prostate functions.

WHAT ARE THE PARTS OF THE PROSTATE?

In a top-down view of a prostate that has been sliced horizontally across the middle and had its top half removed, you would see the urethra at the center. Moving outward, you'd notice many tiny tubelike ducts, akin to a thicket of tree branches, with microscopic glands strewn about the tips like a profusion of leaves.

The portion of the prostate immediately surrounding the urethra is called the **transition zone**. This area of the gland is most infamously known as the site of BPH, which often constricts urinary flow as men age.

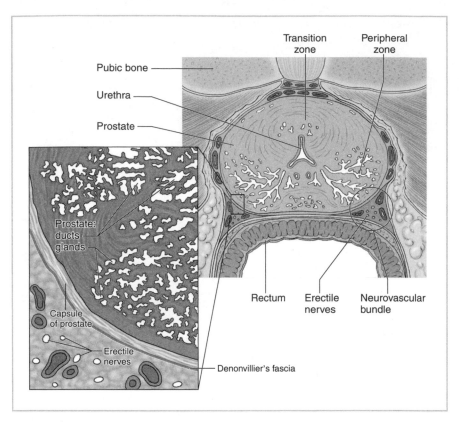

Cross-section through the prostate showing its key parts, the nearby neurovascular bundles (erectile nerves), and the rectum. An enlarged view to the left shows the microscopic ducts and glands.

Continuing out from the transition zone, we come to the **peripheral zone**, which lies beneath the outer covering, or **capsule**, of the gland like an orange rind. In another rich potential source of misunderstanding, the prostate's "capsule" is actually soft and membranous like the skin of a plum, not a hard, impervious barrier as the name might seem to imply. Most prostate cancers arise in the peripheral zone, directly beneath the capsule. If left alone long enough, these tumors tend to spread outward through the capsule into surrounding tissues. Still, about one in four prostate cancers arise in the transition zone. Although the transition zone and the peripheral zone are anatomically distinct, many men with prostate cancer have malignant disease in both zones because prostate cancer often arises in many areas at once.

In addition to these zonal divisions, the prostate can be divided down the middle into left and right lobes, a distinction enhanced by the **median sulcus**, a groove that runs down the rear surface of the gland and can be felt during a DRE. These anatomical landmarks play an important role in describing the location of prostate diseases and in planning for their treatment.

HOW DOES THE PROSTATE GROW?

In a young boy, the minuscule prostate weighs 3 to 6 grams (a nickel weighs 5 grams) and has no known function. At puberty, the gland grows to about 20 grams—the weight of a medium-sized strawberry—and begins to produce part of the seminal fluid. For decades thereafter, the prostate holds steady at this size and goes uneventfully about its business. Except for the problems some have with the inflammation or infection known as prostatitis, most young men remain happily oblivious to the workings of their prostate. Then, with appalling frequency, this formerly innocuous bit player on the reproductive stage begins to grow again in

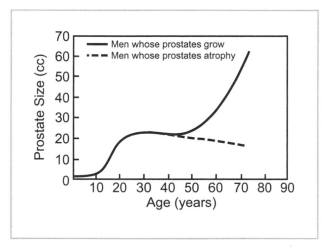

Growth of the Prostate with Age. After most men reach age 40, the prostate begins to enlarge with BPH, but in some men, the gland remains the same size or shrinks (atrophies).

the fifth decade or beyond, developing into a strident, intrusive bully that can seriously erode a man's quality—or even quantity—of life.

WHAT PROBLEMS DEVELOP
IN THE PROSTATE?

The prostate could be considered the biblical Job of internal organs, destined to suffer one crushing misfortune after another. From puberty, the gland is highly susceptible to various forms of acute or chronic **prostatitis**, an infection, inflammation, or enigmatic noninflammatory syndrome that lands many men in the doctor's office in search of relief. One in four men will experience a bout of prostatitis in his lifetime. The problem affects men of all ages. Though it almost never poses a threat to survival, the condition can make men miserable. In the most severe cases, patients have likened the pain, urinary symptoms, and general malaise of prostatitis to the chest pain of angina, the abdominal cramps of inflammatory bowel disease, or the aftermath of a heart attack. (See Chapter 4, Prostatitis.) Prostatitis can also be a serious pain in the wallet. The cost to men suffering from this disease averages $1,760 per year.[1]

Benign prostatic hyperplasia (BPH) is another common source of prostate-induced misery. For reasons we still don't fully understand, the gland, which reaches full size at puberty, frequently undergoes a second growth spurt after age 40 that can provoke a litany of urinary woes. Symptoms may include a slow urinary stream, hesitancy in starting, intermittent voiding (stream stops before the bladder is empty), post-void dribbling, decrease in the size and force of the stream, and the need to get up at night to urinate (**nocturia**). In extreme cases, the urinary obstruction becomes so severe that a man cannot urinate at all (**acute urinary retention**) and requires emergency catheterization or surgery. (See Chapter 5, BPH [Benign Prostatic Hyperplasia].) In addition to benign enlargement, the prostate is also prone to developing malignant tumors (**cancer**) as men age. It is often said, and not far from the truth, that if you're a man and live long enough, you're bound to develop some cancerous cells in your prostate (though many of these are microscopic and would never cause a serious problem if left alone). (See Part Three for a more detailed discussion of prostate cancer.)

WHY DO MEN DEVELOP PROSTATE PROBLEMS?

The prostate's troublemaking potential is unique. No other secondary sex organ develops cancer or enlarges with aging. We almost never see benign or malignant overgrowth in the seminal vesicles, vas deferens, or Cowper's glands, though these organs are exposed to many of the same environmental conditions, genetic factors, and hormonal influences as the prostate.

Despite our best research efforts regarding the prostate's function and what can go wrong with it, questions and conundrums abound. We don't know why the prostate is so prone to benign and cancerous growth or why the gland so often gets infected or inflamed. Nevertheless, we have come a very long way from the meager state of knowledge about the prostate that greeted me thirty years ago when I first became a urologist. We now know that prostate cancer and BPH can run in families.[2] We've identified genes associated with increased risk of prostate cancer. We've learned that some prostate cancers pose little risk to life and health (**indolent** cancers), while others grow rapidly and require aggressive treatment. Perhaps most critically, we've learned that early detection and appropriate intervention can reduce the chances of dying of prostate cancer and often mitigate the symptoms of BPH and prostatitis. We're making steady inroads toward understanding prostate diseases and learning how to treat them with better outcomes and far fewer negative, lasting effects.

IN SUMMARY

The prostate is a small gland with an outsized capacity to cause problems, notably prostate cancer, prostatitis, and BPH, especially as men age. Because of the gland's location, prostate diseases and their treatments carry a risk of damage to urinary, sexual, and bowel functions. Our understanding of the prostate remains incomplete, but our ability to detect and manage prostate problems has evolved remarkably in the past two decades, and the outlook for men with prostate diseases grows brighter all the time.

2

■

Normal Male Function

As a urologist, I specialize in the functions and diseases of the male reproductive organs and in the prevention and treatment of urinary diseases in both males and females. In other words, as Sam Spade might have put it: the genitourinary system is my beat.

Though the penis is the clear sentimental favorite and garners more attention than all of the other male genitourinary organs combined, the quality of its performance depends on things going smoothly behind the scenes. Male urinary, sexual, and reproductive functions are intertwined in many ways. These systems share common ground and are often called upon to work in concert. When something goes wrong in one area, the others may be affected as well. Urinary problems and their treatments can impair sexual and bowel function and damage fertility. Problems with the genital organs—where the prostate, more often than not, is the culprit—can throw urinary and bowel, as well as sexual and reproductive functions, out of whack. To grasp how things go awry, let's look at how genitourinary organs arise and how they are meant to work.

HOW DO MALE ORGANS DEVELOP BEFORE BIRTH?

The embryonic kidneys begin to form in the first month after conception. While still in a highly primitive state, they commence their lifelong function of filtering wastes from the blood and producing urine. By the thirty-seventh day of gestation, when the fetus is about the size of an apple seed, the bladder forms by first expanding out like a bubble from tiny tubes called **ureters**, which branch off from the kidneys, and then coming together to create an elastic, muscular pouch designed to store urine until it is ready to be released.

All embryos have at least one X chromosome, and everyone is female at the outset. During the second month of fetal life, reproductive (germ) cells generate primitive gonads that eventually grow into ovaries in the female and testes in the male. By six weeks into a pregnancy, the testicles' tiny precursors begin to secrete signaling substances that promote the development of the male organs and inhibit their female counterparts. At seven to eight weeks, under the influence of the Y (male) chromosome, specialized **Leydig cells** arise in the testicles. Their job is to secrete testosterone, the primary male hormone. At first, this production is controlled by the pregnancy hormone **HCG (human chorionic gonadotropin)**, which is produced by the mother's placenta. Gradually, the fetal brain takes over this management task. From then on, the hypothalamus and pituitary glands in the brain provide the signals that keep the Leydig cells pumping testosterone throughout a male's life.

Males whose cells are genetically incapable of utilizing testosterone are born with a condition called testicular feminization, aka complete

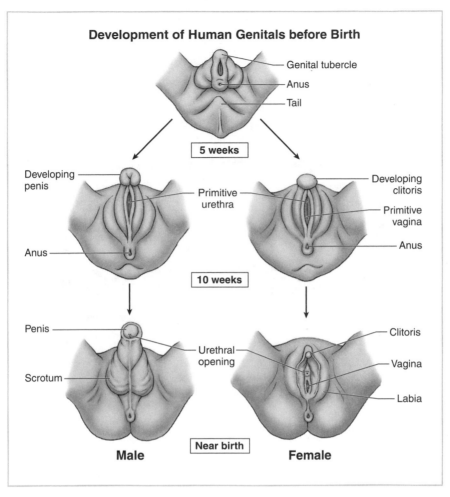

Development of Human Genitals before Birth

Genital tubercle

Anus

Tail

5 weeks

Developing penis

Primitive urethra

Developing clitoris

Primitive vagina

Anus

Anus

10 weeks

Penis

Urethral opening

Clitoris

Scrotum

Vagina

Labia

Near birth

Male

Female

All humans begin life with similar anatomy. Well before birth, a distinctly male or female external appearance develops.

androgen insensitivity syndrome. Externally, they appear to be normal females, but they have undescended testes, lack a uterus and fallopian tubes, do not menstruate, and, obviously, cannot bear children. Famous, and famously beautiful and voluptuous actresses, such as Jamie Lee Curtis and the late Kim Novak, are well-known examples of people with this syndrome.

The external genitalia first appear as a tiny nub, called a **tubercle**, when the embryo is about six weeks old. By ten weeks, the tubercle yields the beginnings of either a penis or a female clitoris (which, like its male counterpart, contains erectile bodies and engorges and enlarges with sexual arousal). Similarly, primitive genital folds develop into either the inner vaginal folds (**labia minora**) or the male urethra. In the female, the labia and urethral tube remain open. In males, the urethra closes to form an extended channel that passes through to the tip of the penis.

The **seminal vesicles** (glands that produce seminal fluid) develop as an outgrowth of the **vas deferens** (tubes that carry sperm from the epididymis [see page 20] to the prostate), while the pea-sized **Cowper's glands**, which lie below the prostate and also secrete part of the seminal fluid, arise from a special fold in the embryo, called the **urogenital sinus**.

At three months, when the fetus is 3 inches long, the testes commence their slow descent through the inguinal canal into the scrotum, where they take up permanent residence. Housing these organs

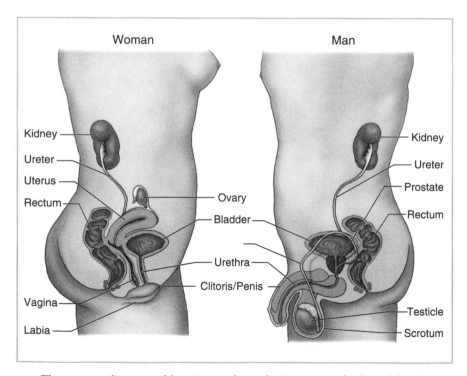

The corresponding parts of the urinary and reproductive systems of males and females.

externally allows their temperature to be carefully modulated, a feature essential to the production of healthy sperm. Elastic ligaments adjust the distance that the testes are held from internal body organs, making sure they are kept cool enough to prevent sperm damage. In severe cold, they are drawn closer to the body, where they can be kept sufficiently warm to protect the sperm. In females the counterparts of the scrotal sac are external vaginal folds, the **labia majora**.

During the twelfth to sixteenth week of gestation, the prostate develops as an offshoot of the urethra. First, many small buds arise from the urinary channel just below the bladder. Gradually they spread and extend to form the prostate's network of ducts and tiny glands (**acini**). These are supported by the gland's fibrous and muscle tissue (**stroma**). At this point, all the essential male equipment is in place.

THE URINARY TRACT

The **urinary tract** functions as a waste management and disposal facility, which helps maintain the body's critical balance of minerals and fluids. First, the kidneys filter the blood of waste products and excess water, which are excreted as urine—anywhere from ½ to 2½ liters per day in a normally hydrated adult. Average voiding output varies widely, depending on a person's size and activity, the ambient temperature and humidity, the amount of fluids consumed, and a host of other factors.

The **bladder** serves as a holding tank. Urine is stored under very low pressure, though when opportunity and need are at loggerheads, it may seem as if your bladder is positively screaming for attention. As it fills, the urinary reservoir relaxes and offers little resistance. While voiding, pressure in the bladder rises, but at its peak it amounts to a paltry 5 percent of the pressure of beer being pumped from a properly chilled keg.

The mild-mannered bladder does little to assert itself until it has been stretched very near its limits. Only then does it transmit frantic signals to the brain that emptying and consequent relief are imperative. In a typical adult, a sensation of bladder fullness kicks in when about 200 cubic centimeters (30 cc equals 1 ounce) of urine have accumulated. When

300 to 400 cc have collected, the urge to void grows powerful. Though maximum bladder capacity varies with size and individual urinary habits, the average is about 400 cc.

A full bladder triggers a voiding reflex, which in infants works as automatically as the irresistible jerking response to the tap of a rubber mallet against your knee. The bladder muscle contracts, pulling the inner sphincter open. All resistance gives way as the outer sphincter relaxes, and the urine flows freely through the urinary channel (**urethra**) to the outside. Toilet training derails this automatic feedback loop, modifying the brain's reaction to messages from the bladder. Once urination comes under voluntary control in early childhood, a person wishing to void must consciously let go, releasing the powerful learned inhibitory response that normally keeps us dry.

A newborn urinates two to six times a day for a total output of 30 to 60 cc. By the time a child passes his tenth birthday, four to five daily voiding episodes produce a whopping 800 to 1,400 cc daily urinary yield (about 1 to 1½ quarts). Adult men continue to urinate four to five times per day on average, as long as nothing, such as an enlarged prostate, interferes with normal function. Women void slightly more often, typically five to six times per day, though their stream tends to be stronger and their bladder empties faster than a man's. Men over 40 often notice a gradual slowing of their stream (measured in the doctor's office as the **urinary flow rate**) as the prostate enlarges.

SEX ORGANS

The central responsibility of male genitalia (the penis, scrotum, and testicles) is reproduction. The **testicles**, aka **testes**, manufacture sperm, which then pass to the adjacent **epididymis**, a long, slender, tightly convoluted tube that runs along the rear of each testicle. Here, during a ten-day storage period, the sperm mature and learn to swim (become motile). These tiny reproductive road warriors are then deployed through the complex mechanisms of emission, ejaculation, and orgasm. The testes also churn out male hormones (**androgens**), principally **testosterone**, which is required for normal development. Testosterone also maintains healthy libido, muscle mass, bone density, body and facial hair, and other characteristics throughout life.

The internal secondary sex organs—including the vas deferens, the seminal vesicles, and the prostate—comprise a critical supporting cast. During sexual climax, these three organs contract vigorously, forcing the sperm and seminal fluid into a staging area within the urethra in a process known as **emission**. To complete ejaculation, the muscles of the urethra and the **perineum** (the area between the scrotum and the rectum) contract rhythmically, propelling the semen out through the penis.

The tasks carried out by the reproductive organs are aided and abetted by a rich blood supply and triggered by carefully choreographed signals from the brain and spinal cord, which in turn rely on the precise action and interplay of many stimulatory and inhibitory nerves. You could liken this to a dazzling theatrical production involving hundreds of dancers, singers, acrobats, and musicians, not to mention props and special effects. The startling fact is not that things occasionally go awry but that they typically proceed without a hitch.

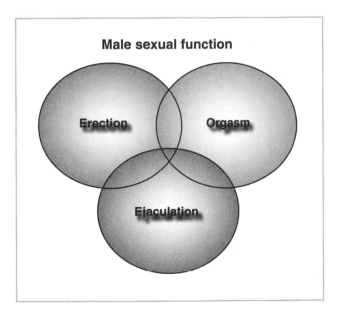

The three parts of male sexual function are interrelated but distinct. For example, orgasm can occur without erection or ejaculation.

THE BASIC ANATOMY OF ERECTION

The penis contains a pair of large erection chambers (**corpora cavernosa**) on top and one smaller chamber (**corpus spongiosum**) surrounding the urethra underneath. When sexual arousal is stimulated by a dream, conscious mental imagery, or a sensory stimulus (touch, sight, taste, sound, or smell), arteries leading to the penis relax, allowing a sudden forceful influx of blood. The erection chambers are nonelastic sacs, like tires on a car, so when they're filled to capacity under the pressure of arterial blood, they become rigid. In this state, the penile veins are compressed in a valvelike action, trapping the blood until orgasm occurs or the stimulus that caused the erection ceases.

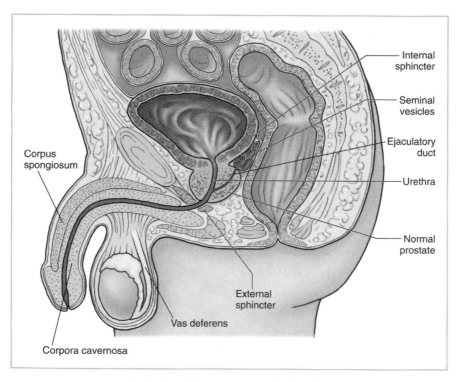

A side view of the normal pelvis in the adult male.

WHAT IS AN ORGASM?

It may surprise you to learn that an orgasm occurs between the ears, not between your legs. The sensation, which lasts about three to five seconds in a man and five to eight seconds in a woman, takes place strictly in the brain, and the brain is the sole organ required to generate the reflexive flood of pleasure and release. Erection is *not* required for orgasm, and a man incapable of having erections or ejaculating can still experience sexual climax as long as his brain is intact. After **simple prostatectomy** (removal of part of the gland) for an enlarged, obstructing prostate, or **radical prostatectomy** (complete removal) to treat prostate cancer, the ability to reach orgasm should not be impaired despite the loss of ejaculation (**dry orgasm**).

WHAT HAPPENS DURING EJACULATION?

Ejaculation involves the powerful expulsion of fluid through the penis at the startling rate of 28 miles per hour, which, by amusing coincidence, is also the top speed a world-class runner can achieve during a sprint. In normal males, each ejaculate measures a scant ½ to 1 teaspoon but still contains a whopping 100 million or more sperm—enough to repopulate all of Mexico! Nevertheless, sperm are so unfathomably tiny that this enormous number accounts for a mere 3 percent of the total ejaculatory volume. The seminal vesicles, Cowper's glands, and prostate contribute the other 97 percent in the form of seminal fluids (semen), which help to preserve and protect sperm. Without semen, sperm would never be able to survive the perilous 12-inch journey from the vagina through the uterus and into the fallopian tubes, where, if all goes according to nature's plan, one or more might succeed in fertilizing an egg.

NOTE: If that 12-inch distance strikes you as no big deal, consider that, given the sperm's minuscule size, the feat is roughly the equivalent of a grueling 70-mile swim for a 6-foot-tall human being.

On their passage through the female reproductive system, sperm, powered by their flickering tail-like **flagellum**, chug along at about 8 inches per hour, which is actually quite a startling burst of speed for such minute travelers. Since they tend to take a tacking course, rather than making a beeline to the target, the trip toward a rendezvous with an ovum can take several exhausting hours. Then, for any surviving sperm that have managed to go the distance, the daunting work of penetrating the egg and negotiating a successful genetic merger begins. This final phase presents its own considerable challenges. An ovum, though still microscopic, is twenty times as long and forty to fifty times as wide as the male reproductive cell. From a sperm's-eye view, the egg is enormous, significantly larger than the gargantuan 100-foot-long blue whale, the world's largest animal, appears to a typical human adult.

IN SUMMARY

The male genital and urinary systems are complex and intertwined. Normal sexual and urinary development and function hinge on all the component parts running smoothly. Of all the organs involved in male function, the aging prostate is most often the culprit when problems occur.

3

■

Changes with Aging

READ THIS CHAPTER TO LEARN:

- How do sexual and urinary functions typically change as men age, and what can you do to age successfully?
- How do aging hormones affect the prostate?
- Is hormone replacement therapy a good idea?

In our youth-obsessed society, we are bombarded by the notion that growing older is undesirable and unattractive. If we can't stop the clock, we will do almost anything to stop its effects on our appearance. The resultant costs are staggering. We spend billions annually on "anti-aging" creams and potions, alleged aging "remedies" and reversers, and cosmetics and surgical procedures that promise to preserve or restore the look of youth.

Still, no matter how we attempt to alter or mask our aging exteriors, no matter how doggedly we pursue eternal youth by popping pills or submitting to the scalpel, our internal clocks tick on. Aging is a universal, inescapable fact for all living creatures. It is also a normal process, and *not* a disease to be treated in a desperate attempt at a cure. Despite the deep-seated fear many people have of getting on in years, aging and well-being can, and often do, go hand in hand. While change over time is inevitable, dysfunction and disability are not.

This is good news for our graying population. Americans are living longer in ever greater numbers. Nearly 13 percent of us are now over 65, up from only 4 percent in 1900. People over 85 represent the fastest-growing segment of our population. It was rare indeed to find a centenarian at the turn of the twentieth century. Today, over 84,000 of our countrymen have passed the 100-year mark, and that number is expected to swell to over 600,000 by the middle of this century. Though this means that many men will reach their century milestone birthday, 80 percent of centenarians are women. For reasons we have yet to uncover, women continue to outlive men by an average of about five years.

Americans are not only living longer—they are living longer in good health, thanks to lifestyle improvements, advances in medical science, and an ever-increasing awareness that successful aging is very different from a futile attempt to imitate youth.

Since it began in 1982, the annual National Long Term Care Survey has documented a steady reduction of 1 to nearly 3 percent per year in the number of people who become disabled with age. Increasingly, older citizens remain capable of performing the activities of daily living (e.g., personal grooming, arranging for meals, and paying the bills) that are necessary for independence. The percentage of elderly Americans requiring supervised living arrangements or home care continues to decline. An ever-decreasing proportion now suffers from chronic diseases such as emphysema, arteriosclerosis, arthritis, dementia, stroke, and high blood pressure. Control of these health problems, when they do occur, has improved greatly, allowing older people to enjoy fewer debilitating side effects and better quality of life. For example, the cholesterol-lowering drugs known as **statins** have been shown to lower many serious health risks, including heart attacks.

While average life expectancy and long-term well-being continue to increase, the maximum limit of human life remains the subject of considerable speculation and debate. Based on cross-species studies, many scientists set the number at about 108 to 120 years old. In almost all animals, the longest observable life span is about six times the number of years it takes to grow from birth to full maturity.

Biologically this may be related to an enzyme called **telomerase**, which is responsible for restoring the ends of DNA that are damaged and lost each time a cell is reproduced. Normal cells grown in a culture dish in the laboratory can replicate themselves about fifty times, and then they expire. In every species, the life span ceiling is determined by how many times cells can resurrect themselves before they give out. All animals eventually succumb to death from "natural causes" if they aren't killed or don't die earlier from accidents or diseases.

To age successfully, it's important to understand the normal changes that occur over time and learn what can be done to maintain optimal function and maximal quality of life.

EFFECTS OF AGING ON MALE ORGANS

For many men, an enlarged prostate (BPH) and the changes in voiding habits that can occur as a result are as much a part of aging as is a gradual loss of vision, hearing, and hair. As the prostate enlarges, the flow of urine often weakens, and urination may be difficult to start. The stream may become intermittent, and some men develop a "nervous" bladder—annoying and unpredictable—that demands frequent emptying, even during the night.

When men reach middle age and beyond, gradual changes typically occur in sexual function as well. Older men often notice decreased **libido**, diminished erections, and reduced staying power during sexual encounters. Orgasm becomes more difficult to achieve. Fertility also slowly declines, and eventually most men lose the ability to father children. (See What Changes Occur in Sexual Function? on page 35 for a more complete discussion.)

These age-related changes are common but not inevitable or universal. Some men breeze through life without urinary problems or any perceptible dwindling of sexual powers. Still, the vast majority of us will have to deal with some or all of these eventually, if we're fortunate enough to live a good long time.

HOW DOES AGING AFFECT MALE HORMONES?

Testosterone, the predominant male hormone circulating throughout a man's body, is responsible for the development and maintenance of male sex organs and characteristics, including body hair, facial hair, and lean muscle mass. This highly productive hormone also spurs the growth of the prostate gland, penis, and testicles at puberty and, from then on, controls the production of sperm by the testes. Testosterone also plays a role in keeping bones strong, regulating mood, and maintaining libido, which we experience as sexual desire.

The amount of testosterone in a man's blood is regulated by a complex feedback loop. Think of a thermostat in which hormones are released or halted in turn in attempts to regulate the level. First, the hypothalamus stimulates the pituitary gland in the brain to secrete a hormone called **luteinizing hormone (LH)**, which acts as a chemical dispatcher. LH in turn sends out marching orders to the Leydig cells in the testicles, which manufacture and release testosterone into the bloodstream. Once testosterone increases, the hypothalamus holds up production of LH until the male hormone level declines again.

Leydig cells discharge testosterone in episodic pulses, so levels of the hormone vary throughout the day. If you have your serum testosterone (amount found in a blood sample) checked, one result may not reflect your actual hormone level. Measures of testosterone level taken in the morning are most accurate and reproducible.

Generally, testosterone levels follow your circadian rhythms, which are natural fluctuations in such bodily functions as alertness, metabolism, and hormone secretion. In humans, these activities tend to run at higher gear in the mornings than in the evenings, which may explain why some men experience greater sexual arousal on awakening than they do later in the day. Circadian rhythms also vary throughout the year. Testosterone levels are higher in the fall and lower in the spring, exactly contrary to popular notions of when human sap rises and, as the poet Alfred Lord Tennyson wrote, "a young man's fancy lightly turns to thoughts of love."

Starting at about age 40, testosterone levels begin to decline. This appears to result from a gradual decrease in the secretion of LH from the pituitary, along with a gradual loss in responsiveness of the testosterone-producing Leydig cells to chemical signals. The result is typically a slow

---

A WORD ABOUT BALDING

While testosterone is the major male hormone circulating in the blood, a higher-octane androgen called **dihydrotestosterone (DHT)** can be found in organs including the prostate and hair follicles. This powerful chemical messenger is produced when a special enzyme, **5 alpha-reductase**, mixes with regular testosterone in the cells. Though testosterone is far better known and gets the banner headlines, it's the relatively obscure DHT that causes the prostate to grow at puberty. DHT also spurs the development of body and facial hair. Over time, 5 alpha-reductase and the DHT it produces are responsible for thickening of the beard, continued growth of the prostate (BPH), and often gradual hair loss that eventually leaves many men with the characteristic horseshoe configuration at the sides and back of the head known as male-pattern baldness.

By blocking the activity of 5 alpha-reductase, the drug finasteride (Propecia), at a dose of 1 mg a day, reduces DHT levels, prevents progressive balding, and even causes regrowth of hair in 90 percent of men. In larger doses (5 mg a day in the form of Proscar), the same drug shrinks the prostate and alleviates the symptoms of BPH (see Chapter 5, BPH [Benign Prostatic Hyperplasia].) New evidence indicates that 5 alpha-reductase inhibitors also prevent prostate cancer. Less than 2 percent of men taking 1 mg of finasteride per day experience sexual side effects, which may involve a loss of libido and/or erectile dysfunction. Reduced ejaculatory volume is common.

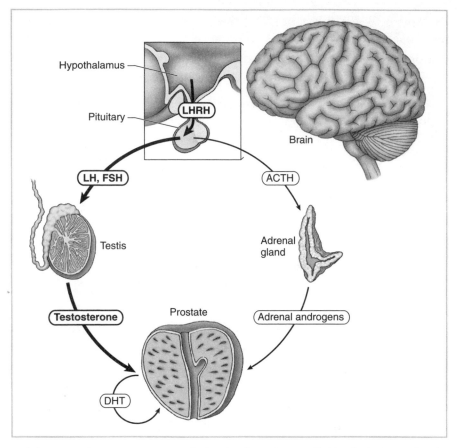

Male hormones (testosterone, DHT, and adrenal androgens), controlled by the brain, regulate the prostate and other sexual functions. Luteinizing hormone-releasing hormone (LHRH), produced by the hypothalamus region of the brain, stimulates the pituitary to release LH, FSH, and adrenocorticotropic hormone (ACTH), causing the testes to release testosterone and the adrenal gland to release other androgens.

but steady reduction in sex drive, arousal, and quality of erections with age. From the beginning of the fifth decade, 10 percent of men report that they no longer have erections adequate for sexual penetration. This percentage increases at the rate of about 1 percent per year, which means 20 percent of men report inadequate erections by age 50, 30 percent by age 60, and 50 percent by age 80 (though it also means that 50 percent of octogenarians are able to function quite well!). Since production of sperm by the testicles also requires testosterone, diminishing male hormone levels also translate into a steady decline over time in the ability to father children. Again, this does *not* mean that infertility is inevitable. There are men who continue to defy the odds.

FSH AND SPERM PRODUCTION

The testicles function like a manufacturing plant with two distinct divisions. On one side of the factory, LH triggers the Leydig cells to pump out testosterone. On the other, **follicle-stimulating hormone (FSH)** triggers sperm production. In women, the same hormones are responsible for estrogen supply and egg production, respectively.

Historically, some men have been known to father children at unusually advanced ages. Actor Cary Grant, whose only child was born when he was 62, was once considered a remarkable example, though given today's high-tech fertility treatments, the male and female biological reproductive clocks can be drastically reset to run for a far longer time. Still, the level of FSH and the consequent production of viable sperm typically decrease with age. After age 50, the number of sperm-producing cells drops to about half the level found in a 20-year-old. Consequently, fertility, especially in the absence of medical intervention, often steadily declines with advancing age.

IS THERE REALLY A "MALE MENOPAUSE"?

In women, menopause, which occurs on average at age 51, involves a dramatic shutdown of the production of ovarian stimulatory hormones (LH and FSH) by the brain. Ovulation and menstruation cease, and a host of other physical changes typically follows. Many women suffer hot flashes or other menopausal symptoms for a time. After the body adjusts to the drastic hormonal change, it's common for women to find that they are prone to the bone loss of osteoporosis, rising cholesterol levels, increased risk of stroke and heart attack, and altered sexual function, including thinning of the vaginal walls and vaginal dryness.

Many women and their physicians embraced hormone replacement therapy (HRT) as a means to "cure" menopausal symptoms. Extravagant claims that this therapy could deliver smoother skin, a healthier heart, stronger bones, greater emotional well-being, and improved mental acuity led to the common belief that the hormonal component of female aging could be slowed, arrested, or even reversed by taking a pill.

Given the profit potential of extending the market to the other half of the population, male menopause soon crept into common parlance, as did its more recently introduced equivalents, Androgen Decline in the Aging Male (ADAM) or Partial Androgen Deficiency in the Aging Male (PADAM). Many health care practitioners, drug companies, and supplement manufacturers would like men to believe that a sudden male hormone decline analogous to female menopause occurs routinely as men age. Symptoms of ADAM and PADAM, said to include diminished muscle mass, reduced libido and sexual function, fatigue, decreased energy level, and depression, are alleged to be cured by testosterone replacements and other substances designed to boost male hormone levels. In fact, such problems could be caused by many things, including physical illnesses, obesity, lack of exercise, alcohol or drug dependency, as well as relationship issues, job problems, or financial stresses.

What Is Your Testosterone Level?

Your testosterone level can be measured with a blood test, but a single result will not tell the whole story. Male hormone levels fluctuate from hour to hour and day to day. To get a true picture, multiple samples must be drawn on different days within four hours of waking. Further complicating matters is that, there are two kinds of testosterone. So-called free testosterone is not bound to a protein known as **sex hormone binding globulin (SHBG)**. Unfettered by this chaperone, the hormone is able to do its intended work of regulating mood and sexual function, maintaining muscle and bone, and so on. To determine whether or not your male hormone levels are abnormally low, you need to know both your total and your free testosterone scores.

Starting at about age 40, the amount of SHBG slowly rises, while total testosterone decreases at about 1 percent per year. As a result, there is less and less active male hormone to conduct business as men age. Nevertheless, it's important to distinguish between normally declining hormone levels and a hormone deficiency that may warrant medical intervention.

Androgen deficiency is defined as a total testosterone level below 325 ng/dl. With proper testing, we find abnormally low testosterone in 20 percent of men in their 60s, 30 percent in their 70s, and 50 percent of octogenarians.

To make an accurate diagnosis, your doctor should consider your test results and symptoms. Testosterone deficiency has been overdiagnosed in many men and unrecognized in others. While it is estimated that 2.5 million men per year between age 40 and 60 have bona fide androgen deficiency with bothersome symptoms, only 500,000 are diagnosed.[1]

Symptoms of androgen deficiency include loss of libido, erectile dysfunction, depression, lethargy, difficulty concentrating, sleep disturbance, and irritability.[2]

SHOULD YOU CONSIDER HORMONE SUPPLEMENTS?

Administered in small doses, testosterone has been shown to boost flagging libidos, improve erections, and increase men's feelings of well-being, but this only works in cases where the problems stem from an abnormally low male hormone level. For men with adequate testosterone, using a gel or patch may sound like an irresistibly easy fix for diminished desire or other natural changes that often accompany aging, but there are significant downsides to these drugs.[3]

Over time, testosterone replacement can shut down the normal hormonal feedback loop, silencing the signals that ordinarily cue the testicles to get to work. Sperm production stops, as does the normal production of testosterone. The testicles can shrink, as they often do in athletes who abuse anabolic steroids to increase performance on the field. Taken long

NOTE: We now know that testosterone replacement therapy can be safe for carefully selected prostate cancer patients with symptomatic testosterone deficiency whose prostate cancers have been treated with surgery or radiation, or those with very favorable cancers on a program of active surveillance. While a threshold amount of testosterone is required for prostate cancer to develop and grow, levels above the threshold do not cause these tumors to progress more quickly. We monitor these patients very closely. If prostate cancer is diagnosed while a man is taking testosterone replacements, the cancer was already present.

For men with advanced prostate cancer, removing all testosterone (medical or surgical castration) is a highly effective therapeutic approach that has been used since the 1940s. These men would not be appropriate candidates for testosterone replacement.

Unfortunately, we do not know the precise threshold level of testosterone necessary for prostate cancer to develop. In a severely hypogonadal man (one with very low testosterone) whose PSA and DRE are normal, a small existent cancer could grow rapidly once hormone levels are increased. Though a biopsy is not mandatory, patients considering testosterone replacement therapy should be evaluated thoroughly for prostate cancer before starting treatment and monitored closely while taking hormones.

Men with breast cancer should not take testosterone replacements. This treatment is also inappropriate for men with a high red blood count, indicative of thickening of the blood, untreated sleep apnea, moderate to severe lower urinary tract symptoms, or severe congestive heart failure.

Though hormone replacement can be safe in some men with prostate cancer, caution is warranted. If you have a PSA over 3, an abnormal digital rectal examination, or a history of prostate cancer, you should be evaluated thoroughly by a urologist before beginning hormone therapy. While on this treatment, men should be tracked regularly with PSA and DRE to identify signs of a progressing cancer.

enough and in large enough doses, testosterone replacements can shut down the testicles permanently, causing irreversible infertility and irrevocably shrunken testes.

Nevertheless, for men with abnormally low testosterone and troubling symptoms, hormone replacement therapy is a reasonable approach that may improve quality of life. The goal should be to bring testosterone to the mid-to-normal range, 350–700 ng/dl, using a patch or gel.

A gradual decline in male hormone levels is an expected part of aging, not a medical condition that requires treatment. By medicalizing menopause, countless women were actually put at *increased* risk of serious medical conditions, including breast cancer and blood clots, along with the heart attacks and strokes they were purported to prevent. Testosterone replacement therapy should be reserved for men with troublesome symptoms and abnormally low testosterone levels, and then taken only after a thorough medical examination and a careful consideration of the pros and cons.[4]

WHAT CHANGES OCCUR IN SEXUAL FUNCTION?

Mr. Jones complained to his doctor that he was not able to make love the way he used to. Checking the chart, the doctor noted that his patient was 92 years old. "When did you first notice this problem?" he asked. "The first time was last night," said Mr. Jones. "And then it happened again this morning."

While the randy nonagenarian may be the stuff of jokes, aging is not, as is commonly presumed, synonymous with sexual disinterest or incapacity. Many men remain sexually active throughout their lives. For those who do not, sexual dysfunction often results from disease, cultural factors, emotional issues, or the lack of a partner, rather than from aging alone.

This is not to say that sexual performance and experience remain unchanged over time. The primary job of male biological machinery is to facilitate reproduction, not to sustain sexual activity into old age.

While there are wide individual variations, most healthy men experience progressive, gradual sexual changes as they get older. The exact mechanism for the common age-related decline in erectile function has yet to be proven, but aging laboratory rats have a reduced ability to produce nitric oxide, the crucial chemical signal that dilates the blood vessels in the penis, allowing the critical inflow of blood that causes rigidity.

DHEA

Dehydroepiandrosterone (DHEA), a steroidal hormone similar to testosterone, is produced naturally by the adrenal glands. Peak production starts to decline in one's early 30s, and sinks to a mere 20 percent of the lifetime maximum by age 75. The function of DHEA in the body remains unclear. All that researchers agree on completely is that the hormone can be converted into either testosterone or estrogen.

A synthetic form of DHEA has been touted as a veritable fountain of youth in handy, over-the-counter pill form. People marketing the drug claim that it improves erectile function, causes weight loss, and increases muscle mass without diet or exercise. Banner ads in the media and on the Internet maintain that this wonder substance cures chronic diseases, including Parkinson's disease, lupus, diabetes, and Alzheimer's. Purveyors also tout DHEA as a cancer preventative, an immune-system booster, and a quick fix for depression and fatigue.

As with anything that sounds too good to be true, there is ample cause for skepticism. Synthetic DHEA is sold as a dietary supplement, not a medication, and is therefore not subject to regulation by the Food and Drug Administration. Despite the hype about its potential to halt or even reverse many signs of aging, the safety and effectiveness of DHEA have not been proven. Also, because the supplements are unregulated, the purity and dosage of what you may be getting are not guaranteed. DHEA supplements may also carry significant health risks, including a possible increase in prostate cancer, worsening of BPH, and liver damage.

In general, older men take longer to achieve erections. Their erections are less rigid than those of young men and do not last as long. Ejaculations tend to become less forceful and lower in volume. The refractory period increases, meaning that it takes more time after orgasm to achieve an erection again. Some researchers have reported decreased tactile sensitivity of the penis with advancing age, and others have noted a reduced incidence of spontaneous nocturnal erections, even in men who continue to have regular intercourse while awake. Young men have an average of four to five erections each night during sleep, each lasting more than thirty minutes. Associated with the REM (rapid eye movement)

Andro

Like DHEA, **androstenedione ("Andro")** is produced by the adrenal glands and can be converted into testosterone. Andro supplements have been promoted as a "natural" alternative to anabolic (muscle-building) steroids for increasing athletic performance. Allegedly, Andro accomplishes this by increasing testosterone levels. St. Louis baseball star Mark McGwire made headline news in the late nineties when he touted his regular ingestion of Andro as a key to his on-field prowess.

In fact, studies have failed to support the extravagant claims of Andro promoters, and no significant increase in testosterone levels has been found in users. The hormone does increase estrogen levels, which could result in heart or pancreas problems. Changes in blood cholesterol have also been observed, with a rise in LDL ("bad") cholesterol and a reduction in HDL ("good") cholesterol, both of which are associated with an increased risk of heart attacks and strokes.

Fortunately, in 1999, McGwire backed off from both his use and support of Andro, likely saving legions of impressionable fans from following his dubious lead in taking such an unproven and potentially risky drug.

NOTE: In 2004 the FDA banned the sale of Andro, and in 2005 it was declared a controlled substance.

sleep that accompanies dreams, these nocturnal erections are thought to help maintain healthy erectile tissue by providing a regular supply of highly oxygenated arterial blood to the penis. Erections during sleep continue throughout the life of a healthy man, but their frequency and duration slowly decline as he gets older.

CAUSES OF AGE-RELATED ERECTILE DYSFUNCTION

THE USUAL SUSPECTS

While the incidence of serious **erectile dysfunction (ED)**, the consistent inability to get or maintain an erection, increases as men age, aging alone is rarely the cause of the problem. Many things, including hormonal imbalances, vascular or neurological problems, smoking, many diseases and the medications used to treat them, psychological factors, and situational issues such as the loss of a partner, can lead to a loss of effective erections. For reasons we don't fully understand, men with lower urinary tract symptoms—frequency, nocturia—are more likely to complain of ED, and vice versa.[5]

PSYCHOLOGICAL FACTORS

The mechanics of erection are extremely complex, and many crucial elements were not recognized or understood until the past decade. Earlier, the majority of erectile dysfunction was thought to be psychological. If no obvious organic cause could be identified, the problem was presumed to reside in the patient's mind. This common misconception arose from studies of nocturnal erections. Many men who complained of erectile problems were put in a lab where their erections were measured during sleep. A strain gauge placed on the penis would register **nocturnal penile tumescence** (penile swelling that occurs during sleep) or—in an odd source of revenue for the postal service—a line of stamps would be placed around the penis. If the stamp "bracelet" broke, it was presumed that an erection had occurred.

Often, using a strain gauge or stamp test, nocturnal tumescence was found to be normal. From this, investigators concluded that there was no physical reason for the reported sexual dysfunction. If a subject had erections while asleep, logic suggested that everything physical was in proper working order.

We now know that the neurological control of nocturnal erection is different from the nerve pathways involved in arousal from physical contact or other sensory stimulation when a man is awake. In addition, the testing of nocturnal erections measures tumescence (swelling), not rigidity. The penis might swell during sleep and still lack sufficient rigidity for sexual penetration. Also, in some men there can be a decrease in arterial blood flow to the penis with active movement, despite the fact that normal blood flow may occur passively during sleep.

Of course, psychological issues can and do affect sexual performance. Depression, relationship problems, anxiety, and stress, all common in the aging male, can lead to loss of erections. Performance anxiety can hamper sexual function at any age, but it can be a greater problem for older men, especially after the loss of a partner (widower's syndrome). The telling difference is that physical problems tend to persist without treatment, while psychological ones are usually temporary and clear up once the underlying issue is resolved.

Vascular Problems

Normal erectile function requires adequate blood flow into and out of the penis. Hardening of the arteries, diabetes, or the cumulative negative effects of smoking, all of which are associated with aging, may impair the necessary influx of blood. The impact of these problems can be considerable. Diabetes results in a fourfold increased risk of erectile problems, and high blood pressure coupled with high cholesterol doubles a man's chances of developing ED.

A venous leak, which allows the blood to escape without being trapped in the penis, may make it impossible to maintain an erection. Injury to penile arteries, which can result from an accident or surgery, can also hinder adequate blood flow. In some male bicyclists, the arteries that feed blood to the penile arteries may be damaged, leading to erectile dysfunction. In one vascular condition, known as pelvic steal syndrome, blood is diverted from the penis to supply necessary circulation to other organs that are more critical for survival.

HORMONE ABNORMALITIES

As discussed above, levels of the male hormones that affect libido and sexual performance decline with age, but many older men continue to enjoy healthy erectile function nonetheless. A loss of erections may signal a hormonal abnormality or imbalance, and checking hormone levels is certainly indicated when erectile problems occur. Abnormally low testosterone or a thyroid imbalance can impair erectile function. Increased prolactin (which spurs milk production in females but has no known function in males) may signal the presence of a prolactin-secreting tumor.

Many effective treatments are available for erectile problems. (See Chapter 18, Sexual Side Effects.)

DISEASES AND THEIR TREATMENTS

Drugs designed to treat hypertension lower blood flow, including the blood flow to the penis that is required for erections. Diabetes can also affect blood flow, as can atherosclerosis (hardening of the arteries). Neurological disorders including Parkinson's disease, stroke, encephalitis, temporal lobe epilepsy, tumors, dementia, and traumatic brain injury can impair sexual function, as can multiple sclerosis, pelvic fracture, and pelvic surgery (colon, bladder, prostate). Medicines used to treat some psychiatric diseases can impair sexual function as well.

Benign Prostatic Hyperplasia (BPH) and Lower Urinary Tract Symptoms (LUTS)

In recent years there has been growing awareness that men with voiding problems (frequent urination, urgency, urinary flow that stops and starts, incomplete voiding, getting up at night to urinate) are twice as likely to have erectile dysfunction as men without these problems. Experts speculate that these men have common vascular or neurological impairments, though the exact connection remains to be proven. Because an association between ED and BPH is so common, doctors have learned to examine both issues when a man complains of problems with either urinary or sexual function. (See Chapter 5, BPH [Benign Prostatic Hyperplasia], for more on the effects of BPH.)

AGING AND THE PROSTATE GLAND

BPH

Beginning at about age 40, the level of male hormones (**androgens**) slowly declines. At the same time, there is a small, gradual increase in female hormones (**estrogens**), which all normal men have in meager amounts. The result is a significant shift in the critical ratio of these two hormones. Current thinking points to this change in hormonal balance as the prime suspect in facilitating benign enlargement of the gland (BPH).

During puberty the prostate grows from its minuscule 3- to 6-gram childhood size to the normal adult range of 20 to 25 grams. Starting in middle age, the gland often begins to grow again, frequently doubling in size. In extreme cases, an older man's prostate can reach ten or even twenty times the size of a gland we'd find in a healthy 20-year-old. The enlarging prostate can narrow the urethra, slow the voiding stream, and may compel men to awaken at night to void or to urinate with increasing frequency and diminished efficiency during the day. Fortunately, if these symptoms become troublesome, they can often be relieved with simple medications. Good surgical interventions can alleviate the problem in more serious our intractable cases. (See Chapter 5, BPH [Benign Prostatic Hyperplasia].)

Prostate Cancer

The incidence of prostate cancer also increases dramatically with age, rising at a faster rate than any other cancer. This represents a major, head-scratching paradox. Since prostate cancers require male hormones to develop, why would they arise with much greater frequency as androgen levels decline and estrogen levels rise?

The prostate's lifetime exposure to testosterone appears to be the cause. From puberty on, the gland is constantly besieged by high levels of male hormones. This is in sharp contrast to women, for whom the menstrual cycle, childbearing, breast-feeding, and menopause create periodic hormonal surges and dips in hormone levels. Still, we have much to learn about the role that androgens play in causing prostate cancer and why prostate cells are so devilishly prone to developing malignant changes over time.

Once a prostate cancer has spread beyond the local area, withdrawal of male hormones (**androgen deprivation therapy**) nearly always puts the tumor into remission. Removal of testosterone through medical means or surgical castration has been the mainstay in treatment of advanced prostate cancer for decades. Unfortunately, these cancers eventually learn how to grow in the absence of testosterone, becoming relatively **hormone refractory, at least to the first attempt to deprive the tumor of androgens**. How long androgen deprivation succeeds in arresting a cancer is related, to some degree, to a man's testosterone level at the time of diagnosis. Prostate cancers in men with higher male hormone levels take longer to become resistant to androgen withdrawal. When prostate cancers arise in men with low testosterone, the tumors have already mastered the way to survive in a hormone-deficient environment. The key suspect in this scenario is the **androgen receptor (AR)**, a molecule that enables male hormones to communicate with cells and tell them what to do. Picture a speaker at a lectern. If he lowers his voice, we can still hear him if he turns up the microphone sufficiently. In similar fashion, when testosterone falls, the volume of the androgen receptor can increase, allowing less male hormone to be equally effective.

This explains why men with elevated androgen receptor levels in their prostate cancers are more likely to have a cancer recurrence after treatment and tend to have a shorter response to hormone ablation therapy. When we reduce testosterone through medical or surgical castration, the androgen receptor levels tend to rise. (See Chapter 21, Treating Advanced Prostate Cancer.)

IN SUMMARY

Aging is a normal process, not a disease. With continued advances in the management of aging-induced changes, such as prostate enlargement, prostate cancer, and erectile dysfunction, we should continue to see an ever-increasing number of men who not only live longer but do so free of urinary miseries, with the ability to enjoy sexual pleasure and satisfaction for the duration of their natural lives.

Part Two

COMMON PROSTATE
PROBLEMS

4

■

Prostatitis

READ THIS CHAPTER TO LEARN:

- What are the different types of prostatitis, and what causes this painful inflammation in the gland?
- How can prostatitis be treated, and what should you do if your symptoms persist?
- How can prostatitis affect your PSA level?
- If your PSA rises but you have no symptoms, do you have prostatitis? Do you need antibiotics?

What's in a name? When the name is prostatitis, the answer is neither simple nor clear. While experts estimate that at some point in their lives a quarter of all men will experience the urinary burning or irritation and pelvic or rectal pain that can result from an inflamed or infected prostate,[1] the condition remains strikingly underresearched, inadequately treated, and poorly understood. Tom Stamey, a Stanford University urologist, summed up the sorry situation aptly when he referred to prostatitis as a "wastebasket of clinical ignorance."[2] In many cases, we remain uncertain about what causes prostatitis, how to prevent it, or what to do to ensure that the symptoms will reliably and permanently resolve.

On a more positive note, recent research efforts have begun to yield some promising answers about this strikingly common complaint. Though we lack strong evidence, some cases of prostatitis may be caused by an underlying bacterial infection that eludes detection by conventional means. Reflux of urine into the prostate may trigger the condition in some men. In other cases the inflammation may result from the body's own dogged, though misguided, attempts to heal itself—the immune system gone awry. Some men with persistent prostatitis-like symptoms actually may have treatable BPH or bladder abnormalities. Many men with symptoms of prostatitis have nothing wrong with the prostate at all—no infection, no inflammation. This vexing condition, known as **chronic pelvic pain syndrome (CPPS)**, is thought to arise from a wide variety of causes. A coordinated national effort is under way to define the various forms of prostatitis more precisely so we can better identify what triggers the problem in any individual case.[3] Recent studies looking at quinolone antibiotics, e.g., ciprofloxacin (Cipro), alpha blockers, COX-2 inhibitors such as celecoxib (Celebrex), and NSAIDs (see pages 303, 497), all failed to show benefits in treating prostatitis, but the trials may have been too small to yield reliable results or may not have addressed the right subset of men with the type of prostatitis that will respond. Larger studies sponsored by the National Institutes of Health are under way, and the results are being reported periodically. Leaders in the field have begun to distinguish specific subtypes of prostatitis that reflect different causes and will respond to different treatments. These studies will increase our understanding of the value of medications and other therapeutic approaches to alleviate symptoms, promote healing, and prevent recurrences.

WHO IS AFFECTED BY PROSTATITIS?

While benign prostate enlargement (BPH) and prostate cancer are rare before age 50, prostatitis can strike at any time after puberty. In adult men, the problem is an equal opportunity oppressor, distributed fairly evenly across ages, races, and nationalities worldwide. At any given time, about 9 to 16 percent of all men will have one or more of the myriad symptoms physicians look for when diagnosing the condition. In this country alone, prostatitis accounts for upward of 2 million outpatient visits to doctors, 8 percent of all visits to urologists, and 1 percent of all visits to primary care physicians, at an annual cost of more than $1 billion.[4] Still, the costs could be better described on the misery scale. The pain and other symptoms of prostatitis can be disabling. The embarrassing nature of the symptoms (painful urination, pain in the penis, scrotum, and anus, and the inability to have sexual activity), the uncertain cause of the illness, and its tendency to recur repeatedly in some men can induce depression and withdrawal that add to the detrimental direct effects of the disease.

THE FOUR TYPES OF PROSTATITIS

In an effort to promote better understanding of this widespread malady, the National Institute of Diabetes and Digestive and Kidney Diseases (NIDDK) convened a workshop on prostatitis in 1995.[5] There, experts examined the current state of knowledge about the disease and devised the following classification scheme:

CATEGORY I

Acute bacterial prostatitis is a sudden-onset infection in the prostate. Several strains of bacteria can be responsible for this form of the disease, which can cause flu-like symptoms, including fever, chills, nausea, muscle aches, and general malaise, along with pain in the pelvic region, genitalia, and/or lower back. Symptoms of a urinary tract infection, such as urinary frequency, urgency, and burning, are also common. Plus, the urine may have a foul smell.

In severe cases, a localized collection of pus (an abscess) forms within the prostate. Before the advent of modern antibiotics, such an abscess could rupture, causing serious, even life-threatening, complications. Today, treatment with powerful antibiotics specific to the bacteria causing

THE FOUR TYPES OF PROSTATITIS

	Category I Acute Bacterial Prostatitis	Category II Chronic Bacterial Prostatitis	Category III CP/CPPS	Category IV Asymptomatic Inflammatory Prostatitis
How common	Rare	Uncommon	Common	Unknown
Risk factors	Old age, compromised immune system, urinary catheter, prostate biopsy	Prior acute prostatitis or urinary infection	STDs*	Unknown
Symptoms	Fever, chills, urinary burning and frequency, sudden pain in the pelvis and genitals	Prolonged pain in the pelvis, genitalia, or anus; urinary burning and frequency	Intermittent pain in the pelvis, genitalia, or rectum; may be debilitating	None
Signs	Infected urine or prostatic fluid; PSA may be markedly elevated	Prostate tenderness, infected urine or fluid; PSA may be elevated	WBC† in prostatic fluid (Type IIIA); PSA may be elevated	Inflammatory cells found in prostate biopsy tissue; mildly elevated PSA
Cause	Bacterial infection	Bacterial infection	Generally unknown, rarely STDs* or other infectious agents; muscle spasms, bladder irritability due to BPH, stricture, stone, or tumor	Unknown
Treatment	Antibiotics (6 weeks), pain medicine	Antibiotics (6 to 12 weeks), pain medicine	Antibiotic trial, short-term anti–inflammatory agents (COX-2 or NSAID), alpha blockers, hot tub baths, stress relief	None needed
Time course	Sudden onset, responds to treatment in hours or days	Gradual onset, intermittent over months or years	Similar to Category II	May be permanent
Relapse	Unlikely	Common	Very common	Unknown

*STD: sexually transmitted disease
†WBC: white blood cells

the infection can kill the germ, relieve the misery, and effect a cure. The error some patients make is discontinuing the medication when symptoms subside. A full six-week course of antibiotics should be prescribed and faithfully completed to minimize the risk of a relapse.[6]

Category I prostatitis is rare, accounting for only 5 percent of cases. It can occur in young men, sometimes related to one of the sexually transmitted diseases, but occurs more often in older men who have had a **Foley catheter** inserted through their penis to drain the bladder for any reason, or following a prostate biopsy (in 1 percent of cases), or in elderly men with compromised immune systems, who are susceptible to a urinary tract infection.

Category II

Chronic bacterial prostatitis, which accounts for 10 percent of prostatitis cases, describes an infection in the prostate that lingers for longer than three months. Though their prostates may be teeming with bacteria, men with this form of the disease may be asymptomatic between acute episodes. Acute urinary tract infection may develop as a result of the disease. Symptoms can include burning or pain on urination, frequent urination, and sometimes fever and chills.

This type of infection, which is localized to the prostate area, generally responds within a few days to antibiotics such as trimethoprim (Trimpex or Proloprim) or fluoroquinolones such as ciprofloxacin (Cipro) or levofloxacin (Levaquin). Still, a longer course of six weeks on one of these medications is essential to minimize the risk of relapse. Some types of bacteria responsible for this type of prostatitis can develop a protective biofilm that makes them resistant to treatment, causing the symptoms to recur again and again. It is very important that the specific bacteria responsible for the infection be identified in order to choose the appropriate antibiotic. This can be done with the **two-glass urine test**. The patient's urine is collected before and after prostate massage. We send both specimens for culture and microscopic examination for evidence of inflammation, bacteria, or white blood cells.

Category III

The grab-bag term **chronic prostatitis/chronic pelvic pain syndrome (CP/CPPS)** accounts for 85 to 90 percent of all prostatitis cases.[7] Debilitating symptoms and pain persist for three months or more, though there is no evidence of bacterial infection in the urine, semen, or prostatic fluid. A standardized questionnaire, the NIH Chronic Prostatitis Symptom Index (see page 62), can be used to evaluate the symptoms and gauge their severity.[8] In 7 to 8 percent of men with this form of the disease, we find trace evidence of troublesome sexually transmitted organisms, such as chlamydia, herpes simplex, human papilloma virus, trichomonas vaginalis, or mycoplasmas, though these are probably coincidental. Most men with this condition report a triggering incident, such as a urinary tract infection or trauma to the prostate area. Category III is sometimes further subdivided into inflammatory and noninflammatory types (though some experts question whether the division makes sense). If there are inflammatory or pus cells in the urine or in the second glass of the two-glass urine test after prostatic massage in a man with Category III prostatitis, we tend to presume that the symptoms are emanating from the inflammation within the gland (Category IIIA, inflammatory CP/CPPS). On the other hand, if a patient has no white cells, pus cells, or evidence of prostatic inflammation, the symptoms are likely caused by something else, such as problems in the bladder or the muscles of the pelvic sidewall (Category IIIB, noninflammatory prostatitis).

In *Category IIIA, inflammatory CP/CPPS,* a significant number of white blood cells (leukocytes) are found in the semen or fluid expressed from the prostate when a doctor massages the gland. Leukocytes are one of the body's major defenses, and their presence signals that a battle against an injury, foreign protein, or bacteria is under way. Oddly, the severity of prostatitis symptoms appears to be unrelated to the number of white cells found in the gland, suggesting that some other mechanism may be the cause.

Whether or not we find white blood cells indicative of an inflammation, further testing is recommended to rule out other conditions that can mimic the symptoms of nonbacterial prostatitis. Men thought to have category III prostatitis should have a full medical evaluation, including a complete history, a physical exam, a urinalysis including a two-glass urine test, and a urine culture. To rule out other conditions that can mimic chronic prostititis, such patients should complete the NIH Chronic Prostatitis Symptom Index (CPSI) questionnaire. They should also have a urinary flow rate test, an ultrasound to measure **post-void residual urine (PVR)**, and have their urine sent for cytological examination. A number of sexually transmitted diseases can cause similar symptoms (see page 50). They can be diagnosed through a history of exposure and cultures of urethral discharge. A urine specimen can be checked for blood or malignant cells to rule out a kidney stone or bladder cancer, both rare causes of prostatitis-like symptoms. A cystoscopic examination is sometimes indicated, especially for men who fail to respond to standard therapy. This exam can determine whether a urethral stricture, stone, or tumor is causing the pain and urinary problems. Other possible causes for such symptoms are benign enlargement of the prostate (BPH), hypertrophy, or thickening of the bladder neck.

In *Category IIIB, noninflammatory CP/CPPS,* few or no white blood cells are found in the semen or **expressed prostatic fluid**. The condition, which used to be called **prostadynia** (literally, "pain in the prostate"), involves the same constellation of urinary symptoms and pain as the inflammatory Category IIIA, but the underlying causes and effective treatments can be even harder to divine.

Though we currently lack hard evidence, Categories IIIA and B may develop differently. Category IIIA may stem from an infection, inflammation, or an autoimmune response (a kind of "friendly fire" in which the body's natural defenses go haywire and launch a misguided attack against its own organs). Category IIIB is probably more akin to a headache of the prostate. It's typically either neurological (**neurogenic**), caused by muscle contractions (**myogenic**), or stress-related (**psychogenic**).

What Are the Treatment Options?
Though we find little or no evidence of active bacterial infection in Category III prostatitis, it is reasonable to try a single three- to six-week

course of antibiotics.[9] Beyond that, antibiotics should not be used. There is no good medical evidence that further antibiotic therapy is effective, and these medications are far from risk-free. Antibiotic use can trigger common side effects such as nausea and vomiting, headache, diarrhea, skin rash, a drug allergy, or a yeast infection. Antibiotic resistance is also a serious concern. Exposure to too many germ-killing drugs can set the stage for an invasion by hard-to-control bacterial infections elsewhere in the body. The National Committee for Quality Assurance in Medical Care has targeted antibiotic use as one of the top twenty areas in need of improvement.

In many cases, prostatitis symptoms clear up spontaneously over the course of a year, making it hard to determine whether a given treatment was effective. Also, the majority of men with prostatitis symptoms have no abnormalities on tests or physical exams. Except for infection in the gland, we lack diagnostic tests to confirm the presence of prostatitis or when it goes away.

If symptoms persist or recur after a course of medication, a more intensive evaluation is indicated. This should involve a comprehensive urinalysis, a blood test for PSA, a two-glass urine test (before and after prostatic massage), an ultrasound to assess whether an abnormal amount of urine remains in your bladder after voiding (measurement of the post-void residual urine), and **urodynamic testing**, which measures bladder capacity, bladder function, and urinary flow. Your physician should also do tests to eliminate other possible reasons for the symptoms, such as enlargement of the prostate (BPH), **bladder outlet obstruction**, or **carcinoma in situ of the bladder** (cancer contained in the cells that line the urinary reservoir). If all these measures fail to expose the root of the problem, a number of second-line therapies may offer some relief.

NOTE: Even when the problem resolves with a course of medication, antibiotics may not be the actual hero in the piece. Symptoms of Category III prostatitis tend to fluctuate over time. You may have seen the same results without any intervention.

Second-Line Medications and Other Therapies

Alpha blockers (e.g., doxazosin, terazosin, tamsulosin, alfuzosin, silodosin, sold in the U.S. as Hytrin, Cardura, Flomax, Uroxatral, and Rapaflo) relax the smooth muscles of the prostate and the bladder neck, allowing urine to flow more freely. Up to 50 percent of men with chronic prostatitis symptoms—especially those with diminished flow rate, post-void residual urine, or bladder outlet obstruction—experience moderate relief with these drugs. For men with typical CP/CPPS, a 12-week course of alpha blockers proved ineffective in a randomized trial.[10] Nevertheless, for men with a diminished urinary stream or high post-void residual urine that results from bladder outlet obstruction, these drugs are worth a try. We're not sure whether the benefits result from a direct effect on prostatitis or from the muscle relaxation these drugs cause. If you try an alpha blocker, stay with it for at least 12 weeks.

5 alpha-reductase inhibitors (e.g., finasteride, dutasteride) can shrink the prostate and alleviate urinary symptoms in men with BPH. Some prostatitis patients have also found these medications helpful, though, once again, they proved ineffective in randomized trials in men with CP/CPPS.[11] We now recognize that many men with prostatitis symptoms also have BPH, and those men may benefit from a 6-month course of finasteride or dutasteride. Pentosan polysulfate, which is FDA-approved to treat bladder pain and symptoms of the painful bladder condition known as interstitial cystitis, has been tested for effects against CP/CPPS in a few small studies. Though the evidence is meager, some promising preliminary results have been reported.[12] Because Category III prostatitis causes so much misery and the symptoms can be so difficult to resolve, many men turn to alternative remedies, including herbs. Quercetin, a bioflavonoid (natural pigments found in vegetables and fruits), and Cernilton, a derivative of pollen, work by reducing inflammation in the prostate. These substances showed some benefit in small placebo-controlled studies. Flaxseed or soy (isoflavones) may also be helpful, though we don't have solid evidence as yet. The effectiveness of other commonly used substances, such as saw palmetto, *Pygeum africanum* (African prune), and zinc, is largely anecdotal and remains to be proven.[13]

In their long and often frustrating quest for symptomatic relief, typical prostatitis sufferers try five or more different approaches. Soaking in a warm bath can relax the prostate and pelvic floor muscles and provide some transient respite. Patients have reported benefits from biofeedback, local applications of heat to the affected area, or acupuncture. In some cases prostatic massage through the rectum has been useful. **Thermal (heat) therapy** delivered through the urethra (**transurethral microwave thermotherapy, or TUMT**) has been advocated by some. Supportive counseling can be very helpful in relieving the depression and anxiety that can accompany intractable malaise.[14]

A new approach views Type III prostatitis as a chronic pain problem. In a pain clinic, men with the syndrome can be treated with nerve blocks, electrical stimulators (e.g., TENS units) that block pain, medications, and other means of controlling persistent discomfort. As yet, none of these has been proven effective in a clinical trial. Where pain is the major problem, tricyclic antidepressants, such as nortriptolene or amitriptolene, can be helpful. There is no evidence that prostatitis, in any of its forms, is caused or relieved by frequency of sexual activity or regularity of ejaculation, despite age-old clinical wisdom to the contrary. Scientifically rigorous trials are still needed to determine which, if any, of the many therapeutic approaches available today offer any real and lasting benefits. Aside from antibiotics to treat known infection in the gland, studies to date have failed to confirm significant benefits of any drug or other therapy for most patients when subjected to the most rigorous scientific testing: a prospective, double-blind, placebo-controlled, randomized trial. Leading experts in CP/CPPS now advocate intense scrutiny of patients who suffer these chronic symptoms to characterize the particular features of the syndrome and individualize treatment accordingly.[15]

CATEGORY IV

Asymptomatic inflammatory prostatitis is a "silent "form of prostate inflammation, meaning there are no symptoms. The condition is discovered by chance when a microscopic examination of prostatic fluid or prostate tissue taken on biopsy or examined after the prostate is removed shows abnormal numbers of inflammatory white blood cells.[16] This type of prostatitis sometimes can be found in prostatic fluid when a man is evaluated for infertility. We may also find evidence of inflammation in a urine specimen after a man has a digital rectal examination for any urological problem or because of an elevated PSA.

We do not have a clear understanding of what causes this inflammation, but the problem is common. Twenty percent of asymptomatic men have inflammatory cells in their prostatic fluid, as do 32 percent of men with prostatitis symptoms. Five percent of men with Category III prostatitis have moderate or severe inflammation on biopsy. There appears to be no correlation between the amount of inflammation found and the severity of symptoms, and inflammation is rarely associated with infection, so antibiotics offer no benefit.

Prostatitis and BPH

Even in the absence of prostatitis pain, if we find inflammatory cells on a biopsy, men with Category IV prostatitis should be evaluated for symptoms of BPH, such as frequency, intermittency, and awakening at night to urinate. Twenty-five percent of men with BPH have inflammation in their prostates. These patients are at increased risk of progressing to acute urinary retention or other complications. They may require medical therapy (alpha blockers or 5 alpha–reductase inhibitors) to treat their prostate enlargement in order to avoid the need for surgery down the road.[17]

The clear distinction we used to make between BPH and prostatitis turns out to be faulty. We now understand that symptoms of the two conditions overlap. Prostatitis is more common in younger men, and BPH tends to strike older men, but there is considerable overlap in age. In one study, 57 percent of men who reported that they had prostatitis also had BPH. Thirty-nine percent of men with BPH in another study had a history of prostatitis. The distinguishing clinical feature of BPH is lower urinary tract obstructive symptoms (slow stream, hesitancy, intermittency, nocturia, or waking at night to urinate). The distinguishing feature of prostatitis is pain, especially on ejaculation, with frequent and urgent urination and burning on urination. In many men, these problems coexist.

Prostatitis and PSA

Though we describe Category IV prostatitis as asymptomatic, inflammation in the gland can cause an elevated PSA. Some researchers believe there may be an association at the cellular level between prostate inflammation, subsequent atrophy in the gland, and the development of prostate cancer.[18]

> NOTE: Having symptoms of prostatitis, or signs or inflammation in the prostate, has not been shown to predispose a man to cancer.

HOW DOES PROSTATITIS AFFECT PSA?

Under normal circumstances, PSA is contained in the prostate, and only minute levels are detectable in blood. The inflammation that accompanies some forms of prostatitis breaks down tissue barriers in the gland, allowing PSA to leak into the circulatory system. This can lead to a much higher number on the screening test for prostate cancer. An acutely inflamed or infected prostate can send the PSA soaring to a stratospheric 50 to 100 ng/ml, or even higher. If there is an active infection (Category I or II), the level should return to normal with effective antibiotic treatment, though it can take up to six months. Those with prostatitis that is not caused by bacterial infection (Category III or IV) can also have an increased PSA level.[19] For Category III patients who have symptoms, we recommend a single 2- to 4-week trial of quinolone antibiotics. For men without symptoms, there is no reason to prescribe antibiotics. Given the risks associated with the use of these drugs, a watch-and-see approach makes more sense. If a biopsy shows inflammation, the problem may clear up on its own, and the PSA will fall to normal. If the elevated PSA persists, a second biopsy may be indicated to rule out cancer.

For very young men in their teens, twenties, or early thirties, a PSA level that is elevated for a brief time is no great cause for concern, and testing men in this age group for prostate cancer is questionable. Prostate cancer is almost never a consideration in this situation, with the rare exception of men in their thirties who have strong family histories of prostate cancer. In men over 40, an elevated PSA is worrisome and calls for complete medical evaluation. An extreme, rapid rise in PSA almost always comes from infection or inflammation in the gland, not prostate cancer. Still, the same man can have both prostatitis and prostate cancer, so abnormally high PSA levels should not be ignored, especially in men over 50.

WARNING: Beware of taking antibiotics for an elevated PSA. Except in the rare instance of a bona fide bacterial infection causing the PSA level to rise, antibiotics are of no value. It is common for doctors to prescribe a course of antibiotics to see if it will reduce PSA, but absent symptoms and signs of infection, there is no reason to take these medications and compelling reasons to avoid taking them unnecessarily.

While antibiotics can influence the course of bacterial prostatitis, 90 percent of symptomatic Category III prostatitis and almost all cases of prostatic inflammation in men with no symptoms (Category IV) are not caused by bacteria. In the absence of a bacterial infection, antibiotics are no more likely to lower PSA or cure the problem than a placebo.

Aside from the expense, antibiotics pose a risk of side effects. Taking these medications can foster the growth of resistant organisms, exposing a patient to a severe, life-threatening infection if the PSA remains elevated and a biopsy becomes necessary.

NOTE: If you have an elevated PSA but no cause can be found, it makes little sense to use medications or herbal remedies to drive the PSA down. Drugs like finasteride or dutasteride will reduce the PSA level and yield more comforting test results, but these medications have no effect on the underlying cause of the elevation. Some men convince themselves that a "normal" PSA, even when achieved by artificially masking the actual level, means that they have no cause for concern. Wise medical decisions depend on careful consideration of all the real and relevant facts.

The real dilemma is what to do when the PSA suddenly rises from normal—say 2—to 6 or 7. Such an increase can cause enormous anxiety, and most men find it hard to wait a month or more before taking action. Nevertheless, if you have an elevated PSA but a normal digital rectal examination, the best course of action is to wait four to six weeks and repeat the blood test. In many cases PSA will return to or trend down toward normal with no treatment.[20] It's important to keep in mind that PSA levels can fluctuate from day to day for no apparent reason by more than 30 percent.[21] An elevated PSA caused by prostate inflammation can be slow to subside, so it's generally prudent to wait four to six weeks and repeat the test before submitting to a biopsy. A prostate biopsy is not a trivial procedure, and it carries a small but definite risk of bleeding or serious infection. The exceptions to this rule are cases where there's another reason to suspect cancer. If your PSA spikes and the doctor feels an abnormality on DRE, having a biopsy makes sense.

If you have urinary symptoms such as a slow stream, hesitancy, or nocturia, you may also have BPH. Men with inflammation and BPH are more likely to progress rapidly and they might need treatment for BPH. (See Chapter 5, BPH [Benign Prostatic Hyperplasia].)

CURRENT STATUS

We have many miles to go on the road toward understanding the causes and establishing reliable cures for the varied and often enigmatic disorder we call prostatitis. Studies sponsored by the National Institutes of Health (NIH) have taken critical first steps by developing a questionnaire that can rate symptoms and objectively gauge the effectiveness of various therapies in managing the disease. (See the NIH Chronic Prostatitis Symptom Index on page 62.)

These studies have also established standardized definitions for various forms of the disease, documented the damaging effect of prostatitis on quality of life, and begun to test the alleged benefits of many treatments commonly used in an attempt to vanquish the vexing symptoms. Unfortunately, the major trials of treatment strategies have failed to identify any effective therapies for the large majority of patients with CP/CPPS.

THE FUTURE

Leading thinkers in the field believe that we may need to reclassify chronic prostatitis patients according to their unique constellation of signs and symptoms—is the problem more neurological, muscular, prostatic, or psychological? This approach (**phenotyping**) may allow us to devise more effective therapeutic regimes. Meanwhile, bear in mind that while prostatitis may cause discomfort, or even misery, with modern treatment it is *not* a dangerous or deadly medical condition. Though living with persistent or recurrent symptoms may be an inescapable fact of life for some men, the way you deal with these symptoms can make all the difference. A positive attitude and equanimity will go a long way toward minimizing the impact of this disease. If chronic prostatitis is pummeling your quality of life, you might want to consider short-term counseling or even long-term psychotherapy to restore your sense of control and keep the condition from looming disproportionately large.

IN SUMMARY

Though a quarter of all men develop prostatitis at some point in their lives, our understanding of the condition remains woefully incomplete. Typically, patients try several treatments in the quest for symptomatic relief, and the process can be difficult and frustrating. Thankfully, given modern medicine, prostatitis is no longer a dangerous or lethal disease.

After ruling out possible medical causes (e.g., BPH, cancer, infection), patients should be open to therapies that address their symptoms directly. Even where the underlying cause cannot be identified, pain management techniques, such as relaxation, psychotherapy, acupuncture, and guided imagery may enhance coping and improve quality of life.

NIH CHRONIC PROSTATITIS SYMPTOM INDEX (NIH-CPSI)

PAIN OR DISCOMFORT

1. In the last week, have you experienced any pain or discomfort in the following areas?

	YES	NO
a. Area between rectum and testicles (perineum)	$\square_1$	$\square_0$
b. Testicles	$\square_1$	$\square_0$
c. Tip of the penis (not related to urination)	$\square_1$	$\square_0$
d. Below your waist, in your pubic or bladder area	$\square_1$	$\square_0$

2. In the last week, have you experienced:
   a. Pain or burning during urination? $\square_1$ $\square_0$
   b. Pain or discomfort during or after sexual climax (ejaculation)? $\square_1$ $\square_0$

3. How often have you had pain or discomfort in any of these areas over the last week?
   $\square_0$ Never
   $\square_1$ Rarely
   $\square_2$ Sometimes
   $\square_3$ Often
   $\square_4$ Usually
   $\square_5$ Always

4. Which number best describes your AVERAGE pain or discomfort on the days that you had it, over the last week?

$\square$	$\square$	$\square$	$\square$	$\square$	$\square$	$\square$	$\square$	$\square$	$\square$	$\square$
0	1	2	3	4	5	6	7	8	9	10

NO PAIN   PAIN AS BAD AS YOU CAN IMAGINE

URINATION

5. How often have you had a sensation of not emptying your bladder completely after you finished urinating, over the last week?
   $\square_0$ Not at all
   $\square_1$ Less than 1 time in 5
   $\square_2$ Less than half the time
   $\square_3$ About half the time
   $\square_4$ More than half the time
   $\square_5$ Almost always

6. How often have you had to urinate again less than two hours after you finished urinating, over the last week?
   $\square_0$ Not at all
   $\square_1$ Less than 1 time in 5
   $\square_2$ Less than half the time
   $\square_3$ About half the time
   $\square_4$ More than half the time
   $\square_5$ Almost always

IMPACT OF SYMPTOMS

7. How much have your symptoms kept you from doing the kinds of things you would usually do, over the last week?
   $\square_0$ None
   $\square_1$ Only a little
   $\square_2$ Some
   $\square_3$ A lot

8. How much did you think about your symptoms, over the last week?
   $\square_0$ None
   $\square_1$ Only a little
   $\square_2$ Some
   $\square_3$ A lot

QUALITY OF LIFE

9. If you were to spend the rest of your life with your symptoms just the way they have been during the last week, how would you feel about that?
   $\square_0$ Delighted
   $\square_1$ Pleased
   $\square_2$ Mostly satisfied
   $\square_3$ Mixed (about equally satisfied and dissatisfied)
   $\square_4$ Mostly dissatisfied
   $\square_5$ Unhappy
   $\square_6$ Terrible

SCORING THE NIH CHRONIC PROSTATITIS SYMPTOM INDEX DOMAINS

Pain: Total of items 1a, 1b, 1c, 1d, 2a, 2b, 3, and 4   = _____

Urinary Symptoms: Total of items 5 and 6   = _____

Quality of Life Impact: Total of items 7, 8, and 9   = _____

The NIH-CPSI is a patient questionnaire developed by the National Institutes of Health (NIH) to measure the severity of symptoms caused by prostatitis or related conditions.

5

∎

BPH (Benign Prostatic Hyperplasia)

READ THIS CHAPTER TO LEARN:

- Why does the prostate enlarge as men age, and what problems can an overgrown prostate cause?
- How can we diagnose and treat BPH?
- What effect does benign prostate enlargement have on PSA?

Benjamin Franklin famously opined that nothing is certain but death and taxes. But if you are a normal male and live long enough, you can add **benign prostatic hyperplasia (BPH)** to the list. BPH is the most common benign neoplasm (abnormal mass of tissue) in American men, and no normal male is immune. In fact, Franklin himself is believed to have suffered from bladder stones, urinary obstruction, and other advanced symptoms of the disease, as did his brother. In a classic case of necessity breeding invention, this resourceful founding father devised the flexible urinary catheter to manage the problem.[1]

The first recorded accounts of attempts to relieve men's urinary blockage date from an Egyptian papyrus, written in the fifteenth century BC. One remedy from that era involved a complex tea brewed from the bark of juniper and cypress trees, and beer.

Despite the best efforts of physicians, little progress in treating the condition was made for the next thousand years. The famous Greek scientist Hippocrates, who became the father of medicine when he founded the discipline in the fifth century BC, expressed extreme pessimism about patients with voiding troubles. He characterized urinary obstruction as a dire condition with a very poor prognosis and held out no hope for permanent relief. Sufferers were forced to rely on the painful insertion of harsh metal catheters of varying composition (depending on a man's financial means), which often caused life-threatening injuries or infections.

Over subsequent millennia, doctors have tried a staggering array of therapies—including heat, irrigation, galvanic cautery, electrical stimulation, injections designed to shrink the prostate, drugs, and acupuncture—in a desperate quest for the elusive cure. Elaborate, expensive, and highly questionable approaches sprang up to solve the frustrating and common condition. In the early twentieth century, a popular regimen prescribed for men with obstructive voiding symptoms involved abundant fresh air, avoidance of sexual excess and constipation, regular holidays in favorable climates, and frequent rounds of golf.[2]

Before the discovery of effective treatments, chronic urinary obstruction could result in permanent bladder and kidney damage and, in extreme cases, death. **Acute urinary retention**, where a man could not urinate at all, was a real and very serious concern. In Victorian times, the condition even spawned a fashion statement. Men with severe urinary blockage carried the catheters they needed to empty their bladders in the hollow shafts of walking sticks or umbrellas or beneath the band of the popular bowler hat. Cowboys tucked them inside their ten-gallon hats when they set out to ride the range.

In 1891, a doctor aptly named George Goodfellow is said to have performed the first **perineal prostatectomy** for urinary obstruction, removing excess prostate tissue through an incision between the scrotum and rectum. In 1895, Eugene Fuller performed the first proce-dure to clear the urinary channel using a lower abdominal "suprapubic" approach. Soon afterward, Hugh Hampton Young—who also pioneered **brachytherapy** (seed implants) and **radical prostatectomy surgery** (to remove the gland) in cases of prostate cancer—devised a punch that could remove the overgrowth through the urethra, eliminating the need for open surgery in most cases. One of Young's most famous patients, "Diamond Jim" Brady, was so grateful for the relief he got from this operation that he funded the Brady Urological Institute at Johns Hop-kins University and the Brady Foundation at Cornell University, both devoted to the study and cure of urological diseases.[3]

Today, a refined **transurethral resection of the prostate (TURP)** is the most common surgery for prostatic enlargement. Medicines that relax or shrink the gland and minimally invasive surgical approaches have transformed this ubiquitous disease from a potentially grave or even fatal condition into a manageable problem whose impact on quality of life can be minimized and often completely overcome.

WHAT IS BPH?

BPH (benign prostatic hyperplasia) can be devilishly difficult to under-stand. Technically, the term refers to microscopic changes in the prostate. "Benign" indicates that the growth is not cancer, which by definition has the ability to escape its organ of origin and spread to other parts of the body. "Hyperplasia" means overgrowth of cells. In BPH, new prostate cells proliferate, while the old ones somehow lose their way and fail to die off as they should. Still, no matter how much BPH a man develops, the abnormal overgrowth remains within the gland. Ironically, because it grows in close quarters, pressing inward on the urethra, BPH often causes bothersome urinary symptoms, while prostate cancer, which can spread outward to other organs, usually causes no symptoms at all until it is well beyond a cure.

BPH *does not* become cancer or predict that a man will develop a malignancy. Though some men are diagnosed with both BPH and

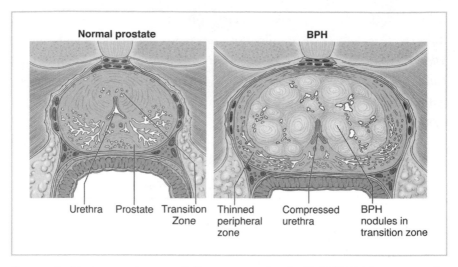

Compared with the normal prostate (left), a prostate enlarged with BPH (right) compresses the peripheral zone and narrows the urethra, causing urinary symptoms.

prostate cancer, the two diseases are distinct and typically arise in different parts of the gland. BPH affects the transition zone, the core of the prostate that surrounds the urethra, while the majority of prostate cancers develop in the peripheral zone, which lies under the outer skin (capsule) of the prostate.[4]

Though BPH actually refers to microscopic overgrowth, doctors also commonly use the term to describe a wide range of physical changes and symptoms that may occur as a result. BPH can cause enlargement of the prostate, lower urinary tract symptoms (LUTS), and bladder outlet obstruction, though any of these conditions can exist without the others. Some men with the disease have enlarged prostates, and some don't. Voiding problems may be mild, involving a slight increase in frequency or a minor decrease in the force of the urinary stream, while other patients experience severe urinary frequency or incontinence. In the worst cases, a man cannot urinate at all (acute urinary retention) and requires emergency catheterization or surgery to relieve the blockage. Though BPH is a chronic, progressive disease, symptoms can vary over time, sometimes clearing up on their own, for no apparent reason.[5]

The severity of urinary problems hinges heavily on where the BPH is located. If the enlargement occurs in the lateral (side) lobes, they may be able to swing away like the flippers on a pinball machine, allowing good urinary flow. On the other hand, an enlarged median (middle) lobe can act like a cork in the neck of a wine bottle, blocking the stream altogether. Eventually, if this benign tumor grows extremely large, it forms strange-looking, knobby protrusions that resemble cauliflower.

NOTE: There is a loose relationship between the size of the prostate and the severity of symptoms. A small prostate can cause vexing urinary problems, while a man with a very large gland may be symptom-free. Doctors often estimate prostate size with a digital rectal exam alone, but accurate measurement requires an imaging study, such as a transrectal or transabdominal ultrasound, or an MRI.

WHAT CAUSES BPH?

HORMONES

We still don't fully understand why BPH develops, but hormones seem to play a leading role. For the 7-year duration of the landmark Prostate Cancer Prevention Trial (PCPT), study subjects had their hormone levels and urinary symptom scores measured regularly. Men with higher male hormone levels and less activity of the enzyme that converts testosterone to its more potent form, DHT, were at less risk of developing BPH. This may explain why BPH occurs as men get older and their male hormone levels naturally decline.[6]

Every normal aging man is at risk of developing BPH. "Normal" is the operative word here. The condition only develops in the presence of circulating male hormones. Men castrated before puberty do not develop BPH. Neither do men with a hereditary enzyme deficiency that affects androgen metabolism.

During the early 1970s, Dr. Julianne Imperato-McGinley, a Cornell epidemiologist, traveled to the Dominican Republic to investigate reports of a tribe in which many female children seemed to develop magically into men at puberty. Called *guevedoces* ("penis at twelve"), these people were genetically male, with an X and a Y chromosome, but they had scant body hair and poorly developed genitalia, with a small penis and only one testicle, which was undescended. Intriguingly, they were also immune from acne and balding. Their prostates never grew to adult size, and they never suffered with benign prostate enlargement later in life.[7]

On examination, these men were found to have a deficiency of the enzyme **5 alpha-reductase**, which is needed to convert testosterone to DHT. Without this enzyme, some male sexual features—the prostate, seminal vesicles, and tendency to baldness—do not develop. This revelation eventually led to the development of a new class of drugs, 5 alpha-reductase inhibitors, that now includes finasteride (Proscar) and dutasteride (Avodart), which shrink the prostate, reduce the need for surgery to alleviate BPH symptoms, and lower the risk of acute urinary retention.[8]

Many men taking the medication reported an unexpected reduction or even a reversal of balding, and studies ensued to test its safety and effectiveness for this use. At a much lower dose than that prescribed for BPH, finasteride, marketed as Propecia, was approved by the FDA in 1997 as the first oral medication for the treatment of hair loss.[9]

AGING

Aging is strongly associated with BPH, and the incidence of the disease increases dramatically as men grow older. While other body parts have the good sense to reach full size at maturity and then remain stable or shrink slowly over time, the prostate undergoes a second growth spurt starting in middle age. After age 40, the prostate grows by an average annual rate of 1.6 percent per year. In men with BPH, the growth rate may accelerate to 3 to 5 percent per year.[10]

As a result, 20 percent of 40-year-olds, 60 percent of 60-year-olds, and 90 percent of men in their 80s have the overgrowth characteristic of

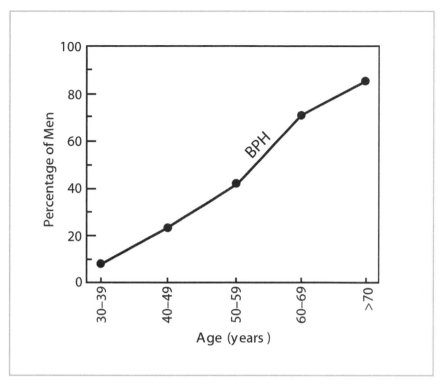

The percentage of men with BPH at each age. Most of these men will have no symptoms.

BPH.[11] In about a quarter of all men, the condition causes urinary symptoms troubling enough to land them in a doctor's office. In this country alone, BPH is responsible for 4.5 million medical visits and 85,000 surgical procedures per year. The annual bill for treating BPH in the United States is estimated to be $9 billion and growing rapidly as the average age of our population continues to rise. By 2020, an estimated 11.2 million American men each year will seek treatment for symptoms of the disease.[12]

INFLAMMATION

While BPH classically has been considered to mean enlargement of the prostate, recent studies suggest that inflammation may play an active role as well. One study of health professionals in the United States found that 57 percent of men with prostatitis also had BPH. Over a third of men who had BPH reported a history of prostatitis. When men with BPH have a prostate biopsy, one half to three quarters are found to have inflammation in the gland.

While BPH is characterized by urinary symptoms and prostatitis is defined by pain, about a quarter of men with obstructive urinary problems report painful ejaculation as well. Men with prostatitis are 2.4 times more likely to be diagnosed with BPH later on and require treatment for the condition. We now suspect that prostatitis may be an early marker that predicts which men will develop BPH.

Inflammation plays a role in BPH progression as well. In one large study (the MTOPS trial), men with inflammation on a prostate biopsy (Category IV prostatitis) were more likely to have worsening symptoms over time that resulted in acute urinary retention and were twice as likely to require surgical intervention for prostate enlargement.[13]

ERECTILE DYSFUNCTION

Men with ED are more likely to have BPH, and men with benign prostate enlargement are more likely to have erectile dysfunction, though we lack evidence that either of these problems causes the other. Both ED and BPH increase significantly with age. But regardless of age, ED and urinary symptoms are strongly associated. Why these two conditions so commonly coexist is the subject of intense investigation. At this point, we can only speculate that vascular or neurological abnormalities affect all the deep pelvic organs, including the bladder, prostate, and penis.[14]

OTHER RISK FACTORS

Researchers have explored a host of possible causes of BPH, including level of sexual activity, general health, race, diet, exercise, exposure to toxins, and presence of other diseases. None of these has been found to correlate significantly with whether a man is likely to develop urinary symptoms.

Family history. In a small percentage of cases, the disease appears to run in families, though we have yet to identify the underlying genetic mechanism.[15] On average, men with a family history of BPH have larger prostates at a younger age. Men with a first–degree family member (father or brother) who has required surgery for BPH are four times more likely to need surgery for the condition themselves.

Diet. In one large study, BPH risk was reduced in men whose diet was heavy in protein and vegetables, and in regular consumers of alcohol. Daily consumers of red meat and men with high dietary fat intake had a higher incidence of the disease.[16]

Other health issues. What's good for the heart seems to be good for the prostate. Heart disease, diabetes, and obesity are all associated with prostate growth and with the severity of BPH in men who have the disease. Exercise is good for general health and for the prostate. Smoking may exacerbate BPH because it stimulates the sympathetic nervous system, making it more difficult to relax the bladder outlet. Men with hypertension are more likely to have BPH. Both conditions are probably related to increased tone in the blood vessels and the bladder opening.

HOW DOES BPH AFFECT URINATION?

The characteristic overgrowth of BPH occurs in the transition zone, the part of the prostate surrounding the urethra, which channels urine from the bladder to the outside. Think of a fist squeezing a drinking straw and you can imagine what happens as the urethra is progressively narrowed. The bladder must work harder and harder to force stored urine past the resistance created by the constricted outlet.

Early on, the bladder compensates by building more muscle so it can contract with sufficient force to void successfully. Over time, this muscular buildup thickens the bladder wall, limiting its ability to expand to store urine. With less and less storage capacity, the bladder must empty more often. As a result, BPH may lead to a constellation of symptoms we call **prostatism**, with frequent urination during the day and awakening to urinate at night (nocturia). This should be distinguished from awakening

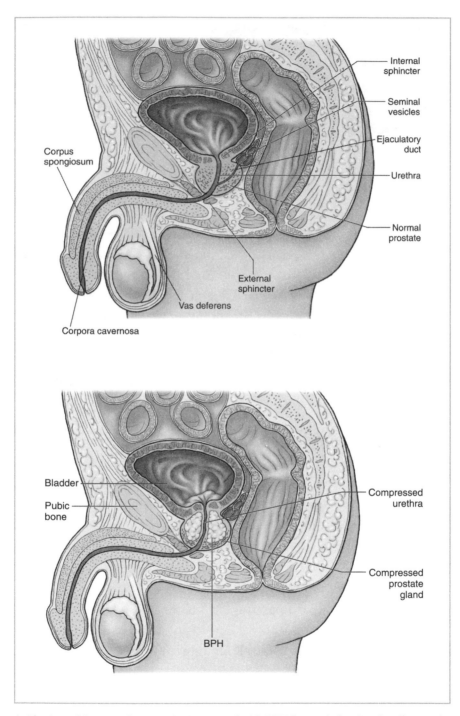

A side view of the normal prostate (top) compared with BPH (bottom), showing the effects on the urethra.

for some other reason and deciding to use the bathroom while you're awake. (See page 76.)

Eventually, the overtaxed bladder gets worn out and weak, a situation known as bladder decompensation. Daytime frequency increases, along with more trips to the bathroom during the night. When you get to the bathroom, it may take a while to get the stream started (hesitancy). This is different from the bashful bladder some men have, characterized by difficulty urinating in public restrooms.

Once urination begins, you might notice a decreased urinary flow rate, which is the equivalent of poor water pressure in the sink. The bladder may not be able to contract forcefully enough to empty all at once, and the stream becomes intermittent. The flow stops and starts again unpredictably, sometimes after you've zipped up (post-void dribbling). As the situation worsens, the bladder might become incapable of emptying completely. The presence of post-void residual urine (PVR) in the bladder leaves less room for new fluid to enter, and some men need to urinate with alarming frequency. Standing urine is a bacterial breeding ground, and a bladder that is never fully emptied sets you up for recurrent urinary tract infections. Painful bladder stones are more likely to form under these conditions as well.

As the bladder overfills, it loses the capacity to hold additional urine. Some patients develop **overflow incontinence**. Like **stress incontinence**, this causes leakage when you cough, strain, or stand. The bladder is so full—even though you may not be aware of it—that urine is forced out with any increase in abdominal pressure. Other men develop **urge incontinence**. When they feel the need to go, it has to be *immediately*. They may plan their lives around the availability of a bathroom and still can't always make it on time.

Today, with modern medical management, the most common serious complication of BPH is **acute urinary retention (AUR)**, a medical emergency that requires immediate drainage with a urinary catheter and often leads to surgical intervention. Over a 5-year period, 8 percent of men with BPH will suffer an episode of acute retention.

NOTE: The urethra in males has two distinct sections. (See illustration on page 72, the normal prostate.) The part of the urethra that runs through the penis is a tube. The prostatic urethra is a channel, carved like a tunnel through the gland and covered by protective lining (epithelial cells). When the prostate is removed to treat cancer, a new end-to-end connection (anastomosis) is sewn between the bladder and the tube that leads to the outside. A urethral catheter keeps the channel clear while the connection heals and the lining regrows.

NOTE: **Prostatism** refers to the urinary symptoms of BPH, including a weak stream, hesitancy, intermittency, frequent urination, and awakening at night to urinate (nocturia). **Prostatitis** (see Chapter 4) is an inflammation or infection in the gland, or a chronic syndrome that can cause pain in the **perineum** (the area between scrotum and rectum), lower abdominal pain, pain in the tip of the penis, and urinary symptoms such as frequency or urgency of, and pain on, urination.

HOW DO YOU KNOW YOU HAVE BPH?

Troublesome urinary symptoms call for a careful medical evaluation. Your doctor should take a focused medical and surgical history to rule out conditions like diabetes, Parkinson's disease, and stroke that can cause symptoms similar to those of BPH. The physical checkup includes a digital rectal exam to check for abnormalities that might signal the presence of prostate cancer or prostatitis. If you've ever had surgery or injury to the area or had a catheter inserted for any reason, a **urethral stricture** (narrowing of the urethra by scar tissue) could be causing your symptoms. To check for this, the doctor can examine the urethra by inserting a thin, flexible **cystoscope** through the penis under local anesthetic. Certain sexually transmitted diseases (STDs), such as gonorrhea, can also cause a stricture, and testing for such conditions should be part of the visit if you are at risk.

INTERNATIONAL PROSTATE SYMPTOM SCORE (IPSS)

Name: _____ Date: _____

	Not at all	Less than 1 time in 5	Less than half the time	About half the time	More than half the time	Almost always	Your score
Incomplete emptying Over the past month, how often have you had a sensation of not emptying your bladder completely after you finish urinating?	0	1	2	3	4	5	
Frequency Over the past month, how often have you had to urinate again less than two hours after you finished urinating?	0	1	2	3	4	5	
Intermittency Over the past month, how often have you found you stopped and started again several times when you urinated?	0	1	2	3	4	5	
Urgency Over the past month, how difficult have you found it to postpone urination?	0	1	2	3	4	5	
Weak stream Over the past month, how often have you had a weak urinary stream?	0	1	2	3	4	5	
Straining Over the past month, how often have you had to push or strain to begin urination?	0	1	2	3	4	5	

INTERNATIONAL PROSTATE SYMPTOM SCORE (IPSS) *(continued)*

	None	1 time	2 times	3 times	4 times	5 times or more	Your score
Nocturia Over the past month, how many times did you most typically get up to urinate from the time you went to bed until the time you got up in the morning?	0	1	2	3	4	5	
						Total IPSS score _____	

Total score: 0–7 mildly symptomatic; 8–19 moderately symptomatic; 20–35 severely symptomatic

	Delighted	Pleased	Mostly Satisfied	Mixed— About Equally Satisfied and Dissatisfied	Mostly Dissatisfied	Unhappy	Terrible
Quality of life due to urinary symptoms If you were to spend the rest of your life with your urinary condition the way it is now, how would you feel about that?	0	1	2	3	4	5	6

Symptom scores range from 0 to 35. A score of 7 or less would be considered within normal limits. Eight to 19 indicates moderate obstruction, 20 to 35 means severe symptoms of BPH.

The BPH workup includes filling out an International Prostate Symptom Score (IPSS) questionnaire to assess which symptoms you have and how troublesome they are.[17]

We also do a urinalysis to rule out urinary tract infection, prostatitis, or bladder cancer. We check the PSA for warning signs of prostate cancer and take a blood creatinine level, which can alert us to abnormalities in kidney function.

A number of simple, noninvasive tests can confirm the presence and degree of urinary obstruction. To check **urinary flow rate (uroflow-metry)**, a patient urinates into an electromechanical device that measures the force of the stream throughout urination. Ultrasound can determine the presence of post-void residual urine, a sign that the bladder isn't being emptied completely. To really measure the size of the prostate, the digital rectal exam is not accurate. An imaging study, such as an abdominal or transrectal ultrasound or an MRI, is the only way to determine how large the gland really is.

Urodynamic testing, which measures the function of the bladder and other parts of the lower urinary tract, is more invasive and expensive, and we generally reserve it for men with confusing or intractable symptoms.

DOES BPH AFFECT PSA?

A larger prostate is a bigger manufacturing plant, which predictably churns out more PSA (prostate specific antigen). Prostate diseases, including BPH, can break down normal tissue barriers, allowing PSA to leak out of the gland where it belongs and into the bloodstream. This can translate into a high or rising number on the PSA screening test for prostate cancer.[18] In general, the larger the prostate, the higher the PSA level will be.

The major issue is what to do about an elevated PSA, since higher levels signal a greater risk of having prostate cancer. An elevated level for your age or a steadily rising PSA will generally trigger a recommendation for a prostate biopsy to determine whether cancer is the cause. Any PSA level over 10 certainly justifies a biopsy. But when to have a biopsy for a PSA less than 10 is complicated. For more on how PSA testing is used to screen for cancer, see Chapter 8, Detecting Prostate Cancer with PSA and Other Tests.

While 4 used to be considered the upper limit of normal, thinking in the field has changed. The higher the PSA, the greater is the risk you have cancer, but cancers can also be found in men with low PSAs. Four is an artificial cut point, no longer considered absolute. Your risk of cancer depends on your age and the size of your prostate, as well as your PSA level and how much it has changed in recent years.

If BPH is the culprit, you could be put through the discomfort and anxiety of a prostate biopsy only to discover that you don't have cancer at all. Still, if cancer is the cause, we'd want to find it while it is still contained and curable. You and your doctor will have to decide whether a biopsy is justified based on your test findings and PSA history.

The tests for **PSA density (PSAD)** and **percent of free PSA (%fPSA)** were devised in an attempt to improve our ability to predict whether an elevated PSA is caused by BPH or prostate cancer. To determine PSA density, we measure prostate size in grams by an imaging study, usually a transrectal ultrasound, and then divide the PSA by that number. If BPH is causing the elevation, we'd expect the PSA to be directly proportional to the size of the prostate, i.e. a bigger gland equals a higher number. PSA density greater than 0.07 is suspicious, and a level over 0.15 indicates an increased likelihood that prostate cancer is present. Free PSA (PSA in the bloodstream that is not bound to protein) is secreted mainly by BPH cells, not cancer. A low percentage of free PSA (under 10 percent) means you're more likely to have a malignancy. Still, these measures are not perfect, and relying on them too heavily to rule out a cancer is unwise. If your PSA level is elevated for your age or the size of your prostate or has risen rapidly over the last few years, it's important to have a careful evaluation by a urologist.

After successful treatment for BPH with surgery, your PSA level should fall markedly within six to twelve weeks. If the level remains elevated (most doctors would define this as greater than 1 ng/ml), your doctor should be alert to the possibility that something else, including prostate cancer, may be responsible. Some BPH treatments—such as finasteride and dutasteride, which shrink the prostate, as well as any therapy that lowers male hormone levels—can lower PSA levels artificially. Finasteride (including low-dose finasteride, sold as Propecia to treat male-pattern baldness) or dutasteride typically drops PSA production to about half the previous level but does not seem to affect the ratio of free to total PSA (%fPSA).

Despite their effects on PSA levels, the ability of PSA and DRE to detect prostate cancer is actually better when men are on finasteride or dutasteride. These drugs shrink the benign prostate and reduce the background PSA level, but they do not affect the PSA produced by any cancer that might arise. Consequently, it's easier to detect a rising PSA or a new nodule that can be felt on DRE due to cancer in men taking these drugs.[19] If you are taking finasteride or dutasteride, be sure to notify your doctor, because these drugs do affect your PSA.

THE BOTTOM LINE

If you have an elevated PSA, regardless of BPH, you need a medical evaluation to assess how probable it is that you have cancer. Both cancer and benign prostate enlargement can cause a rise in PSA, so it is difficult to distinguish one from the other without a biopsy. While free PSA and PSA density can be helpful clues to whether or not a malignancy is present, only a biopsy can determine whether or not you have cancer. Of course, you should discuss the pros and cons of a biopsy with your doctor. Though it may detect a serious cancer, a biopsy can also lead to unnecessary treatment for a small, innocent tumor that may never have caused a problem if left undetected.

NOTE: Some people mistakenly assume that having surgery for BPH means that you can no longer get prostate cancer. In fact, after a simple prostatectomy for BPH, the peripheral zone, where prostate cancer most often arises, is left in place, and prostate cancer remains a very real possibility. No matter what treatment you have for symptoms of an enlarged prostate, you should continue to have digital rectal exams, have your PSA tested regularly, and take appropriate action if the numbers are steadily rising or abnormally high.

WHEN SHOULD BPH BE TREATED?

Tolerance for BPH symptoms is highly individual. One man might find leaking even a few drops of urine unbearable, while another may consider this an acceptable or even expected fact of life. Getting up during the night to urinate may strike you as a minor annoyance, a major disruption, or a nonissue. Increased frequency could have a very different meaning for a man with a desk job and a bathroom down the hall and for a long-haul truck driver.

You alone can judge what impact your symptoms are having on your quality of life. If you are bothered by urinary changes, it's probably time to see a doctor and explore your treatment options. The International Prostate Symptom Score (IPSS) (see page 75) is specifically designed to assess how bothersome your symptoms are. If you have severe symptoms, such as blood in your urine, recurrent urinary tract infections, bladder stones, or trouble emptying your bladder, toughing it out is *not* a good idea.

Once a man has symptomatic BPH, the likelihood is that symptoms will progress over time.[20] In large studies that tested 5 alpha-reductase inhibitors and alpha blockers as medical therapy for BPH, about 3 to 4 percent of participants per year reported worsening symptoms (an increase in the IPSS score by 3 or more). After five years, 1 man in 4 reported substantially worse symptoms, and 1 in 20 developed acute urinary retention (AUR) or needed surgical intervention. One in 3 got better in the short run without treatment, but in most cases the symptoms progressed over time.[21] The risk of progression is higher in those with a bigger prostate (more than 30 g), a PSA greater than 1.6, a urinary flow test less than 10, or residual urine greater than 40 cc. In addition, symptom progression seems to worsen with age.[22]

In a modern medical care system, the risk of permanent bladder or kidney damage from BPH is very low, although it can cause urinary tract infections, blood in the urine, and bladder stones, and if left untreated, eventually can block the kidneys and cause renal failure.[23]

Appropriate medical or surgical intervention often resolves bothersome symptoms and may avert more serious problems later on. Mild or moderate

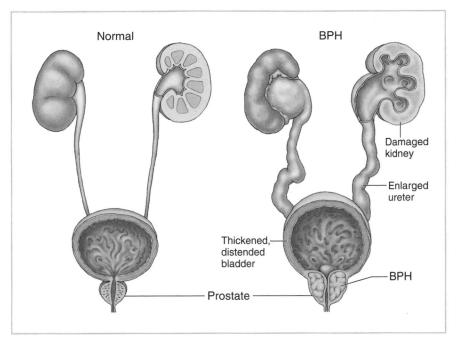

Advanced BPH can cause severe urinary obstruction. The blocked ureters become dilated, and the kidneys are damaged. Given modern treatment, this need not occur.

cases of BPH can generally be managed by more conservative, less aggressive and invasive measures that carry a lower risk of side effects.

WHAT ARE THE TREATMENT OPTIONS FOR BPH?

WATCHFUL WAITING

Whether, when, and how we treat BPH depend on the severity of the symptoms it causes and the impact those symptoms have on a patient's quality of life. Men with minimal symptoms (a score of 7 or less) and those with moderate symptoms (8 to 19) on the **International Prostate Symptom Score (IPSS)** (see page 75) and a small prostate (less than 30 cc) can be managed best with **watchful waiting**. Simple lifestyle changes, such as restricting liquids a couple of hours before bedtime and taking care to empty the bladder before a movie or long car ride, may be enough to alleviate the situation. In men with an enlarged prostate and moderate symptoms or those with severe, bothersome symptoms, active treatment is the wiser course, both to reduce urinary problems and to prevent progressive urinary obstruction.[24]

MEDICAL TREATMENTS

Until twenty years ago, surgery was the only treatment we had for troubling symptoms of prostate enlargement. The first BPH medication was approved in the late 1980s. At that time, it was considered remarkable that we could decrease urinary symptoms with medicine alone. Now we focus more on long-term treatment of this disease. When does it make sense to stay on medications, and when is it best to move to surgery? Studies are now under way to measure the long-term effects of drugs used to treat BPH.[25] Our goal is to prevent worsening symptoms over time.

Alpha Blockers

Alpha blockers, such as **doxazosin** (Cardura) or **terazosin** (Hytrin), were originally developed to treat high blood pressure by relaxing smooth muscles in blood vessel walls. By the same action, these drugs can lower muscle tension in the prostate, bladder neck, and urethra, allowing urine to flow more freely. Newer agents, like **tamsulosin** (Flomax), **alfuzosin** (Uroxatral), or silodosin (Rapaflo) have a more specific effect on relaxing only the prostate and may have fewer side effects. Alpha blockers take effect quickly, providing relief in a matter of days or weeks. They work best in patients with small prostates whose BPH nodules largely arise from the smooth muscle tissue of the gland, though they can be effective regardless of prostate size. Unlike earlier alpha blockers, these newer drugs do not need to be built up gradually to find the appropriate dose. All of the alpha blockers in current use appear to be equally effective.[26] About two thirds of men with symptomatic BPH experience a mild to moderate reduction in voiding problems with the use of these drugs. Five to 10 percent of men taking these drugs experience unpleasant side effects, including fatigue, headache, nasal stuffiness, and **postural hypotension**, where a change in position causes a sudden drop in blood pressure with resultant dizziness. **Retrograde ejaculation**, where the sperm is harmlessly discharged up into the bladder on orgasm, rather than out through the penis, and decreased ejaculatory volume may also occur.

Long-term effects vary, since these drugs do not alter the usual growth of the prostate over time. In clinical trials, alfuzosin reduced the risk of overall symptom progression but did not reduce the risk of urinary retention or the need for surgery over two years. Doxazosin provided durable relief over four years. Overall, alpha blockers have proven effective over a period of one to four years.

5 Alpha-Reductase Inhibitors

The 5 alpha-reductase inhibitors finasteride (Proscar) and dutasteride (Avodart) gradually shrink the prostate by blocking production of 5 alpha-reductase, the enzyme that converts testosterone into its more powerful form, dihydrotestosterone (DHT), within the prostate. These medications reduce the level of effective testosterone in the prostate while raising male hormone levels in the bloodstream, so they rarely cause symptoms of androgen deficiency such as reduced libido or erections. For men whose symptoms are caused by an enlarged prostate, these drugs have been proven highly effective in reducing symptoms and preventing the development of acute urinary retention and the need for surgery to alleviate bladder blockage down the road. Finasteride and dutasteride take longer to work than alpha blockers, so a trial of at least six months on the drug may be necessary to gauge its effects.[27]

NOTE: The 5 alpha-reductase enzyme comes in two forms. Finasteride blocks type II of the enzyme. Dutasteride blocks both type I and type II. So far, no studies have shown that one form of the drug is better than another at relieving symptoms of BPH.

The Medical Therapy of Prostatic Symptoms (MTOPS) study, a large, randomized trial, compared the effectiveness of finasteride taken alone, the alpha blocker doxazosin taken alone, and both of these drugs used in combination. Using both of these medications proved superior in halting progression of the disease and relieving symptoms, but of the two, finasteride was more effective.[28]

5 alpha-reductase inhibitors are approved for the treatment of BPH, but we have also speculated that they might prevent prostate cancer. Indeed, the Prostate Cancer Prevention Trial (PCPT), published in 2003, demonstrated that finasteride can reduce the risk of developing prostate cancer by 25 percent.[29] Though early evidence suggested that the drug might increase risk of more high-grade, potentially aggressive cancers, subsequent studies resolved the issue, and it is now clear that 5 alpha-reductase inhibitors can safely be used for cancer prevention, especially in men with symptomatic BPH or those at high risk of prostate cancer. (See Chapter 7, Risk Factors and Prevention.)[30]

Of course, anyone on finasteride or dutasteride should inform his doctor, since it has an effect on PSA.

NOTE: While 5 alpha-reductase inhibitors reduce the risk that a man with BPH will need surgery over time, the reduction among all men treated was small, from about 10 percent to 5 percent requiring surgery over four years.[31] We need better ways to determine which high-risk patients would benefit most by taking medication permanently, so the other men can avoid the side effects and expense of the drugs. Men with a large prostate (greater than 30 grams), a higher PSA (greater than 1.6 ng/ml) or worse symptoms (IPSS greater than 15) and with inflammation on prostate biopsy are at increased risk, and nomograms (mathematical models) have been developed to quantitate this risk.[32] (For more information about nomograms, see the Resources section at the end of this book or visit www.nomograms.org.)

Four percent of patients who take 5 alpha-reductase inhibitors experience a loss of libido, erectile dysfunction, or both. Reduced ejaculatory volume is common, some men report breast swelling or tenderness, and some have allergic reactions. In most cases, the symptoms resolve promptly when the drug is stopped.

Medications for BPH can cost up to $5 per day, and their effectiveness depends on taking the recommended dose regularly.

Phytotherapy and Nutritional Supplements

These supplements, derived from plant extracts, have not been proven effective in managing the urinary symptoms of BPH. Despite extravagant claims, some of these substances may, in fact, do nothing more than shrink the size of your wallet. Some patients report symptomatic relief when taking such herbal remedies as saw palmetto, but studies have found this substance no more effective than a placebo. Other substances touted to treat BPH, such as African plum, African star grass, stinging nettle, rye pollen and beta sitosterol, have also shown no proven benefit.

Supplements can cause harm. Men who took zinc for macular degeneration experienced worsening of urological symptoms, including BPH, kidney stones, and urinary tract infections.

Keep in mind that these agents are unregulated and not subject to manufacturing oversight. Purity and quality can vary widely, and there is no guarantee of safety. If you try any of them, be sure to let your doctor know. Certain supplements can artificially lower your PSA, altering the results on the screening tests for cancer. Also, there is always a possibility of drug interactions, even with nonprescription "natural" or herbal substances.[33]

Diet

Heart health and prostate health go hand in hand.[34] A diet rich in soy, fruits, and vegetables may reduce the risk of BPH or progression of symptoms in men who have the disease. Caffeine in coffee, tea, or soft drinks may make symptoms worse.

SURGICAL TREATMENTS

If your symptoms persist or worsen on medications, if symptoms severely affect your normal activities, or if you develop recurrent urinary tract infections, repeated blood in the urine, bladder stones, or acute urinary retention, you should strongly consider surgical treatment for your BPH. In general, surgery is recommended for men with bothersome moderate or severe symptoms whose prostate glands are larger than 30 grams.

Many men are reluctant to give up medical therapy, even if drugs fail to alleviate symptoms. If, despite your taking medication, urinary problems are affecting your quality of life, I would encourage you to consider a surgical alternative. Surgery for BPH is safe, can offer permanent relief of troubling symptoms, and allows you to stop the medications and avoid their side effects and cost.

Surgery Designed to Remove BPH Tissue

TRANSURETHRAL RESECTION OF THE PROSTATE (TURP)   Long considered the surgical gold standard, **TURP** (sometimes colloquially known as "Roto-Rooter" surgery) accounts for 95 percent of the surgical procedures done to relieve the symptoms of BPH. Though the development of medicines to treat the disease has reduced the number of TURPs by 60 percent in the past decade, it remains one of the most commonly performed operations in the United States, over 100,000 per year.

TURP is dramatically effective and can restore your urinary tract to the way it functioned when you were 18 years old.[35] Under general, epidural, or spinal anesthesia, a small electric loop is introduced into the urethra through the penis. Excess tissue blocking the urinary channel is chipped away, and then electrical current is applied to cauterize the wound. TURP requires a hospital stay of one to three days.

Side Effects and Complications. Immediate complications include bleeding that may require transfusion in about 4 percent of cases, acute urinary retention (in 6 to 7 percent of cases), and infections in 2 percent. **TURP syndrome**, a very rare and serious, though highly treatable, complication, can cause mental confusion, visual and digestive disturbances, and cardiac symptoms. Men with prostates larger than 60 grams, who require a longer time on the operating table and more fluids introduced to flush out the excised tissue, are at greater risk for TURP syndrome. Experienced surgeons know how to avoid the problem.

Although reported in about 13 percent of cases, a properly performed TURP should not cause erectile dysfunction. About 5 percent of patients develop a urinary stricture, and about 1 percent report some incontinence. Over half of men treated with TURP develop retrograde ejaculation, where semen is harmlessly expelled into the bladder rather than out through the penis during orgasm. As a result, most men are infertile after the procedure. If this is of concern, plan to bank sperm before the operation.

Though TURP often proves to be a permanent fix, about 1 percent of patients per year experience a recurrence of symptoms, requiring further treatment.

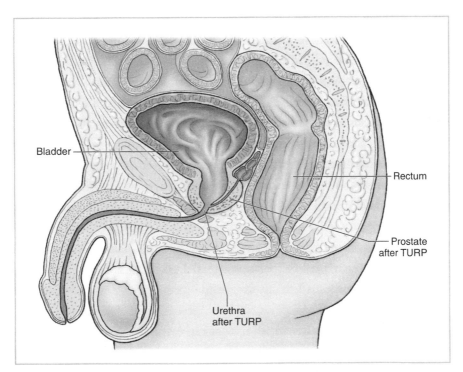

With TURP, laser prostatectomy, or traditional open surgery, the goal is to remove all the BPH tissue obstructing the urinary tract. The normal prostate gland (peripheral zone) is not removed.

NOTE: All the surgical approaches to BPH involve some trade-off. Not surprisingly, the more effective and durable the treatment, the greater the risk of side effects.[36]

LASER PROSTATECTOMY   During the past decade, several laser delivery systems have been developed to vaporize and cauterize prostate tissue.

The KTP Laser. The new KTP high-energy ("green light") laser has become a particularly popular means to relieve urinary symptoms with a lower risk of bleeding.[37] A caveat: The operation is slow. A doctor can only remove about 1 g of tissue per minute, so for men with very large prostate glands, the operation can take several hours. Also, in some men, irritative voiding symptoms such as burning, frequency and urgency can persist indefinitely and be difficult to treat.

The laser can be used on men who are taking blood thinners or anticoagulants, because it immediately seals the blood vessels. But with this procedure, no tissue is removed for examination. Any man with a suspicion of cancer needs a needle biopsy of the prostate before or during this treatment. Cancer has traditionally been detected in 10 to 25 percent of men who have a TURP to treat prostate enlargement.

Laser prostatectomy involves a shorter hospital stay, generally overnight, and more rapid removal of the catheter than TURP. The procedure carries a low risk of blood loss requiring a transfusion. This is especially important for patients with congestive heart failure or medical conditions requiring blood thinners or anticoagulants, who may be more vulnerable to the risks of traditional TURP. Other complications such as incontinence and strictures are uncommon, just as they are after traditional TURP

Symptom improvement in the short term appears to be comparable to TURP, but we don't yet have long-term results.

The Holmium YAG Laser. The Holmium YAG laser uses a different approach. This type of laser allows the doctor to cut out the nodular overgrowth in the prostate, push it up into the bladder, and remove the tissue in pieces as we do in a TURP. This type of laser can be used on large prostates, and it is much quicker than green-light. But the surgery is challenging and requires a skilled surgeon. A doctor must have enormous skill and finesse to avoid cutting too deeply and causing bleeding or damage to surrounding tissues. As with a TURP, Holmium YAG treatment leaves us with tissue to examine for evidence of prostate cancer.[38]

Side Effects and Complications: The side effects vary depending on the type of laser used, the means by which the energy is delivered, and the skill and experience of the surgeon. Some patients have irritative voiding symptoms for a month or two as tissue destroyed by the procedure is sloughed off. About 11 percent experience painful urination (dysuria) for a longer time. Rarely, this persists. Retrograde ejaculation seems less common than with TURP, though it still occurs in a third of men after KTP laser prostatectomy. Loss of erections is rare.

Open (Simple) Prostatectomy

In men with very large prostate glands or those for whom hip or other medical problems preclude the physical positioning required (legs spread and elevated) during TURP surgery, excess prostate tissue can be removed through an incision in the abdomen, using either traditional open surgery or laparoscopic and robotically assisted laparoscopic technique. Although it is as effective as TURP in relieving symptoms, open prostatectomy results in a longer hospital stay and increases the risk of bleeding that requires a transfusion. With the robotically assisted procedure, hospital stays and bleeding are reduced, but major complications have been reported, and its role is not yet clear.

With modern laser procedures, open prostatectomy is becoming rare in technologically advanced countries.

Side Effects and Complications. Retrograde ejaculation (see TURP complications above) occurs in 80 to 90 percent of patients after simple prostatectomy, and 2 to 3 percent of men develop erectile dysfunction or a narrowing of the bladder neck. Simple prostatectomy also carries a small risk of more serious surgical complications, such as pulmonary embolism, deep vein thrombosis, heart attack, or stroke.

The Bottom Line

Complete removal of all BPH is the goal of these surgical procedures. To the extent that each is done successfully, relief of urinary obstruction is comparable, as are side effects. None of these treatments, properly performed, should cause a loss of erections. The erectile nerves lie outside the peripheral zone of the gland, which is not removed to treat BPH. Incontinence should be rare, since the external urinary sphincter is left intact. In all cases, there's a risk of retrograde ejaculation. The more thorough the removal of BPH, especially from the bladder neck, the greater the incidence of retrograde ejaculation. Blood loss and the need for transfusions seem less with the laser procedures, and recovery appears to be a bit quicker. The KTP laser is a good alternative to more traditional surgery, though for a man with a large prostate, the procedure is very time-consuming and can result in significant blood loss.

If you need surgical relief of BPH, my advice is to seek a highly experienced, trustworthy surgeon and have the procedure with which he or she is most comfortable.

SURGICAL PROCEDURES DESIGNED TO IMPROVE SYMPTOMS WITHOUT REMOVING ALL THE BPH

Transurethral Incision of the Prostate (TUIP)

For men with prostates smaller than 30 grams, **TUIP** may be a good, less invasive alternative. Under general or spinal anesthetic, the surgeon passes a special scope through the urethra and uses electrical current or laser energy to make small incisions in the prostate near the bladder neck that allow urine to flow more freely.

Typically, TUIP requires a shorter hospital stay than TURP, and it can sometimes be done on an outpatient basis. A catheter remains in place for one to three days until the area heals. About 80 percent of men report an improvement in urinary symptoms. On the downside, TUIP offers less improvement in urinary flow rate and other BPH symptoms than does TURP, and it carries a greater risk of symptom recurrence with the need for additional procedures.[39]

Side Effects and Complications. Blood loss is low, and only 1 percent of patients require transfusion. Retrograde ejaculation is low as well, affecting only 10 percent. About 1 percent of men develop urinary incontinence.

Transurethral Microwave Thermotherapy (TUMT)

In **TUMT**, the prostate is heated by microwave energy, which is delivered via an antenna inserted through a catheter in the penis. Cooling fluid protects the urethra during this simple procedure, which can be done on an outpatient basis and takes about thirty minutes to an hour. Excess prostate tissue is effectively cooked. Full effects are seen after the dead tissue sloughs off, generally in three to six months.[40]

At that point, more than 50 percent of men experience symptomatic improvement that lasts for up to three years. Longer-term effects are questionable. The procedure works best for men with prostates smaller than 30 grams.

Because tissue is simply heated and not destroyed, TUMT does not cause retrograde ejaculation. Bleeding is kept to a minimum, as are surgical complications and side effects. The trade-off is a greater risk that symptoms will recur and further surgery will be required.

Side Effects and Complications. Complications include a high incidence of acute urinary retention (70 to 80 percent) for up to two weeks after the procedure, requiring the use of a catheter. As the dead tissue is sloughed away, it can get lodged in the urethra, creating the equivalent of a plugged drain. Some patients have blood in the urine or urinary tract infections, and some men have sexual dysfunction after TUMT. In rare cases, if this approach is improperly performed, severe damage to the penis or urethra can result.

Transurethral Needle Ablation (TUNA)

In **Transurethral Needle Ablation (TUNA)**, the prostate is heated by microwave needles that are placed into the BPH nodules through a cystoscope. The operation can be done under local anesthetic or sedation in the doctor's office or in the hospital. The precise placement of the needles requires a transrectal ultrasound for treatment planning. The heated tissue sloughs off slowly over days or weeks. Maximum symptom improvement is generally seen after one to two months. Because the technique is fairly new, we don't have good evidence that it offers a durable, long-term effect.[41]

Side Effects and Complications. Because urinary retention is common right after the operation, patients go home with a urethral catheter that remains in place for three to seven days, depending on the size of the gland. Other immediate complications may include painful urination, which is often worse for men with chronic prostatitis. Some men have mild urinary bleeding for 24 to 36 hours, and some develop acute urinary retention or a urinary tract infection.

A third of men develop retrograde ejaculation. A small percentage have erectile dysfunction, and less than 1 percent of men develop some degree of urinary incontinence.

High-Intensity Focused Ultrasound (HIFU)

In this approach, **High-Intensity Focused Ultrasound (HIFU)** quickly cooks prostate tissue. An ultrasound transducer placed in the rectum heats the prostate overgrowth to 80 to 90°C for about a second. The procedure must be done under heavy sedation or general anesthetic.[42]

Fifty percent of men experience some symptomatic improvement, but results are modest and not very durable. Ten percent of patients per year require re-treatment. HIFU equipment is expensive, and the procedure requires considerable training. Good comparative studies to other treatments are not yet available.

OTHER PROCEDURES DESIGNED TO OFFER MECHANICAL RELIEF

Prostatic Stents

For elderly patients or men with serious medical conditions, who are not good candidates for other surgical interventions, inserting a stent can relieve urinary obstruction and improve voiding. Basically, this is a mechanical metal-mesh device, which is inserted into the portion of the urethra that runs through the prostate and keeps the channel clear.

On the downside, stents have to be replaced periodically and can become encrusted with stones, so this fix is only temporary.

THE FUTURE

Now that we know that alpha-blocking drugs like alfuzosin, tamsulosin, and silodosin relieve symptoms of BPH and that 5 alpha-reductase inhibitors like finasteride and dutasteride lower the risk that BPH will progress to cause urinary blockage and the need for surgery, further studies are needed to see which men with BPH are most likely to benefit from taking these drugs. We are working on new mathematical models (nomograms) to predict the long-term risks for patients with BPH, so we can identify those who most need medication. New blood tests such as bPSA (PSA produced by BPH) and proPSA may help us find patients at high risk for acute urinary retention as well as help us distinguish between BPH and prostate cancer.

Further studies are needed to determine the long-term benefits of alpha blockers and the optimal combination of drugs for BPH. New studies are also needed to determine which men with BPH are likely to benefit from each type of drug therapy and when surgical intervention is most appropriate.

If patients stop taking 5 alpha-reductase inhibitors, the prostate regrows and symptoms reappear. Could there be a permanent way to block the abnormal overgrowth that causes BPH? To answer this question, we need to learn much more about the fundamental biology of the prostate. Will minimally invasive procedures be refined so that all men with budding BPH could have their transition zone ablated at an early age without causing retrograde ejaculation or other unpleasant side effects?

Newer antiandrogens may prove even more effective than 5 alpha-reductase in shrinking large prostate glands. With hope, we'll soon better understand the role of inflammation in BPH. This could lead to better diagnostic tests and new approaches to therapy for prostate enlargement. Ultimately, more effective prevention and treatment will depend on understanding the fundamental cause of this disease.

IN SUMMARY

Benign enlargement of the prostate is remarkably common as men age. Effective treatment with drugs or, if need be, surgery can alleviate urinary symptoms caused by BPH and prevent permanent bladder or kidney damage. Often, early medical treatment can avert the need for surgical intervention. But surgery can dramatically improve quality of life when medicines are no longer effective.

Part Three

PROSTATE CANCER

6

■

Prostate Cancer Facts

READ THIS CHAPTER TO LEARN:

- How common is prostate cancer?
- Who is most likely to get this disease?
- What is cancer?
- How does prostate cancer develop, progress, and spread?

HOW COMMON IS PROSTATE CANCER?

Prostate cancer strikes with remarkable frequency. In 2008, 192,280 new cases were diagnosed in the United States, and 27,360 men died of the disease, making it the most common internal cancer in American men and the second leading cause of male cancer deaths (after lung cancer). This pattern holds true throughout most of the developed world.[1]

Prostate tumors account for one fourth of all internal cancers diagnosed in men, and the lifetime risk of the disease is greater than that of breast cancer in women. One man in six will be diagnosed with prostate cancer in his lifetime, while a woman's risk of developing a malignancy in the breast is 1 in 8. The five-year survival rates for early prostate or breast cancer are nearly identical, as are the survival rates for breast or prostate cancer patients with distant spread of the disease. Though we don't fully understand the cause of either cancer, we can now prevent many prostate cancers and we can detect most prostate and breast cancers early, before they have spread, reducing the risk of death substantially. Mortality from prostate cancer is dropping more quickly (4 percent per year) than that for breast cancer (2.2 percent per year). Though it remains a serious disease, the death rate from prostate cancer is now at its lowest level since the 1970s.

WHO GETS PROSTATE CANCER, AND WHY?

Nobody knows precisely why prostate cancer develops, but a prime suspect is the male hormone testosterone. Prostate cancer only develops in men, and males castrated before puberty rarely, if ever, develop the disease. Several other factors may work individually or in concert to cause normal cells in the gland to undergo malignant changes. One man's prostate cancer may have a strong genetic component, while another case might stem primarily from high levels of dietary fat, exposure to infections, or both. Still, though we can't point the finger at any single universal cause, age, diet, race and ethnicity, genetic predisposition, and certain environmental factors all appear to play a significant role.

THE AGING CONNECTION

Prostate cancer and aging go hand in hand. Though I see an increasing number of patients with malignant prostate tumors in their 30s and 40s, less than 1 percent of all prostate cancers are diagnosed before age 45, and the disease is relatively rare before age 50. The median age at prostate cancer diagnosis is 68, and after that, the numbers begin to spike dramatically. In men over 70, the incidence increases faster than that of any other cancer. Since the average age of men in industrialized countries

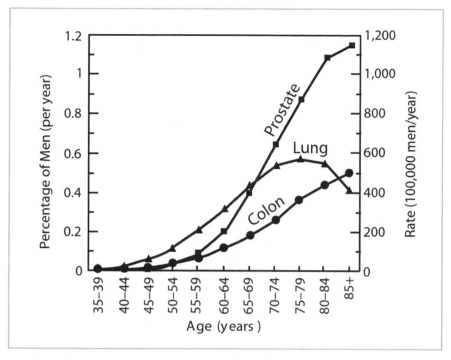

The incidence of prostate cancer increases with age faster than that of any other cancer.

is rising steadily, prostate cancer is a burgeoning problem throughout the developed world. In 2005, an estimated 190,000 men were newly diagnosed in the greater EU with prostate cancer, and 80,000 died of the disease.

THE ROLE OF DIET

Though all the relevant factors have yet to be proven, a lack of adequate exercise coupled with excessive fat and caloric intake and the resultant epidemic of overweight and obesity are all prime suspects in the frequency of this disease. A diet-and-workout regime that is heart-healthy may promote prostate health as well.[2]

The evidence for a nutritional link is compelling. Prostate cancer is ten times more common in the United States than it is in Japan. When Japanese men move to the U.S. and trade their traditional low-fat, soy-rich

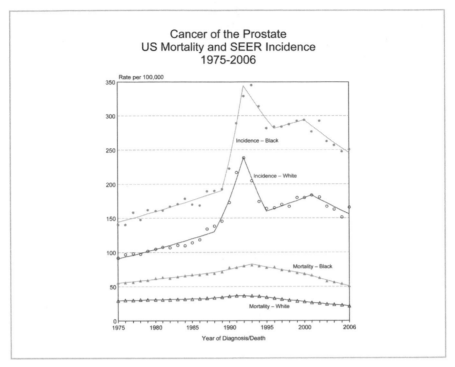

The incidence of prostate cancer by year, corrected for age. Note that the incidence (number of cases per 100,000 men per year) increased markedly in the late 1980s with the introduction of PSA testing, and then declined as many existing cases were discovered, rose again after 1995, and has been declining since. African-Americans are more than twice as likely to die of prostate cancer at any given age. Modified from M. J. Horner et al., eds., "SEER Cancer Statistics Review, 1975–2006." National Cancer Institute, Bethesda, MD, http://seer.cancer.gov/csr/1975_2006/, based on November 2008 SEER data submission, posted to the SEER website, 2009.

diet for fatty American favorites such as pizza, burgers, and fries, their risk of developing the disease soon escalates. By the next generation, the incidence shoots up markedly, and the adult grandchildren of Japanese-Americans develop prostate cancer only slightly less often than the average American man of European descent.

RACE AND DEMOGRAPHICS

Race and ethnicity appear to play a role as well. A 50-year-old European-American has a 16 percent chance of developing prostate cancer in his remaining lifetime and a 3.6 percent chance of dying of the disease. African-Americans have the highest prostate cancer incidence in the world. Their risk of developing and dying from the disease is more than twice as high as it is in European-Americans.[3] Though the causes remain unproven, genetic factors, coupled with less aggressive screening and treatment, are likely to blame. It is noteworthy that prostate cancer is less prevalent in black Africans than in African-Americans, pointing to a possible dietary or other lifestyle link rather than genetics alone. Asians run the lowest risk of developing the disease, and among Asian countries, Koreans have the lowest occurrence of all. The risk is lower for Hispanics than non-Hispanic whites. These differences can be dramatic. The average African-American has a seven times greater risk of having a positive prostate biopsy than does a recent Korean immigrant to the United States.

Geographic differences are evident as well. Men in Sweden have nearly double the prostate cancer incidence of German men, who, in turn, have a far higher risk than Israelis of developing the disease. A host of variables may be responsible, including diet, the amount of selenium in the soil, and sun exposure, which affects the levels of vitamin D. (See Chapter 7, Risk Factors and Prevention, for a further discussion of the factors that affect prostate cancer risk.)

Family History and Genetic Factors

Family history has long been known to be a risk factor for developing prostate cancer. Men who have a first-degree relative (father or brother) with the disease are two to three times more likely to be diagnosed. But since families live, work, and eat together, it has always been difficult to distinguish to what degree a familial tendency represents shared environmental exposure (e.g. diet) versus an inherited predisposition. Many genes have been associated with an increased risk for prostate cancer, but none is very common and none has turned into a useful diagnostic test for the disease similar to BRCA 1 or 2 for breast cancer.

Recently, researchers discovered that an abnormal "fusion" gene called

TMPRSS-2 (pronounced *tem-press*) exists in half of all prostate cancers. Fusion genes had been seen in some rare cancers, but they had never been found in common cancers like breast, lung, or prostate. "Fusion" genes occur when parts of two separate genes combine to form a new entity. In the prostate cancer fusion gene, one part enables the prostate cancer cells to respond to male hormones and the other part signals them to grow. Fortunately, fusion genes require yet another cancer-promoting gene to trigger their action and cause cancers to spread.[4]

The significance of TMPRSS-2 is under intensive study. Once we better understand how it works and its role in promoting prostate cancer, we may be able to use it to devise new, more sensitive diagnostic tests for this disease. A test to measure TMPRSS fusion genes in the urine is under active development.

What Do Fred and Fido Have in Common?

The only species known to develop prostate cancer are men and domestic dogs. Anecdotal evidence suggests that the culprit is diet. Domestic dogs often dine on human table scraps. Hans Lilja, a researcher at MSKCC, discovered that they are also the only mammals aside from men who have the genes for PSA and its close relative, hK2. Both are members of a family of enzymes called kallikreins, and both are strongly suspected of playing a role in the development of prostate cancer.

WHAT IS CANCER?

The disease we call cancer has two distinctive features: uncontrolled growth and the capacity to escape the area in which it arose and invade other parts of the body.

For organs to maintain health, old cells must step aside to create the space new ones require to grow and thrive. Normal cells have a limited life span and then undergo a process of programmed cell death called **apoptosis**. This phenomenon is dramatically evident in nature when autumn leaves explode with vivid color and then fade and wither. What we see as a glorious show of foliage is in fact an example of the cyclical death of old leaves required to make eventual room for new ones. In the life of cells, this process happens without such fanfare, but it is crucial nonetheless. Cancer cells, profoundly resistant to apoptosis, are virtually immortal.

Having lost the critical balance of cell birth and death, cancer grows exponentially. One cell becomes two; two yield four; four spawn eight, etc. If one cell doubles ten times, 1,024 cells result. Double that number ten more times, and the total is over a million. We refer to the rate of this geometric proliferation as a cancer's **doubling time**. The faster a malignant tumor doubles in size, the more dangerous and difficult it is to control. Some highly virulent brain tumors double in size in as little as twelve days. Early prostate cancers have an average doubling time of two to four years, though some grow far more slowly, and others, which we refer to as **high-grade** or **poorly differentiated**, typically run a far swifter and more perilous course (see Chapter 9, Biopsy). Keep in mind that doubling times may not remain constant. As a tumor progresses, its growth rate often accelerates.

The faster a cancer grows, the sooner it's likely to spread. By the time some very rapidly doubling cancers trigger positive test results or cause symptoms, many have already spread to distant organs (metastasized) and are beyond our ability to cure with surgery or radiation. Systemic treatment with hormones, chemotherapy, immune therapy, or experimental approaches would be our only hope of controlling or delaying the progress of the disease at that point.

In addition to unregulated growth, cancers eventually develop the ability to invade and spread, penetrating normal barriers in the body, such as the capsule around an organ or the wall of a blood vessel. Normal cells are like peaceable neighbors who respect property lines and keep to their side of the fence. **Benign** tumors can grow, but no matter how large they become, they are not capable of escaping the organ in which they arise. A benign kidney tumor remains in the kidney. A **malignant** kidney tumor, if left untreated long enough, eventually escapes.

Cancer cells act like greedy, land-grabbing marauders. Their pattern of invasion can be straightforward or unpredictable. As a malignant tumor grows, it may break through biological fences such as the capsule of the prostate and spread into the adjacent seminal vesicles or erectile nerves. Alternatively, some of the cancer cells may enter the blood or lymphatic systems, which circulate throughout the body. If they survive in the circulation, these malignant cells eventually attach themselves to lymph nodes, bones, or other distant organs, where they thrive as metastases. No matter where they are in the body, these cells retain their identity as prostate cancer cells. They don't become bone cancer, even though they attach themselves to bone.

Observing cancer cells under a microscope yields valuable clues about how a tumor is likely to behave. Compared with their normal counterparts, malignant cells look odd, irregular, or even bizarre. Cancers arise from mutations that alter the cell's genetic blueprint, also known as DNA. Imagine a builder working from an abstract sketch by Picasso, and you get the sense of what strange structures might result. Cancer cells have striking abnormalities, including enlarged, irregular nuclei and a generally disorganized appearance. As the disease progresses, the cells become ever wilder. The architecture of the tissue is increasingly disrupted, like a building that has been sacked and abandoned for many years. The more

NOTE: Like normal cells, cancer cells depend on blood to deliver the oxygen and nourishment they need. Without an adequate blood supply, a tumor cannot grow beyond the size of a BB (about ⅛ inch). To survive at all, cancer cells must be in extremely close proximity to blood vessels, no farther away than the width of a grain of sand. Cancers recruit the blood vessels they need through a complex process called **angiogenesis**.[5] A major new strategy for treating cancer is the development of anti-angiogenesis drugs. Thalidomide and bevasizumab (Avastin) are good examples of drugs designed to arrest this process.

abnormal (poorly differentiated) the cancer looks, the more abnormally and aggressively it's likely to behave. So-called "high-grade" cancers, which bear little or no resemblance to normal cells, tend to grow rapidly and metastasize.

THE MOLECULAR BIOLOGY OF CANCER

Cancers result from changes inside cells at the molecular level. Two fundamental mechanisms, analogous to the accelerator and brakes in a car, are responsible. The accelerators, known as **oncogenes**, cause cells to shed their normal inhibitions and grow wildly. Tumor suppressor genes counteract this unregulated growth. In a well-functioning car, you can work the gas and the brakes as needed to regulate your speed and remain in control. But imagine if, no matter what you did, the accelerator kept running at full tilt or the brakes ceased to work. When an oncogene is switched on permanently or a tumor suppressor gene is permanently switched off, cells run amok.

A major current research goal is to identify the molecular changes that are most common in prostate cancer. Scientists are working to identify the specific mechanisms that have gone awry in any given patient's tumor, so we can design the most effective therapy. In other cancers, uncovering these mechanisms has led to breakthroughs in diagnosis and treatment.

While we can observe many genetic changes in cancer cells, it is devilishly difficult to determine which are promoting growth (accelerators), which are allowing malignant changes to occur (permissive), and which are innocent bystanders. Often, the molecular changes we see are a result rather than the cause of the cancer.

The Androgen Receptor in Prostate Cancer

Hormones are chemical signals that control such bodily functions as growth, reproduction, and mood. To take up these signals, cells must have a specialized receptor molecule. Male hormones (androgens) in the bloodstream diffuse into prostate cells and bind to the so-called **androgen**

receptor (AR), forming a "hormone receptor complex." This new entity is able to enter the cell's command center in the nucleus and get to work. In the prostate gland, an enzyme called 5 alpha–reductase boosts the effects of androgens by converting testosterone into DHT, a form of male hormone that is 100 times more powerful than testosterone at binding to and stimulating the AR.

We now recognize that small changes in the level of androgen receptors in cells can drastically increase the cell's response to signaling hormones. To understand how this works, imagine a radio wave traveling through the air. Without a receiver, you hear nothing. If the signal is weak, a receiver coupled with powerful amplifier might enable you to pick it up. On the other hand, you could hear a very powerful signal without amplification.

The androgen receptor is incredibly sensitive. As little as a threefold change in AR levels can drastically alter a cancer cell's response to male hormones.[6] In some early-stage prostate cancers, the AR level is already elevated. These tumors tend to behave more aggressively, and they do not respond as well later in their course, when hormones are withdrawn through medical or surgical castration.

Given increased AR levels, a prostate cancer cell eventually can learn to thrive despite hormone ablation by using the tiny amounts of androgens made by the adrenal glands or elsewhere in the body.[7] In some advanced cancers, the prostate tumor produces male hormones on its own. A number of promising new treatments involve more powerful antiandrogens. One such drug, abiraterone, blocks all androgens everywhere in the body, including the tumor.[8] Another drug, MDV3100, in the final stages of testing, binds to and blocks the AR, rendering it ineffective.[9]

ARE ALL PROSTATE CANCERS SERIOUS?

Conventional wisdom holds that any man who lives long enough will develop prostate cancer at some point. This statement is based on the presence of minuscule clusters of malignant cancer cells found so commonly when the prostate is examined during an autopsy in men who die with no known prostate cancer. Tiny clusters of cancer cells would be found in one third of men over 50 if their prostates were removed and examined under the microscope.[10] The presence of these microscopic cancers rises dramatically among men in their 80s and 90s, when as many as two thirds have what we call autopsy or **incidental** cancers, names designed to indicate that these tiny malignant tumors are found only by chance when prostate tissue is examined after it is removed on autopsy or during surgery to treat urinary obstruction. Incidental also means that because these cancers are so minuscule, they have no effect on one's health. Another term we use to describe these small, early tumors that pose no current or immediate risk is **indolent** (sometimes referred to as clinically unimportant).[11]

The high frequency of malignant cells in the prostates of older men leads some people to view the disease as inevitable and to adopt an attitude of potentially dangerous apathy: *Everyone gets this,* they think, *so I may as well simply ignore it and hope for the best.* The oft-repeated statement that more men die *with* prostate cancer than *of* it can reinforce the risky notion that a laissez-faire approach to the disease is as good as any.

While many prostate cancers found on biopsy are large and aggressive, some are tiny, indolent tumors, discovered incidentally, that pose little or no threat to life or health. In populations like the U.S., where screening for prostate cancer is common, about a quarter to one half of prostate cancers found on biopsy today are small enough to be considered indolent. A major challenge when a man is diagnosed with prostate cancer is determining the seriousness of the threat it poses. (See Chapter 10, Understanding Your Cancer.) The level of treatment should match the risk posed by the cancer.

It takes a long time for a tiny acorn to yield a giant oak tree, and the same holds true for prostate cancers. Because this disease is typically slow-growing, most indolent cancers never grow large enough to pose a threat to health or life.

Still, finding tiny cancer clusters in the prostate does raise the risk that a man will eventually develop a serious cancer in the gland. About 1 in

12 incidental cancers do eventually grow, develop the capacity to spread beyond the prostate, and turn lethal. While active treatment for these tiny cancers is typically unnecessary at the time they are discovered, ignoring them is not a good idea. Regular PSA tests, digital rectal exams, and repeat biopsies should provide ample time to successfully detect and treat a growing tumor.[12] (See Chapter 13, Watchful Waiting [Active Surveillance].)

The picture is considerably worse for men whose biopsy results lead to a diagnosis of clinical cancer. Without the benefits of modern intervention, 20 percent will eventually die of the disease.[13] You don't want to be on the losing end of that statistic. Prostate cancer can be a fearsome adversary whose lethal potential should not be underestimated. If you are healthy, with a life expectancy of more than ten years, your best defense is to have regular screening with PSA and DRE, so we can catch the disease early in its course, understand how aggressive it is, and treat it at a time when it can still be cured.

LIFETIME RISK OF DEVELOPING OR DYING OF PROSTATE CANCER FOR A 50-YEAR-OLD MAN IN THE UNITED STATES			
LIFETIME RISK OF	RISK (%)	RISK RATIO	PROPORTIONAL RISK
Developing incidental cancer	42	11.7	100
Developing clinical cancer	16.7	4.4	38
Dying of prostate cancer	3.6	1	8.6

For every 100 men who develop cancer cells in their prostate during their lifetime, only 38 will ever be diagnosed with prostate cancer by biopsy, and only 8.6 are at risk of dying of prostate cancer.

CANCER IN OTHER MALE ORGANS

One question that continues to confound scientists is why the prostate is so prone to developing cancers, while other similar organs are virtually immune to tumor development. Cancers almost never arise in the seminal vesicles or Cowper's glands, though, like the prostate, both secrete seminal fluid and both come in regular contact with testosterone. Cancers do develop in reproductive cells in the testicles, but not because of male hormones. Testicular cancers are markedly different from prostate cancers. They do not respond to hormone withdrawal as prostate cancers do, but are exquisitely sensitive to chemotherapy, which has become a part of the prostate cancer treatment arsenal only recently, and thus far with limited effects. Penile cancers, which occur rarely in this country, have no hormonal basis either. Infections with the human papilloma virus and poor hygiene in uncircumcised men are seen as probable causes.

Something about the prostate gland makes it uniquely vulnerable to the effects of male hormones, and once we determine what that is, we may finally be able to unravel the mystery of why this disease develops with such staggering frequency and learn how to stop it before it starts.

WHERE DOES CANCER DEVELOP IN THE PROSTATE, AND HOW DOES IT SPREAD?

Seventy-five percent of all prostate cancers and 90 percent of serious ones develop in the **peripheral zone**, which lies just beneath the outer rim or capsule of the gland like an orange rind.[14] As they grow, these tumors spread out toward the capsule as well as inward toward the urethra. Because many are located within millimeters of the rectal wall, peripheral zone tumors—if they are **large** enough—can be felt during a digital rectal exam.

Eighty-five percent of prostate cancers are multifocal, meaning they arise in several parts of the gland at once. In about 85 percent of cases, **adenocarcinomas** (the type of cancer most common in the prostate) are found on both sides (**lobes**) of the prostate. This explains why many men have positive biopsies on both sides of the gland. It also explains why we treat the entire prostate gland, with either radiation or surgery, when we treat a serious cancer.

Though this disease is typically multifocal, the greatest threat usually lies in the largest cancer detected, often called the **index cancer**. In a new, experimental approach to treatment, targeted (focal) therapy treats the area of the prostate containing the largest cancer, leaving the rest of the gland intact. If smaller remaining cancers are present or grow in the future, the patient can be retreated.[15] This approach is most appropriate in men with small, low-risk cancers, but may eventually become feasible for more aggressive cancers as well.

Note: Many patients, and their partners, worry that prostate cancer could be transmitted during sexual activity. Fortunately, this has never happened. Prostate cancer cells retain the immune identity that all cells have. They cannot grow in another individual and would be rejected, just as a skin graft would. There is no danger of spread during sexual activity.

About 25 percent of prostate cancers start in the **anterior (front) half of the prostate gland, typically in the transition zone**, which encircles the urethra and is the part of the gland that develops BPH. Transition-zone tumors tend to be less aggressive and less likely to metastasize than peripheral zone cancers, but they are also trickier to diagnose.[16] Anterior cancers often arise in the part of the prostate that is farthest away from the rectum, toward the front of the body (anterior), so they are often missed on digital rectal exam and biopsy. On ultrasound or MRI, such cancers can be hidden by or confused with BPH. Still, as standard practice shifts toward sampling an increased number of biopsy cores, more and more transition-zone cancers are being discovered. (See Chapter 9, Biopsy.) I am particularly suspicious that a man has an anterior cancer if his PSA is high for the size of his prostate, and one or two previous biopsies have found no tumor or have found only a cancer that is too small to account for the PSA elevation.

In addition to being difficult to detect, transition-zone cancers are challenging to treat, no matter what method is chosen. A surgeon must take extra care to excise the cancer completely and avoid cutting into it, resulting in a **positive surgical margin**, which means that cancer cells are present at the edge of the tissue that is removed. To avoid damaging the urethra, seed implants tend to focus on the outer peripheral portion of the prostate, and the radiation dose they deliver may be inadequate to destroy a more centrally located transition-zone cancer. With transition-zone cancers becoming increasingly common, treatment must focus on the whole gland, not just the rear or peripheral zones.

If prostate cancer grows unchecked, it may spread to the seminal vesicles, which are soft, fluid-filled sacs above the prostate. **Seminal vesicle invasion (SVI)** is an ominous sign, signaling a locally advanced cancer. (See Chapter 10, Understanding Your Cancer.) While malignant cells can migrate to the seminal vesicles from anywhere in the prostate, most cancers invade these sacs by direct extension from the base (top) of the prostate. Because SVI can be difficult to detect, the seminal vesicles should be included in the radiation field or surgically removed whenever a prostate cancer is treated.

Eventually, untreated prostate cancers invade lymphatic and blood channels, sending cells off to colonize in **lymph nodes**, bones, or other sites. While breast cancer spreads on a predictable pathway to nearby "sentinel" lymph nodes, the area of prostate cancer spread to the lymph nodes can be diffuse. Recent studies have shown that it may be possible to detect the primary sites of lymph node drainage and cancer spread by injecting dye or radioactive material into the prostate before surgery to remove the gland, highlighting the first landing site in the pelvic lymph nodes by nuclear medicine scans or in the operating room by Geiger counters held over the involved lymph nodes.[17]

Spread to lymph nodes is overlooked by many doctors treating men with prostate cancer today. With earlier detection of these cancers and the limited, localized lymph node dissection so often performed, doctors expect to find spread to the nodes in only 2 to 3 percent of patients. As a result, most surgeons, especially those performing robotic prostatectomy, omit the lymph node dissection. This is a serious mistake. The limited node dissection currently used by many surgeons only detects about a third of cases in which cancer has spread to the nodes. A thorough, properly performed node dissection will find cancer in 6 to 8 percent of all cases and in 13 to 15 percent of men with intermediate- or high-risk cancers.

New data shows that 15 to 20 percent of men with microscopic

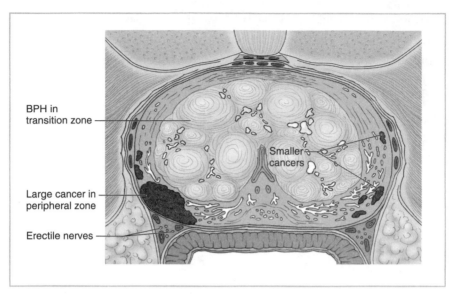

BPH in
transition zone

Smaller
cancers

Large cancer in
peripheral zone

Erectile nerves

Cancer typically develops at several sites at once within the peripheral zone of the prostate, which lies just inside the capsule. Large, peripheral-zone cancers can usually be felt during a DRE.

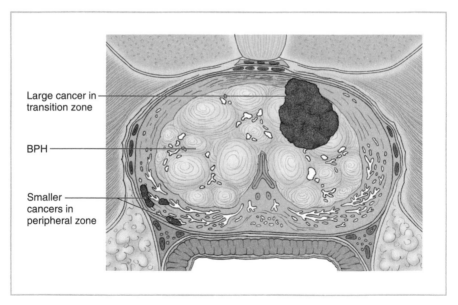

Large cancer in
transition zone

BPH

Smaller
cancers in
peripheral zone

About 1 in 4 prostate cancers arise in the transition zone, the area where BPH arises. Because they are at the front of the prostate, they usually cannot be felt during a DRE or seen on ultrasound or MRI. Transition-zone cancers are often accompanied by smaller but more aggressive cancers in the peripheral zone.

spread to lymph nodes will live out their lives without recurrence if the nodes are removed or irradiated. Treating spread to lymph nodes may improve disease–free survival rates and lower recurrence rates in prostate cancer.[18,19]

By growing directly into blood vessels, a tumor may travel through the circulation to bones in the hips or spine without ever involving the lymph nodes, so finding no cancer in the pelvic lymph nodes does not guarantee that the cancer has not spread. Bones are a prime target for prostate cancer metastases. Like enriched soil, bone marrow appears to provide a particularly hospitable environment in which these malignant cells can settle and thrive.

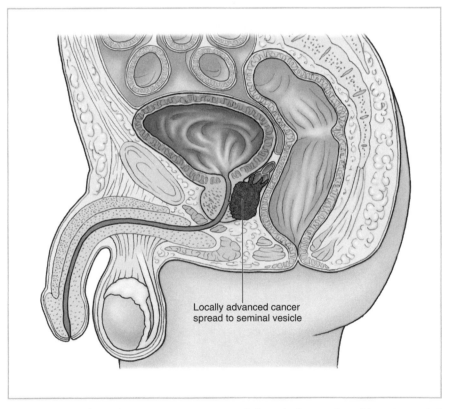

Locally advanced cancer
spread to seminal vesicle

A large, locally advanced prostate cancer may spread through the capsule and into the seminal vesicles.

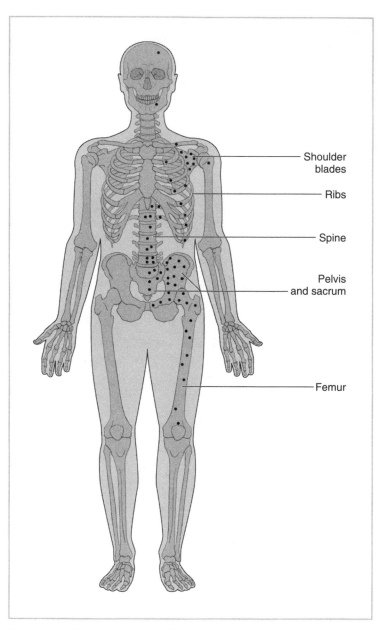

Bones, especially the spine, hips, and ribs, are the most common sites of spread when prostate cancer metastasizes.

THE SYMPTOMS OF PROSTATE CANCER

Prostate cancer is typically slow-growing and can take years, or even decades, to cause serious problems. More like the fabled tortoise than the hare, it tends to run a steady, persistent course. The disease is highly curable while still localized but difficult to interrupt once spreading cells become firmly established beyond the gland.

Early prostate cancer is silent, meaning it offers no warning in the form of symptoms. As the tumor grows, however, it can trigger a variety of problems. Once the disease is advanced enough to cause symptoms, it has spread beyond the local area and is no longer curable.

Urinary symptoms of locally advanced prostate cancer may include diminished size or force of the stream, a sense of incomplete emptying of the bladder, or the need to get up during the night to urinate. If cancer is the culprit, these symptoms tend to develop rapidly, over six months or less, compared with the slowly worsening urinary problems that are more characteristic of BPH. As prostate cancer progresses, some patients develop acute urinary retention, requiring emergency catheterization or surgery. The disease sometimes causes bleeding in the urine (**hematuria**), typically at the beginning or end of the stream. If there is blood in the urine throughout voiding, bladder or kidney problems are more likely the cause.

Blood in the semen (**hematospermia**) is rarely a sign of prostate cancer, though if it occurs, you should consult with a doctor to rule out a different malignancy or other serious condition. Usually, the problem is a ruptured varicose vein within the prostate or an infection or trauma to the area.

As a tumor grows within the prostate, it may extend upward and block the ureters, the small tubes that carry urine from the kidneys to the bladder. Ureteral obstruction can cause flank or abdominal pain, or fever and chills if the blockage leads to infection or signs of reduced kidney function such as an increased blood creatinine level. The problem puts a patient at risk for kidney damage or even kidney failure. Treatment may involve the insertion of a stent or tube to open up the channel and restore the flow.

If prostate cancer spreads to the lymph nodes, obstruction of the lymphatic drainage system may result. This can lead to intractable swelling of the scrotum, penis, feet, and legs. In the pelvis, a spreading cancer can surround nerves and cause sciatic-like pain.

Bone pain is the most common symptom of advanced prostate cancer. In addition to causing discomfort, metastases in the hips and vertebrae can lead to spontaneous fractures (see page 484). Some patients experience sudden weakness or radiating pain to the legs that can signal spinal cord compression. *Immediate* medical intervention is essential to avoid permanent paralysis.

Advanced prostate cancer can also metastasize to other sites, including lymph nodes in the abdomen or chest, the liver, and the lungs. Anemia caused by invasion of cancer into the bone marrow may also accompany advanced disease, as can appetite changes, fatigue, and increased susceptibility to infections. When men die of prostate cancer, it's usually due to a constellation of system failures.

> NOTE: Prostate cancer spreads to central skeletal bones in the hips and spine, not to peripheral bones like those of the hands and feet.

HOW FAST DOES PROSTATE CANCER GROW AND SPREAD?

Early prostate cancers grow very slowly, typically taking two to four years to double in size. Over time, as the tumor grows and the cells become wilder and more aggressive, the growth rate accelerates. Think of a small, peaceful assembly of protesters that attracts a steadily spreading groundswell of support and eventually spawns a huge, uncontrollable mob.

If we don't treat prostate cancer while it is still curable, the disease will take an average of ten to twelve years to metastasize and fifteen to seventeen years to cause death.[20] If the tumor is large and locally advanced, invading the seminal vesicles or surrounding organs, life expectancy drops to the eight- to twelve-year range. If the lymph nodes are grossly involved, meaning they are recognizably enlarged on a CT scan or MRI, or seen as enlarged by the surgeon in the operating room, the cancer generally takes six to eight years to cause death. Once there are bone metastases, the average patient lives about five to six years.

NOTE: All these figures are averages. Actual outcomes vary widely for individuals, depending on the features of their particular cancer— including stage, grade, PSA level, and so on—so you should not view statistical averages as literally predictive of what will happen to you. (See Chapter 10, Understanding Your Cancer.)

THE FUTURE

Recent findings suggest that PSA can signal the probability that a man will get prostate cancer, decades in advance of diagnosis. This challenges us to determine which of the cancers found on biopsy need immediate treatment and which can be observed over time and treated later if they show signs of becoming more aggressive. Many will never need treatment.

The steady drop in prostate cancer incidence and mortality should continue as more men, especially those at high risk, take finasteride or dutasteride, which have been shown to prevent the disease. And the dramatic decline in mortality rates should continue as aggressive, life-threatening cancers are detected earlier and treated more effectively. (See Chapter 7, Risk Factors and Prevention.)

With widespread screening and earlier diagnosis, the prostate cancer timeline is getting longer. If only a few metastatic spots are found in the lymph nodes at the time of radical prostatectomy, the average man survives this cancer for 15 to 20 years. The goal of a treatment program is to cure the disease when possible, but if it is not curable, to control it for as long as possible, hopefully for the remainder of a man's natural life.

With this objective in mind, our philosophy at Memorial Sloan-Kettering Cancer Center is to treat a serious cancer in the prostate even if the disease has spread to other areas. If lymph nodes are found to contain cancer during surgery, we still recommend removing the gland. Doing so will stop further metastatic spread from the primary tumor and avoid debilitating symptoms that can come from a cancer growing deep in the pelvis.

Modern radical prostatectomy and radiation therapy have far fewer side effects than they did fifteen to twenty years ago. Further refinements in surgical technique (see Chapter 14, Surgery) and radiation delivery (see Chapter 15, Radiation Therapy) are constantly being introduced.

Because prostate cancer has a tendency to spread to bones, one important research focus is on bone-protective agents. Another is chemotherapy. While chemotherapeutic drugs have commonly been used to treat many cancers, they have not traditionally been part of the treatment protocol for prostate cancer. That is changing as emerging studies show that certain drugs, such as docetaxel, are in fact effective against this disease.

We're learning more about the molecular biology of prostate cancer and which cellular mechanisms enable it to grow and spread. With greater understanding of the critical role that male hormones play in this disease, an important research focus is on measuring the level of androgen receptors in prostate cancers. Drugs that block or target the androgen receptor for destruction are extremely promising and are now in clinical trials.

Researchers are also looking at novel treatments such as vaccines, gene therapies, monoclonal antibodies, and variations in the way we administer hormone therapy that may slow or even arrest the progression of advanced prostate cancer, while maintaining the best possible quality of life.

IN SUMMARY

Prostate cancer is the most common internal cancer in men and the second leading cause of male cancer deaths. One man in six will eventually develop the disease, though not all cases need to be treated. Fortunately, this malignancy is typically very slow-growing and highly curable while it is still locally contained. Awareness and vigilance can ensure that we will catch the disease before it takes a lethal turn.

7

Risk Factors and Prevention

READ THIS CHAPTER TO LEARN:

- What are the risk factors for prostate cancer?
- Should you take a pill to prevent prostate cancer?
- What other steps can you take to lower your risks?

If you have prostate cancer, you may be asking: *Why me?* If you are worried about developing the disease someday or living with the anxiety of an elevated PSA of uncertain origin, you may be wondering: *What, if anything, can I do to prevent it?*

Being concerned about prostate cancer is completely understandable. If you are an American man, your lifetime risk of being diagnosed with the disease is 1 in 6, and the chance that you'll subsequently die of it is 1 in 28. In stark contrast, only 1 person in 4,000 is killed in an automobile accident, 1 in 30,000 succumbs to drowning, 1 in 100,000 dies in an airplane disaster, and lightning claims a mere 1 in 2,000,000 (though fear of flying and anxiety about being struck during a lightning storm far exceed those rare-as-hen's-teeth odds).[1]

Of course, the risks are not equal for everyone. A stunt pilot is far more likely to die in a plane crash than someone who flies frequently on large commercial airliners. The regular business flyer in turn is obviously at greater risk than a traveler who always drives. That said, road warriors on wheels trade the slim possibility of an airline crash for an increased probability of a fender-bender.

Certain risk factors, such as an inherited predisposition to develop an illness, might be difficult, if not impossible, to circumvent. Someday, manipulations of our genes may allow us to simply reprogram or disarm our genetic time bombs, but that remains a distant dream. Other risks can be reduced, and perhaps eliminated, by simple lifestyle changes. Standing under a tree in a thunderstorm is asking for trouble. If you want to avoid a lightning strike, you can simply seek appropriate shelter until the danger passes. If the storm you're trying to escape is death from prostate cancer, crucial first steps include understanding your risk of developing the disease and learning the facts about prevention, early detection, and treatment alternatives.

WHAT PUTS A MAN AT RISK FOR PROSTATE CANCER?

GENDER AND HORMONES

Every normal man is at risk for developing prostate cancer. The disease does not develop in the absence of male hormones, so men castrated before puberty and those born with severe androgen deficiencies are not susceptible. Without the most common male hormone, testosterone, or 5 alpha-reductase, the enzyme required to convert testosterone into its more potent form, DHT, the prostate will never grow to normal size, enlarge with aging, or become malignant.

Androgens are manufactured by the testicles. They circulate in the bloodstream and then attach to special receptors in organs that rely on these hormones, including the penis, prostate, skeletal muscles, and hair follicles. The degree of hormone exposure depends on how much testosterone is floating in the circulation and on how efficient a man's cells are at taking it up and using it.

NOTE: This is not to suggest that a testosterone drought is desirable. Male hormones play a crucial role in lean muscle development, bone growth and health, virility, libido, and mood.

RACE AND NATIONALITY

African-American men have the highest prostate cancer incidence in the world. They are seven times more likely to be diagnosed with the disease than Asian men, who run the lowest risk. African-Americans have positive prostate biopsies 70 percent more often than do white Americans. On average, their cancers are detected at younger ages. They are more likely to present with advanced disease, and their mortality rate is more than twice as high as whites'.[2] Several factors may account for these racial differences. Young African-American men tend to have higher levels of prostate cancer–promoting testosterone than whites, whose levels are higher, in turn, than Asians. In addition, many blacks have a quirk in their androgen receptor genes, called a **short CAG repeat**, which renders them more vulnerable to testosterone's effects, including the promotion of prostate cancer. Other prime suspects in the more ominous picture for African-American males include high levels of dietary fat, low vitamin D synthesis (see page 134), and less access to medical care.

North American and northwest European countries have the highest rates of prostate cancer, while far fewer men develop the disease in South and Central America, Africa, and Asia. Though geographic variations may be partially due to genetics, environmental factors such as diet, sunshine, and soil selenium content (see page 134) may be responsible for some of the differences as well.

AGE

The incidence and death rate from prostate cancer rise faster with age than any other malignancy.[3] Though I have treated a 29-year-old with prostate cancer,[4] and men in their 40s are now a regular part of my practice, the overall percentage of new cases rises sharply after age 50 and skyrockets in men over 70. The median age at diagnosis is 68, as opposed to age 63 for breast cancer. The median age for prostate cancer death is 77. With breast cancer, fatalities rise dramatically through a woman's 50s, 60s, and early 70s, and then steadily decline.

Age and prostate cancer appear to be bound together in some fundamental biological way that we don't yet understand. Either through a cancer-promoting factor, an alteration in hormones, or a reduction in the body's normal ability to inhibit cancer development, nearly all men eventually develop some microscopic cancers in their prostates if they live long enough. Many of these are never detected, and most will never grow large enough to present a real risk or cause problems in a man's lifetime, but some pose a highly significant danger, and we must make every effort to detect and treat them before they get out of hand.

> NOTE: "Median" means that half the men are over and half are under this age.

DIET

Prostate cancer is far less common in countries like Japan, where the diet is low in fat and rich in soy. When Japanese men immigrate to America and adopt a typical meat-and-potatoes Western diet, their risk of prostate malignancy soon increases. Their sons have an even higher incidence, and their grandsons develop the disease at a rate much closer to that seen in Americans of European descent.[5]

Such epidemiological evidence suggests that greater fat consumption is strongly associated with a higher risk of prostate cancer. Still, we can't leap from this observation to the conclusion that eating fat is ill-advised or that reducing fat intake will solve the prostate-cancer problem. In heart disease, the issue is not simply the overall amount of fat in the diet but the particular type of fats consumed. Saturated and trans fats—found in foods like margarine—have been implicated in elevating the risk of atherosclerosis and heart attacks, while certain unsaturated fats, such as olive oil and omega-3 fatty acids, are thought to be protective. Fat intake itself may increase the risk of prostate cancer, or the crucial link may be the total number of calories consumed or the higher ratio of weight to height—also known as body mass index (BMI)—that often results from a diet laden with high-calorie fatty foods, especially in the absence of an exercise program to burn them off.[6]

Being overweight also affects how well men fare once they get the disease. A recent large, long-term study found that the mortality rate for prostate cancer increased in direct proportion to body mass. The heaviest subjects were nearly 30 percent more likely to die of their cancers than were patients whose weight/height ratio fell within normal limits.[7] The relationship between obesity and prostate cancer is complex. Some studies point to obesity as increasing the risk of developing aggressive prostate cancer, but like race and nationality, weight may have little to do with the age-related development of small insignificant clusters of cancer cells within the prostate. These tend to be present regardless of body mass index. Hormones may play a role as well.

Being overweight dilutes the PSA level, so heavier men have lower PSAs than thinner men given the same size prostate and risk of cancer. They also tend to have larger prostates. As a result, their prostate cancers are likely to be detected later in the course of the disease when the chance of a cure is reduced.

Diet and exercise seem to be promoting, rather than initiating agents in prostate cancer. Men with higher body mass index may actually have a reduced incidence of low-risk prostate cancer, but if they develop the disease, it's likely to be more serious, with a higher mortality rate.[8]

Genetic factors render certain men more susceptible than others to the effects of dietary fat and obesity. The cholesterol in animal fats is converted to testosterone through the action of an enzyme called CYP17, which some men produce in greater than average quantity.[9]

There is some evidence that a diet low in protective antioxidants such as vitamin E and selenium may increase prostate cancer risk, while a regime rich in fruits and vegetables might help ward off the disease. (See Prevention, starting on page 128.)

FAMILY HISTORY

Having close family members with prostate cancer considerably increases your risk of developing the disease. If a first-degree relative (your father or brother) has had the disease, you are two to three times more likely to be diagnosed with prostate cancer and four times more likely to have a serious cancer. With two first-degree relatives, your risk of developing the disease soars to five to ten times higher than that of a man with no family history. Three first-degree relatives elevate your risk by a multiple of eleven. Closer relatives increase your odds of getting the disease more than distant ones do, but a strong familial strand, even among uncles and cousins, may be significant nevertheless.[10]

About one of every eleven men with prostate cancer reports that a family member also has had the disease. These patients have what we consider to be familial prostate cancer. By studying identical twins who have been reared apart, researchers have determined that about 40 percent of familial cases of prostate cancer are caused by inherited genes.[11] On the basis of this finding, only 1 in 28 men with prostate cancer—less than 4 percent—have an inherited form of the disease, which is somewhat less than the percentage of women with inherited breast cancer.

To date, human genome studies have identified more than a dozen separate genes that appear to have some correlation with prostate cancer, though none has proven as important or as prevalent as the mutated BRCA1 and BRCA2 genes, which are strongly predictive of breast cancer and can be identified through a simple blood test. None of the prostate cancer genes accounts for more than about 1 percent of cases, and to date we have no reliable means to screen for them.[12] Prostate cancer, whether inherited, familial, or **sporadic**, as we call all other cases, seems to develop through multiple pathways. Just as it took a combination of bad loans, a mountain of debt, plummeting consumer confidence, and a host of other adverse conditions to trigger the worldwide recession that began in 2007, prostate cancer requires a confluence of events within a man's cells.

NOTE: Prostate cancer is inherited just as often via the maternal side, so if your mother's father, uncles, or brothers were diagnosed with a malignancy in the gland, extra vigilance is in order. Many studies have sought a link between breast and prostate cancer inheritance, but so far the association is weak.

NOTE: Families tend to be exposed to similar environmental, lifestyle, and dietary influences. Many cases of familial prostate cancer appear to result from exposure to these shared factors, rather than genes. For example, familial prostate cancers might result when all men in the family eat the same high-fat diet or live in a northern climate where they are rarely exposed to the sunshine required to produce vitamin D. The inherited form of the disease, resulting from mutated genes, affects far fewer men. As a consequence of the interaction between environmental and genetic factors, identical twins reared apart may not have the same risk of getting the disease.

NOTE: Men with a strong family history tend to develop prostate cancer at younger and younger ages in succeeding generations. In patients diagnosed with the disease below the age of 55, half are thought to have the familial form. One of my patients, diagnosed at 62, has three sons in their 30s with prostate cancer. If your family tree hangs heavy with prostate cancer, your male blood relatives should begin to check the PSA as early as age 30. (See Chapter 8, Detecting Prostate Cancer with PSA and Other Tests.)

OTHER RISK FACTORS

SEXUAL FUNCTION

Studies attempting to demonstrate a link between prostate cancer and various sexual issues have generally struck out. We have found no association between the incidence of the disease and the age at which a man reached puberty. The same is true of sexual behavior, including frequency of sexual encounters, frequency of masturbation or orgasm, number of partners, types of sexual activities, sexual orientation, or marital status.[13] The risk is no different for heterosexual and homosexual men. Celibate priests get the disease just as often as men who have frequent sex with multiple partners.

For a time, it appeared that having a vasectomy might somehow increase a man's risk of getting prostate cancer. After further, more carefully designed studies, researchers concluded that the link was strictly coincidental. Men who had vasectomies were simply being checked by urologists more often, and that extra scrutiny led to the detection of more cancers.

> NOTE: Sexually transmitted diseases (STDs) such as gonorrhea may increase the risk of inflammation or prostatitis, but there is no evidence that they raise the odds of developing prostate cancer.

LIFESTYLE

Rodeo cowboys, motorcycle riders, long-distance cyclists, and long-haul truck drivers all put extra stress on their prostates, but while that can result in the perineal or pelvic pain typical of prostatitis, none of these activities has been found to contribute to the development of BPH or prostate cancer.[14]

A sedentary lifestyle contributes to increased body mass—a prime suspect both in promoting prostate cancer and in increasing the risk of dying from the disease. Regular exercise makes sense for many reasons, and reducing your risk of dying from prostate cancer may well be one of them.

NOTE: Researchers have found some evidence that inflammation at the molecular level may contribute to malignant changes in prostate cells, but whether these findings will translate into a causative link between inflammation and prostate cancer remains to be seen.[15]

EXPOSURE TO TOXINS

A few early studies suggested that workers exposed to the heavy metal cadmium in mining or in nickel cadmium battery manufacturing plants ran an increased prostate cancer risk. Cadmium is a known carcinogen that is weakly associated with the risk of developing lung cancer, but more recent, more extensive investigations have failed to confirm any causative link to prostate cancer.[16]

Dioxin is a toxic by-product of Agent Orange, which was widely used as an herbicide during the Vietnam War. Though the issue of whether or not dioxin causes prostate cancer has not been resolved, the government provides benefits for veterans who were exposed to Agent Orange and subsequently developed the disease.[17]

Studies have failed to confirm anecdotal observations that smoking and/or heavy alcohol consumption might increase prostate cancer risk, though avoiding both is wise for many other health reasons.

Anabolic steroids were developed in the 1930s to treat testosterone deficiencies. Today, they are frequently abused by athletes attempting to boost their performance or beef up their appearance. Some of these drugs, including DHEA, are legally and readily available without a prescription, though they may cause heart disease, testicular shrinkage, breast enlargement, mania, depression, violent behavior, severe acne, and cancers of the kidney, liver, and prostate. In recognition of its dangers, androstenedione was declared a controlled substance by the FDA in 2005. While the precise level of risk posed by anabolic steroids has not been fully documented, androgens are such a powerful stimulus for prostate cancer, and this disease is such a significant risk for all men, that I strongly recommend against using these bodybuilding substances.[18]

THE FIRST LINE OF DEFENSE: PREVENTION

In the public health field, prevention describes a three-pronged assault on a targeted disease. As with a security system, the primary goal is to keep trouble at bay, i.e. maintain health. If that frontline defense fails to work, the aim is to minimize negative effects by catching the problem quickly through early detection and intervention and to resolve it before it can wreak major havoc. If that fails, we seek the most effective, least disruptive means to minimize deaths from the disease and reduce side effects, medically known as **morbidities**. If fireproofing fails, the sprinkler system douses the blaze before it can destroy the building. Once the fire is out, we repair any smoke, heat, or water damage with minimal disruption at the lowest possible cost.

WHAT IS DISEASE PREVENTION?

Primary prevention refers to strategies aimed at keeping people from contracting or developing an illness in the first place. Anti-smoking campaigns that discourage teenagers from taking up the virulent habit are geared toward preventing lung cancer, heart disease, and emphysema down the road. Pesticides are sprayed to kill off the ticks that cause Lyme disease or the mosquitoes that carry West Nile virus. Clean needle exchanges, public education efforts, and condom giveaways endeavor to stem the pandemic spread of HIV.

While many studies in the test tube or with experimental mice suggest a variety of effective preventive strategies, proving that they work in humans is a major challenge. Gaining approval of a drug or treatment by the FDA requires studies lasting seven to fifteen years, at a cost of tens of millions of dollars or more. Fortunately, we now have compelling evidence that the risk of prostate cancer can be reduced with a simple medication.

5 Alpha-reductase Inhibitors

Finasteride and its chemical cousin dutasteride inhibit the activity of 5 alpha-reductase, the enzyme that converts testosterone to dihydrotestosterone (DHT), its more potent form. Men born with a genetic lack of this enzyme never develop BPH or prostate cancer. The Prostate Cancer Prevention Trial (PCPT) sponsored by the National Cancer Institute enrolled over 18,000 healthy men over the age of 55 and followed them for nearly seven years. This study found that use of finasteride reduced the overall incidence of prostate cancer from 24.4 percent to 18 percent, an overall reduction of 25 percent when compared with a placebo.[19]

Despite its astounding success, the study failed to engender widespread acceptance of finasteride to prevent prostate cancer. In the initial report in 2003, it appeared that while they had less prostate cancer overall, the men who took finasteride in this study developed a higher number and disturbing percentage of high-grade cancers (see Chapter 9, Biopsy), the kind that pose a serious risk to life and health. Doctors worried that 5 alpha-reductase inhibitors might prevent the small, insignificant cancers that posed little threat, while allowing, or even stimulating, more aggressive cancers to grow.[20]

We now know that finasteride and dutasteride really work to prevent prostate cancer and cause no increase in high-grade cancers. Further investigation of the patients in the original finasteride study proved that the drug reduced the risk for prostate cancer by an even greater margin, over 30 percent. There turned out to be no real increase in intermediate or high-grade cancers. In fact, the overall risk of these serious tumors was lower in the group receiving the drug.[21] The confusion stemmed from the way the original study was designed and evaluated.[22] A second large study, using dutasteride, confirmed the beneficial effect of 5 alpha-reductase inhibitors, ending the confusion. We can now advocate prevention of prostate cancer with two readily available drugs that clearly work.[23]

Nevertheless, because of their poor start, many doctors remain reluctant to prescribe these drugs. I recommend that men at increased risk of developing prostate cancer (African-American men and those with a family history of the disease or an elevated PSA with a negative biopsy) discuss the pros and cons with their physician and consider taking a 5 alpha-reductase inhibitor. In men with symptoms of BPH, these drugs are particularly appropriate, regardless of their other risk factors.

The side effects of 5 alpha-reductase inhibitors are low (see Chapter 5, BPH [Benign Prostatic Hyperplasia]), but these drugs often reduce the volume of semen, occasionally affect sexual function, and in rare cases cause breast enlargement or pain. These side effects are reversible if the drug is stopped.

> NOTE: Dutasteride (Avodart), a more recently approved 5-alpha reductase inhibitor, blocks the action of both forms of the enzyme and is also effective in preventing prostate cancer. (See page 55 for more on dutasteride.)

Diet

A heart-healthy diet may be prostate healthy as well. The dietary guidelines set forth by the American Heart Association will reduce your risk of heart disease—the leading cause of death for adult men. Even though we lack hard scientific evidence that such a regime reduces your chance of developing prostate cancer, it's a good idea to minimize your intake of salt, excess calories, saturated fats, trans fats (e.g., margarine), and cholesterol. At the same time, be sure to consume plenty of fresh fruits, vegetables, unsaturated oils, low-fat proteins, and grains. Soy, a major element in the Asian diet that seems to yield lower prostate cancer rates, may be useful. Finally, if you consume alcohol, do so in moderation.[24]

Some small studies suggest that vegetable consumption may protect against prostate cancer. Cruciferous greens, such as broccoli and cabbage, and cooked tomatoes are thought to provide the best defense, though eating a wide variety of vegetables has been well-established as making sound nutritional sense.

A recent trial of men with low-risk prostate cancer on active surveillance who chose to defer treatment found that a complex regimen consisting of a diet high in fruits, vegetables, whole grains, legumes, and soy, 30 minutes of moderate aerobic activity six days a week, and daily stress reduction (e.g., breathing, meditation, imagery) favorably altered gene profiles and other molecular features associated with cancer, when the men were compared with a group that made no lifestyle changes,[25] and whose PSA increased slightly over a one-year period.[26] We can't say for certain what this means in terms of reducing the risks of the disease over a lifetime, but, one hopes, further studies will determine the value of such lifestyle changes.

Vitamins and Other Supplements[27]

Selenium and Vitamin E. Antioxidants counteract the damaging effects of oxygen in tissues. Selenium and vitamin E are antioxidants that were thought to work in combination to prevent the development of prostate cancer and impede the growth of the tumors that arose. In studies aimed at documenting the beneficial effects of selenium supplements on other cancers, notably melanoma, an unexpected finding was a substantial reduction in prostate cancer deaths.

Selenium is a trace mineral, meaning that the body requires only minuscule amounts to maintain health. Still, researchers have observed that low selenium levels in the soil, which translate into less of the mineral in the food supply, are associated with an increase in cancers and many other diseases. Heavy rainfall tends to wash selenium out of the soil, so people in areas prone to rainy weather could be deficient in this nutrient. A simple toenail clipping can be used to assess selenium levels.

Vitamin E (tocopherol) has been shown to inhibit the growth of prostate cancer cells in the laboratory. Place this vitamin in a dish occupied by tumor cells, and the cells beat a dramatic retreat. A large study of Finnish male smokers initially found that men who took small, 50 IU daily supplements of vitamin E were less likely to develop prostate cancer and less likely to die of the cancers that arose, but further follow-up found the effect to be insignificant. Any beneficial effect on prostate cancer incidence or mortality remains to be established.

The SELECT trial, the largest prostate cancer prevention study to date, involving 32,000 men, sought to discover whether these two nutrients could reduce the incidence of or mortality from the disease. Unfortunately, the trial found no beneficial effect in a 5-year period.[28]

> NOTE: Both of these antioxidants can cause harm in large doses. Be cautious when taking any nutritional supplements or "nutraceuticals."

Phytoestrogens and other herbal antioxidants. A modern cancer-prevention buzzword, **phytoestrogens** (isoflavones, isoflavonoids) are naturally occurring female hormone–like substances found in plant products such as flaxseed and soy products, such as miso, soy milk and cheese, and tofu. In Japan and other countries where the diet is rich in soy, the incidence of breast and prostate cancers is strikingly low (though the Japanese have an alarmingly high incidence of stomach cancer, possibly linked to a different dietary factor, yet to be identified). Epidemiological studies have shown that Asians who drink large amounts of soy milk (more than one glass a day) reduce their risk of prostate cancer by 70 percent. There is some evidence that Asians may have a better ability to convert the active ingredients in soy (genistein and daidzein) to the more active form (equol) and concentrate it in the prostate.

Preliminary laboratory studies suggest that phytoestrogens may reduce tumor-promoting effects of male hormones or even inhibit the blood supply that existing prostate tumors need to grow. While not yet sufficiently proven, a diet high in soy or other phytoestrogens, found in such foods and spices as alfalfa, red clover, wild yam, and fennel seeds, appears to be safe and may help reduce prostate cancer risk.

Soy has also been shown to diminish the incidence of hot flashes in menopausal women. A current study is investigating whether men taking hormone ablation therapy for prostate cancer, which can cause debilitating hot flashes, might enjoy the same symptomatic relief.

A current National Cancer Institute trial is looking at whether dietary soy may reduce the risk of prostate cancer in men with elevated PSA levels. A Canadian trial is studying whether soy plus vitamin E and selenium may reduce the risk of progressing to prostate cancer in men with high-grade PIN. To date, no beneficial effects of soy have been demonstrated in a controlled trial.

Other phytochemicals with antioxidant properties are under intensive study, including **resveratrol**, which is found in grapes, red wine, peanuts, among other foods, and **indole-3-carbinol**, found in cruciferous vegetables such as cauliflower and broccoli. These substances have properties similar to those of phytoestrogens when tested in a laboratory dish, but we have limited evidence in animal studies and no clinical trials showing human benefits.

Silymarin, a flavenoid derived from milk thistle that slows the growth of cells, may have particular activity against prostate cancer, because it inhibits effects of the androgen receptor and blocks some of the specific growth-promoting properties in prostate cancer. Animal studies and limited clinical trials suggest that silymarin, along with a variety of other supplements, may slow the rise in PSA in men with a cancer recurrence after prostate cancer surgery or radiation therapy.

Lycopene. A diet rich in this powerful antioxidant, found in tomatoes and certain other fruits, is under study as a possible means of prostate cancer prevention. The form of ingestion seems to be important, since oil promotes lycopene absorption. Consequently, tomato sauce and pizza would theoretically be more effective than tomato juice. Epidemiological studies have found an association between a diet high in cooked tomatoes and a lower risk of prostate cancer. Nevertheless, no studies to date have proven that if men ingest tomatoes, much less lycopene supplements, they can reduce their prostate cancer risk. There have been conflicting studies about the effects of a tomato-rich diet on men with established prostate cancer, but no evidence that lycopene supplements alter the growth of cancer.

Vitamin D. It's possible that a deficiency in this antioxidant might increase prostate cancer risk, while some believe high levels may be preventive. In the lab, vitamin D markedly reduces the growth rate of prostate cancer cells. The same phenomenon has been observed in animal studies, though a similar effect in humans has yet to be demonstrated.

Dark-skinned African-American men, who have the world's highest incidence of prostate cancer, absorb less sunlight and therefore have lower levels of vitamin D than do people with fair skin. People of all skin tones living in the north, where sun exposure and vitamin D synthesis are generally low, have higher rates of prostate cancer than those living in sunny southern climes. With age, the body's ability to manufacture vitamin D diminishes, while the incidence of prostate cancer increases. Studies are being conducted to test whether these correlations mean that vitamin D offers some protection against the disease and, if so, whether the vitamin is most effectively ingested in foods, given as a supplement, or boosted by some minimal amount of controlled sun exposure that would not increase the health risks associated with sun damage.

While early studies suggested that vitamin D slowed the growth of advanced prostate cancers, more recent, rigorous randomized trials have found no beneficial effect. In one trial, men with advanced prostate cancer who took vitamin D in addition to chemotherapy did worse than those on chemotherapy alone.

Vitamin A. Beta-carotene is the best known of a large group of yellow and red pigments called carotenoids, which are stored in the liver, where they are converted into vitamin A. Foods rich in beta-carotene, such as carrots, and those rich in vitamin A, including dried apricots and spinach, may have a direct protective effect against some cancers, or the benefit may simply derive from eating more fruits and vegetables and less animal fat. Supplements of vitamin A and beta-carotene have never been shown to reduce the risk of prostate cancer. In fact, in the study of male smokers in Finland, beta-carotene supplements actually appeared to increase both the risk of developing prostate cancer and the likelihood of dying from it. Vitamin A should not be used by smokers.

Saw Palmetto. This extract of the American dwarf palm has been widely touted to reduce lower urinary tract symptoms due to BPH. However, in a large prospective randomized trial, this supplement proved no more beneficial than a placebo. Also, despite widespread marketing claims, we have no evidence that saw palmetto has any effect on preventing prostate cancer or lowering PSA.

Green Tea. In Asian countries, where the consumption of green tea is high, the incidence of prostate cancer is low. Epidemiological evidence suggests that prostate cancer risk decreases as the quantity and duration of green tea consumption goes up. Antioxidant compounds in green tea, known as polyphenols, seem to inhibit the growth of tumor cells and induce them to die off. While we need large prospective trials to prove these beneficial effects, adding a cup or two of green tea to your daily diet might be a good idea. It is interesting to note that tea is second only to water as the most consumed beverage in the world.

NOTE: All vitamin supplements, as well as so-called "natural" and herbal medicines, carry a risk of damaging side effects, and many can prove toxic, especially in large amounts. Widely embraced substances such as ephedra, commonly known as herbal ecstasy, which was touted as an appetite suppressant, have turned out to carry significant health risks. You would be wise to discuss with your doctor the pros and cons, as well as the recommended dosage and administration, of *any* supplements before taking them. Also, be sure to advise your doctor of everything you take, no matter how innocuous it may seem. Some supplements or over-the-counter remedies can cause hazardous drug and anesthesia interactions.[29]

NOTE: Medical studies showing no benefit from certain supplements have failed to reduce consumer use of these compounds. Studies showing harm do lower consumer demand.

Pomegranate is also a rich source of polyphenols, containing more antioxidants than green tea and red wine. In animal studies, pomegranate has shown effects against prostate cancer. In one small trial, it seemed to reduce the rate of rise of PSA, but there are no large studies confirming a beneficial effect.

THE SECOND LINE OF DEFENSE: CURE

Our second line of defense is early detection and effective treatment to catch a cancer before it spreads or causes needless adverse effects. PAP smears have dramatically reduced deaths from cervical cancer. In prostate cancer, PSA screening, along with modern, ultrasound-guided biopsy, represent a home run in secondary prevention. Today, we discover these cancers far earlier in their natural history, while the vast majority are localized to the prostate and can be cured with surgery or radiation. The downside has been overdetection and unnecessary treatment of small, nonthreatening cancers. Further advances in PSA interpretation and the development of other, better markers of this disease are essential if we are to better distinguish the cancers that pose a serious risk from those that are unlikely to do harm or require treatment, at least in the short term. (See Chapter 8, Detecting Prostate Cancer with PSA and Other Tests, and Chapter 10, Understanding Your Cancer.)

THE THIRD LINE OF DEFENSE: MINIMIZING SIDE EFFECTS AND COMPLICATIONS

On the prostate cancer front, great strides have been made in reducing death from the disease, as well as the risk and severity of treatment side effects. Modern radiation and surgery have dramatically lowered the incidence of damage to bowel, urinary, and sexual function, and excellent treatments are available for many of the problems that do occur. Improvements in hormone therapy and advances in chemotherapy, along with earlier detection of metastases for men with advanced disease, have doubled the life expectancy for men with metastatic prostate cancer. With these gains, the mortality rate from prostate cancer in this country has dropped more than 40 percent since 1993.

After such excellent progress, a current focus is on finding ways to slow the progression of prostate cancers that are no longer curable. If high body mass index seems to worsen a man's prognosis, might diet, exercise, and resultant weight loss delay cancer spread and metastases? In recent years two studies have shown a decrease in the rate of rise of PSA in men whose cancers have recurred after radiation or surgery. Both trials used a combination approach that included diet, exercise and nutritional supplements or medication. Both found a small but measurable decrease in PSA velocity. Large, prospective, randomized trials would be necessary to confirm the effectiveness of such regimens. Until we have these studies, it is impossible to make firm recommendations about what, if anything, might halt or slow progression of this disease. It's important to note that there is no reliable evidence that anyone has ever been cured of prostate cancer as a result of these lifestyle changes.

THE FUTURE

New antiandrogens are being discovered that may prove to be even more effective than finasteride or dutasteride in preventing cancer. The REDEEM trial is testing whether 5 alpha-reductase inhibitors can suppress tumor growth in men who have been diagnosed with prostate cancer. If the answer is yes, men with early, favorable, low-risk cancers may be able to slow the progression of the cancer and avoid the side effects of surgery, radiation, or hormone therapy by taking one of these safe, established drugs.

IN SUMMARY

While all normal men are at risk for developing prostate cancer, a variety of factors may increase or lower your odds. Men at high risk, including African-American men and those with a strong family history of the disease, should be more vigilant and begin screening earlier than standard guidelines suggest.

Hope springs eternal for simple solutions to prostate cancer, but the only proven, effective preventive agents so far are the 5 alpha-reductase inhibitors, finasteride and dutasteride. If you are seriously concerned about prostate cancer or you are at high risk for the disease, speak with your doctor about the wisdom of taking these drugs.

8

■

Detecting Prostate Cancer with PSA and Other Tests

READ THIS CHAPTER TO LEARN:

- How do we screen men for prostate cancer?
- Why is screening controversial, and should you be screened?
- How do we interpret screening results?

PROSTATE CANCER SCREENING: PROS AND CONS

Though we've had the PSA screening test that can signal the possible presence of cancer in the gland for two decades, public health policy experts and medical professionals continue to debate whether diagnosing these cancers early yields more benefit or harm.

Screening proponents point out that early detection has led to a dramatic nearly 50 percent reduction in prostate cancer death rates. Since PSA testing came into widespread use in the late 1980s, there has also been a major change in the prostate cancer patient population. In the pre-PSA era, men typically were not diagnosed until their tumors had advanced to the point of causing urinary symptoms or bone pain from metastases. At that stage, cancer cure was no longer possible, and treatment focused on easing symptoms and attempting to prolong life. Given widespread PSA screening, we now see patients far earlier in the course of this disease, while their cancers are still localized and—in the vast majority of cases—curable with surgery to remove the gland or radiation to kill the tumor. Also thanks to PSA testing, we now discover prostate cancers far more often in young, healthy men, who can be treated successfully with modern therapies that carry a much lower risk of serious or lasting side effects.[1] Indeed, the large European screening trial, which compared screening every four years with PSA with a control population of unscreened men, found a 20 percent reduction in the risk of death from prostate cancer over ten years.[2]

Skeptics counter that early detection is a decidedly double-edged sword. Though the PSA test can help ferret out clinically significant prostate cancers while they are still curable, it can also trigger unnecessary biopsies and lead to the overdetection of clusters of cancer cells that often lurk in the prostates of older men and would likely never cause any problems if left alone. Discovering these early cancers can expose patients to unnecessary invasive tests and treatments, and the risk of serious complications as well as adverse effects on sexual, urinary, and bowel function.[3]

To support their argument, screening opponents point to the PLCO trial, a large, prospective, randomized trial conducted in the U.S. that compared annual screening with PSA and DRE for five years with a control population that was advised not to have these tests. After seven years, there was no difference in prostate cancer deaths between these two groups.[4]

Given the flaws in these trials, their conclusions remain unconvincing. We cannot say with conviction whether or not all men should be screened for prostate cancer. Perhaps further evaluation and follow-up of the men in these two large, expensive studies will provide the answer. Until then, screening remains an individual decision.

THE SCREENING TRIALS

Critics site many problems with both of the large, randomized studies that tested the benefits of screening for prostate cancer with PSA. The European trial found a benefit—20 percent fewer deaths from cancer—but this came at the cost of treating forty-eight patients for every death that was prevented. The PLCO trial, which showed no benefit to screening, allowed men to enroll even though 43 percent had been screened with PSA before the study, culling out many with serious cancers. In the control arm, over 50 percent of the men advised not to have screening tests did so anyway, while in the screening arm, 15 percent of the men refused testing. No survival difference was found at seven years, but given the typically slow progress of this disease, we would not expect to see many deaths in that short time course.

Despite major advances, our knowledge of prostate cancer remains incomplete. To date, we lack unequivocal scientific proof that catching the disease early confers a survival advantage, though we do have compelling statistics to bolster that conclusion (the aforementioned 50 percent reduction in prostate cancer deaths since PSA screening began in the late 1980s). Still, just as screening advocates can cite impressive reductions in prostate cancer deaths, those opposed to early detection can name studies that failed to find a significant survival difference between men who were diagnosed and treated early and those who were not. Scientific trials often yield such frustrating inconsistencies. Many factors can affect results. (See Chapter 21, Treating Advanced Prostate Cancer, for a discussion of clinical trials.)

Nevertheless, certain facts are indisputable. We *do know* that every year almost 30,000 men in the United States and 80,000 in the greater European Union die of prostate cancer. In developing countries, deaths from prostate cancer are already beginning to rise and are expected to rise more rapidly as the average age of citizens in a those countries goes up. We know that once established, this disease is a formidable foe that causes debilitating symptoms and, eventually, death. We know that cancers have the capacity to change over time, and that it can be difficult to tell at the time of diagnosis which small, seemingly harmless tumors might eventually prove to be aggressive and dangerous. We also know that once prostate cancer spreads to organs beyond the prostate, it becomes far more difficult to control and is often lethal. Screening allows us to find these cancers far earlier in their natural course, when they are still curable. Modern treatment for prostate cancer is generally safe, with a low risk of mortality. Though the side effects of surgery and radiation can be unpleasant and affect quality of life for some men, the problems are often transient and, if not, are generally treatable and remediable.

So, should you be screened for prostate cancer? That depends.[5]

Prostate cancer is a highly heterogeneous disease, and the men who develop these tumors have widely varying personal needs and medical profiles. For older patients in poor health whose life expectancy is less than ten years, screening is most often unnecessary and probably inadvisable. In fact, the U.S. Preventive Service Task Force, the most prestigious group that assesses the benefits and risks of screening for diseases, specifically recommends against screening of men for prostate cancer after age 75. It is unlikely that this slow-growing cancer would cause any problems in their remaining lifetime. For most men in that age group, learning that they have the disease would only cause needless anxiety.[6]

Healthy younger men need to assess whether the risks inherent in treating some cancers unnecessarily are outweighed by the benefits of catching potentially aggressive, life-threatening tumors before they can spread and do harm. Men at high risk for developing prostate cancer, including African-Americans and those with a family history of the disease, have additional issues to factor into the equation. Because of their increased risk, they are typically advised to start screening earlier than the general population.

Given the persistent controversy about prostate cancer screening, it's unsurprising that the guidelines from major health organizations are at odds. The American College of Preventive Medicine (ACPM) suggests that doctors inform men age 50 or older, with a life expectancy of ten years or longer, about the potential positives and downsides of screening and help patients make their own informed decisions about whether to undergo PSA and DRE exams. Testing is not routinely recommended.[7]

The American Urological Association (AUA) and the American Cancer Society (ACS) are more positive about the benefits of screening. They advise physicians to offer men annual digital rectal exams and PSA testing starting at age 50 (and for those at high risk, age 45) as long as the patient's life expectancy is at least ten years. These groups recommend that doctors present comprehensive information about screening so that men can make an informed decision.[8]

Such generalizations are expected and unavoidable from health policy makers, but they don't necessarily speak to what's right for you. The best way to make that highly personal determination is through a careful, reasoned discussion with a physician who fully understands your particular situation and has knowledge of the ins and outs of this complex disease. Together, you can gauge the risk/benefit ratio of screening in your case and, if it seems appropriate, when to start and how often you should have testing done.

I'd urge you to make sure you're fully informed before deciding to forgo screening for prostate cancer. Blinders are a poor defense against a potentially lethal disease. Certainly, you don't want to undergo unnecessary, invasive treatment, but neither would you wish to die an unnecessary death from a disease that is highly curable if detected in time. Detecting a cancer does not mean you're compelled to have it treated. Many small prostate cancers are best monitored until there are clear signs the tumor has become aggressive enough to warrant active intervention. (See Chapter 13, Watchful Waiting [Active Surveillance].)

HOW PSA AND DIGITAL RECTAL EXAMINATIONS HELP TO DETECT PROSTATE CANCER

In the early 1970s, scientists discovered a previously unknown component of human seminal fluid and traced its origins to the prostate gland. One early investigator speculated that this new marker might prove to be a sort of semen signature, unique in each man, that could prove useful in identifying rape suspects. (Though this theory did not hold up in later studies, PSA did play a role in proving whether semen was present in the vagina.)

In the early 1980s, researchers found a way to detect minute quantities of this substance in blood, as little as 0.1 nanograms/milliliter. (To get an idea of how astonishingly tiny this is, a mosquito weighs in at a relatively corpulent 2,000 to 2,500 nanograms.)

Scientists observed that while men normally had low levels of what had come to be called PSA, 68 percent of patients with benign enlargement of the gland, up to 79 percent of men with localized prostate cancer, and as many as 86 percent of men with advanced cancer showed elevated concentrations. Finally we had a marker to alert us to the presence of possible prostate cancer while it was still in an early, curable stage!

PSA, which stands for **prostate-specific antigen**, is produced by the prostate and released as part of the ejaculate. Under normal circumstances, the only two places we expect to find significant amounts of PSA are in the prostate gland and in the seminal fluid. Detecting elevated levels in the bloodstream is a sign that something could be amiss. When things are functioning according to plan, the concentration of PSA in semen is a startling millionfold higher than the minuscule trace there would be in a blood sample.[10]

The term "prostate-specific" highlights the fact that the prostate gland is the sole organ that manufactures a significant amount of PSA (though, in fact, a tiny bit is produced by the salivary glands). An antigen is a substance capable of provoking a response by the body's immune defenses, as PSA can do when damage or disease in the gland allows it to leak into the bloodstream. Because it causes a chemical reaction, PSA also qualifies as an enzyme. And by chemical composition, it can be classified as a glycoprotein, meaning that it is a sugar and a protein combined.

Though we still have much to learn about PSA, Dr. Hans Lilja discovered in 1985 that it plays an important role in human reproduction. Soon after ejaculation, semen coagulates. PSA returns seminal fluid to liquid form in a process called **proteolysis**, freeing the sperm it contains to go about their business.

We expect to find PSA in the ejaculate. But under ordinary circumstances, this hefty molecule is far too large to penetrate tissue barriers in

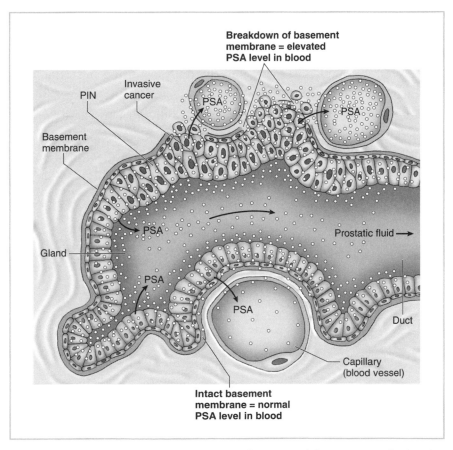

As cancer invades through the barrier (basement membrane) around the microscopic glands within the prostate, PSA can leak freely into the blood vessels, causing an elevated level on the PSA test.

the prostate and find its way into the bloodstream. Discovering a measurable amount of PSA in a blood sample indicates that something has gone awry in the gland, causing those natural defenses to break down.

Anything below 4 ng/ml (referred to as a PSA of 4) used to be considered insignificant, but it is now clear that cancer can be found in men with a PSA at any level (though the higher the level, the greater the risk that we'll find cancer on biopsy),[11] and levels as low as 2 are associated with an increased risk of cancer. (See the table on page 147.) It's reasonable to adjust for age when evaluating PSA (see page 78 for a discussion of BPH-related PSA-level increase). My suspicions might be raised if a 45-year-old man with a strong family history of prostate cancer had a PSA over 1, while a level of 5.5 in a 75-year-old with an enlarged prostate may not sound a serious alarm.[12]

During a digital rectal exam (DRE), the doctor inserts a gloved finger into the rectum to examine the rear of the prostate for abnormalities. Many men, and some physicians, find the test off-putting and would just as soon avoid it. The DRE is also highly subjective. A physician examines you and draws an impression about the probability that you have prostate cancer. The level of suspicion and the way a given doctor responds to that suspicion can vary enormously. What one doctor considers an alarming

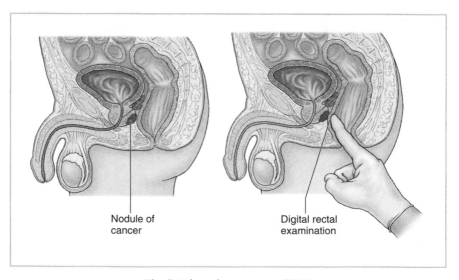

Nodule of
cancer

Digital rectal
examination

The digital rectal examination (DRE).

nodule another might judge to be a harmless, meaningless irregularity in the gland. The DRE is a difficult test to master, and doing so requires a great deal of practice. If a urologist sees fifty or sixty men a day, three or four days a week in the office, it might take six months or more before he really understands all the nuances of this exam. Given all that, you might wonder why we persist in recommending the test at all, especially given the existence of PSA.

PSA is far from perfect. While the test can help to detect prostate cancer, studies that compared screening methods found that one of every five cancers were detected because of an abnormal DRE in patients who had a normal PSA.[13] Part of the reason lies in the uncertain definition of "normal." We've known for years, and the PCPT results confirmed, that cancer can be found in some men with a PSA well below the traditional cutoff of 4. In many cases, the cancer is too small to make enough PSA to push the level that high. Sometimes the cancer is large enough, but there is so little PSA made by the rest of the prostate that the threshold of normal is not passed. In rare cases, a high-grade cancer functions so abnormally that the cells, ironically, make very little PSA.

Probability of Finding Cancer on Biopsy According to a Man's PSA Level and DRE Result		
PSA Level	**DRE Result**	**Probability of Cancer**
0 – 0.5		7%
0.6 – 1.0		10%
1.1 – 2.0		17%
2.1 – 3.0		24%
3.1 – 4.0		27%
4 – 10	Normal	25%
	Abnormal*	45%
>10	Normal	50%
	Abnormal*	75%
Abnormal means modular or suspicious of cancer		

NOTE: While PSA produced by a cancer and PSA made by normal prostate cells are identical, we can distinguish to some degree between these two diseases that raise PSA levels using PSA density, PSA velocity, and the free PSA test. Newer tests for molecular forms of PSA and related antigens are likely to improve our ability to make this distinction in the future.[14]

Recent European studies have focused on relying entirely on PSA for prostate cancer screening. If the test result falls below a predetermined level of 1.5 to 2.5 (depending on the trial), no further testing is done. If the PSA is above the threshold, follow-up with a DRE and a prostate biopsy is recommended. Advocates of this approach argue that cancers found by DRE in men with a very low PSA are rarely dangerous. Theoretically, if they are missed during this screening process, any cancers will be picked up in the next go-round in ample time to treat the tumor successfully.

In this country, we still advocate PSA plus a DRE as the most effective way to detect prostate cancer early.

DRE results can play an important role in treatment planning. If the doctor felt an abnormality, how extensive was it? Did it distort the normal border of the gland? Did it appear to protrude through the capsule? The answers to all these questions will have implications for

NOTE: If you have both tests regularly, it's almost guaranteed that any prostate cancer you develop will be detected while it is still localized and curable.

NOTE: While a small percentage of general physicians are excellent DRE interpreters, urologists, in general, have more experience and expertise. If you're at high risk for prostate cancer, if your doctor found an abnormality in your prostate, or if your PSA is creeping up, having a prostate exam by an experienced urologist is probably a good idea.

PROBABILITY OF FINDING CANCER ON BIOPSY ACCORDING TO A MAN'S DRE RESULT AND PSA LEVEL

	PSA (NG/ML)		
DRE Result	2–4	4–10	>10
Normal	15%	25%	50%
*Abnormal**	20%	45%	>75%

*"Abnormal" means nodular or suspicious for cancer.

whether or not you should have a biopsy and, if you do, how it should be done.

If a biopsy confirms that you have prostate cancer, the DRE you had before the biopsy is critically important in determining the stage of your tumor and how it might best be treated. Following a biopsy, the prostate area may be tender and uncomfortable, and the doctor may be reluctant to do a full exam that could provoke bleeding. Also, due to swelling from the biopsy needles, the prostate might not feel normal.

OTHER THAN CANCER, WHAT CAN CAUSE YOUR PSA TO RISE OR FALL?

With benign prostatic hyperplasia (BPH), the gland enlarges, and a larger prostate produces more PSA. Though BPH is not cancer, it is often accompanied by inflammation and can cause the same breakdown of tissue barriers in the gland that we see with malignant disease. (See the figure on page 50.) PSA leaks into the bloodstream and registers as a higher number on the prostate cancer screening test.

The inflammation or infection of prostatitis can cause a dramatic increase in PSA. By compromising prostate tissues, prostatitis also allows PSA to escape the gland and slip into circulation. With active infection in the prostate, or even with a urinary tract infection, PSA levels can sky-rocket. Men who have acute urinary retention (e.g., after hernia surgery) and need catheterization can have a dramatic rise in PSA that resolves within a few weeks once the catheter is removed.

In addition, transient increases in PSA can result from inflammation caused by a prostate biopsy or a cystoscopic examination of the urethra or bladder through a tube inserted in the penis. Testing for PSA should be postponed for at least three to six weeks after such procedures, to allow the PSA to return to its baseline level.

NOTE: You *should not* take powerful antibiotics such as Cipro or Levaquin just because you have an unexpected rise in your PSA. There is no medical evidence to support this common, unfortunate practice, unless you have a bona fide urinary tract infection or bacterial prostatitis. A rising PSA itself is no indication that you have prostatitis. (See Chapter 4, Prostatitis.) Instead, we look for signs or symptoms such as an abnormal urinalysis, a positive culture, or characteristic pain. In the absence of signs or symptoms of infection, there is no value in taking a course of antibiotics for an unexplained, elevated PSA.[15]

Some medications, most notably finasteride and dutasteride (see Chapter 5, BPH [Benign Prostatic Hyperplasia]), can lower the PSA by reducing androgens within the prostate. Surgical or medical castration for prostate cancer will markedly depress the PSA by lowering the androgen level throughout the body. Be sure to mention to your doctor any medications or supplements you're taking, or planning to take, whether they appear relevant to your prostate or not.

NOTE: Studies have failed to support the common belief that ejaculation or manipulation of the prostate during DRE causes the PSA to rise.[16] Though some doctors caution men to avoid ejaculation for several days before PSA screening and to delay the test for some time after a DRE, I've seen no evidence that either of these practices is necessary.

HOW RELIABLE IS THE PSA TEST?

Though it helps us to catch prostate cancers while they are curable, PSA testing is far from an exact science. In 70 to 80 percent of cases, an elevated PSA that triggers a biopsy uncovers no evidence of cancer. For every man found to have a malignant tumor in the gland, four men are subjected to a biopsy needlessly. Perhaps more distressing, some prostate cancers would be missed if doctors relied on PSA results alone without performing a DRE.[17]

In fact, we now know that there's no such thing as a "normal" PSA. The traditional cutoff of 4 no longer obtains. From the PCPT trial, in which a large group of men had a prostate biopsy regardless of their PSA, we learned that men can have prostate cancer, even a high-grade one, at any PSA level. More like cholesterol, PSA is indicative of risk. The higher the level, the greater is the risk of having a cancer.[18]

To make matters worse, PSA can fluctuate by as much as 30 percent from week to week, for no identifiable reason. If your PSA rises in the absence of other red flags, such as an abnormal digital rectal exam, it's wise to repeat the test in a few weeks before submitting to a prostate biopsy.[19]

This is not to suggest that we should abandon PSA testing. Despite some recent warnings to the contrary, the PSA test, properly used, remains the best indicator of a prostate cancer's presence. In fact, recent studies confirm that a man's PSA level in his 40s powerfully predicts whether he will ever develop a prostate cancer in his lifetime.[20] The test's ability to detect prostate cancer is better than mammography at warning us of the possible presence of breast cancer.[21] Unfortunately, measuring PSA is not very specific, meaning it does a good job of alerting us to the fact that there's a problem, but it's far less adept at telling us what kind. Where there's smoke, there may be fire, but it's also possible that an overcooked dinner, a roomful of cigar enthusiasts, wood chips in a roaring barbecue, or even a special-effects machine might be responsible instead.

FREE PSA

PSA comes in several varieties. Complex PSA circulates with a companion protein. **Free PSA** is a sort of bachelor antigen that travels on its own. This unbound form of PSA comes from BPH, not prostate cancer.

The widely available test for free PSA (**%fPSA**) indicates what percentage of your total PSA comes from benign enlargement of the gland. From this, we can predict the likelihood that a man with an elevated PSA would be found to have prostate cancer if we performed a biopsy. The test is especially useful for men whose PSA falls between 2.5 and 10, a gray area where either BPH or prostate cancer might be responsible for

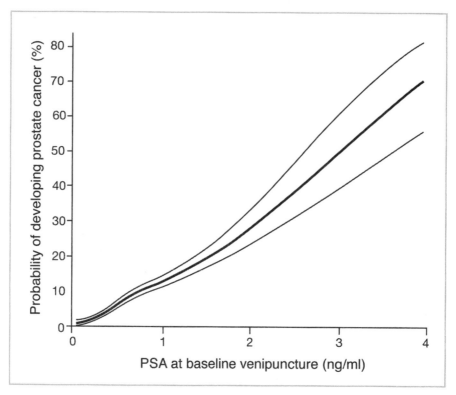

The probability that a man will be diagnosed with prostate cancer by age 75 according to his PSA level at age 44–50. The average lifetime risk is 10%. Note that the median PSA level for men at this age is only 0.55 ng/ml. Modified from H. Lilja et al., "Prostate-Specific Antigen and Prostate Cancer: Prediction, Detection and Monitoring." *Nature Reviews Cancer* 8 (2008): 266.

the increase. Testing for free PSA improves our ability to predict whether cancer is the cause of an elevated PSA by 20 to 40 percent, yet reduces by only about 5 percent the cancers we would otherwise fail to detect. The measure can also be useful in characterizing a cancer after it has been diagnosed.

Readings over 25 percent suggest that the elevated PSA is caused largely by BPH and the probability of having any cancer is small (about 8 percent). Also, any cancer present is more likely to be early and confined to the gland.[22] On the other hand, having a free PSA under 10 percent makes it much more likely that your PSA is elevated by cancer (50 percent probability). Any cancer present is likely to be large and require active, aggressive treatment.[23] In general, the lower the free PSA, the greater the cause for concern. (See the table below.)

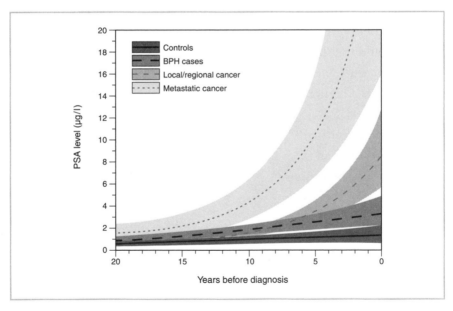

PSA levels in the blood test begin to rise many years before local/regional or metastatic prostate cancer can otherwise be detected. The rate of rise (called **PSA velocity** or **PSA doubling time**) is much faster in men with cancer than in those with BPH or a normal prostate.*

---

*Source: Modified from H. B. Carter et al., "Longitudinal Evaluation of Prostate-Specific Antigen Levels in Men with and Without Prostate Disease," *JAMA* 267, no. 16 (1992): 2218, fig. 3. © 1992 American Medical Association.

PSA Density

PSA density (PSAD) looks at the ratio of PSA to prostate size. Because BPH causes the PSA level to rise, the larger the gland, the higher we would expect PSA to be. To calculate PSAD, simply divide your PSA by the size of your prostate, as measured by ultrasound or MRI. The digital rectal exam is *not* the best way to judge how large your gland may be. In fact, it is notoriously inaccurate. Doctors can only feel the side of the prostate that rests against the rectum. Ultrasound, which is also used to guide the needles for your biopsy, measures prostate shape and volume far more accurately, in three dimensions. If you've had a biopsy, you should be able to get a report of your ultrasound results, which would include the size of your prostate.

If your PSA is 6 and your prostate weighs 30 grams, you would divide 30 into 6 and find that your PSA density is 0.2. A PSA of 4 in a 60-gram prostate would translate into 4 divided by 60, or a density of 0.067.

Higher density, meaning more PSA per cubic centimeter of prostate tissue, suggests a higher likelihood that cancer is the cause. We view PSA density under 0.07 as a safe level that strongly suggests that the elevated PSA is coming from BPH; between 0.07 and 0.15 is uncertain. If your density is greater than 0.15, I would be highly suspicious that a cancer is present and may be serious.[24]

PSA Velocity and Doubling Time

Medical professionals commonly believe that if an elevated PSA can be compared to a smoke detector, a rapidly rising PSA is more akin to a fire detector, sounding the alarm that a prostate cancer is present, and a dangerous one at that. While it is true that over many years the rate of rise (**PSA velocity or PSAV**) is faster in men with cancer than in those with BPH or a normal prostate,[25] PSA velocity adds little to our ability to predict if a man has cancer or, if a cancer is present, how serious it may be.[26]

The problem is the inherent variability of PSA. Test results can differ so much from week to week for no apparent reason that detecting a genuine rise in the short term can be tricky. Different labs use different methods, which can yield different results. Measuring PSA velocity requires at least three reliable PSA tests performed over a year and a half, preferably in the same lab using the same assay (particular way of measuring). Also, the rate of change is reliable only in men with very low PSA levels. At higher levels, there tend to be more false positives, where the increase in PSA results from inflammation, infection, or benign enlargement of the gland, not cancer.

Studies now confirm that your PSA level is more important than the rate of rise in determining how likely it is that you have a cancer.[27] With a higher PSA the probability is greater that you'll have a positive biopsy.

NOTE: PSA velocity is commonly reported as ng/ml/year. For example, if your PSA goes from 2 to 4 over a year, the velocity would be 2 ng/ml/year. Changes in PSA, often referred to as PSA dynamics or kinetics, are also frequently described as **PSA doubling time (PSADT)**, which is commonly expressed as a number of months. If we look at the same 2 to 4 ng/ml/year increase over a year, the doubling time would be 12 months. Higher velocities and shorter doubling times mean PSA level is changing more rapidly.

While PSA velocity and doubling time are not helpful before diagnosis, when the prostate gland is in place, they are critically important in judging the behavior of a cancer that has been treated with surgery, radiation, hormone therapy, or chemotherapy. (See Chapter 20, Rising PSA After Surgery, Radiation, or Other Therapy, and Chapter 21, Treating Advanced Prostate Cancer.)

NEW DIAGNOSTIC TESTS FOR PROSTATE CANCER

Prostate cancer cells find their way into prostatic fluid, which drains into the urethra and gets mixed with urine. Until recently, it was difficult to distinguish prostate cancer cells from look-alike normal cells in a urine specimen. But scientists can now identify the presence of abnormal DNA or RNA associated with cancer in these cells.

PCA3. A promising new urine test for prostate cancer called **PCA3** is being studied. During a digital rectal exam, the gland is massaged to express prostatic fluid into the urethra. The urine is then collected and tested for the presence of the gene for PCA3, which is 100 times more prevalent in prostate cancer cells than in normal cells. This test also measures the ratio of expressed genes for PCA3 to those for PSA. The higher the level of PCA3 relative to PSA, the greater the risk that the patient has cancer. A higher level also predicts a higher Gleason grade if cancer is present. (For a full discussion of the Gleason grading system, see Chapter 9, Biopsy.) The test can be useful in deciding whether to repeat a biopsy in men who have had a negative prostate biopsy.[28]

Genetic polymorphism study. A **genetic polymorphism** is a normal variant in a gene, similar to a blood type. You can live a healthy life with any blood type, but each one has slightly different implications. For example, one study found that people with Type O blood were more likely to contract SARS when exposed to the disease. In another study, Type O seemed to be protective against the bacteria that cause stomach ulcers.

Some genetic polymorphisms increase a man's risk for developing prostate cancer; others do not. By developing a test that measures the variant each man has of five genes, researchers developed a test that produced a genetic profile of prostate cancer risk.[29] Men found to have all five genes, as well as close relatives with prostate cancer, were nine times more likely to get the disease than men with none of these genes and no family history of prostate cancer. The test is not in common use because family history alone provides most of the information, and the genetic component adds little.

THE FUTURE

Scientists are seeking more reliable markers to help us predict the presence and extent of prostate cancers. While PSA remains the cornerstone of prostate-cancer detection, the free PSA test has proven valuable, especially in men with enlarged prostates or those who have had one or two biopsies that have found no cancer.

Another promising test measures **human kallikrein (hK2)**, a protein that is closely related to PSA and present in minute quantities in blood. HK2 begins to rise years before cancer would be detected by DRE, and it may eventually be used to supplement PSA as a screening measure for prostate cancer. In one recent study, hK2 showed promise in distinguishing between cancers that were confined to the gland and those that were not. By combining a number of tumor markers like PSA and hK2, or tracking their levels over time, our ability to detect prostate cancer early and to distinguish potentially dangerous cancers from those likely to remain harmless should be far better in the future.[30] There are more than fifteen genes in the kallikrein family. ProPSA is the unactivated precursor form of PSA and may be particularly promising when combined with PSA and other kallikreins.

In addition to PCA 3, urinary tests are being developed to detect the presence of the fusion genes, such as TMPRSS-2-ETS, to detect prostate cancer risk.

Thanks to remarkable biomedical advances, we are able to produce powerful "high throughput gene arrays," which allow us to analyze tens of thousands of genes on a single chip. Nanotechnology experts at the California Institute of Technology and other institutions are developing chips capable of measuring tens of thousands of proteins from a fingerstick blood sample in a few minutes. These exciting and powerful new technologies are likely to lead to more sophisticated diagnostic tools that can help detect prostate cancer and determine its aggressiveness.

IN SUMMARY

While early detection with PSA and DRE has enabled us to catch prostate cancer while it is still curable and has reduced the prostate cancer death rate by nearly 50 percent in the last fifteen years, screening remains a mixed blessing. Countless men with tiny prostate cancers that would never have harmed them have gone through unnecessary treatment with all its medical risks and effects on quality of life. Until large randomized trials demonstrate whether screening provides more benefit than harm, we have to approach it with caution, making sure that men are fully informed. With hope, in time new markers will allow us to characterize prostate cancers better and determine which are serious and require immediate treatment and which can be safely monitored.

9

■

Biopsy

READ THIS CHAPTER TO LEARN:

- Why are prostate biopsies done, and when might you need one?
- What is the Gleason grade, and what does it mean?
- Why do you need a second read of your biopsy slides?

WHEN MIGHT YOU NEED A PROSTATE BIOPSY?

An elevated PSA level is a warning sign that something might be wrong. The same holds true for an abnormality on a digital rectal exam. Like a storm watch, these tests alert us to potential problems. Still, just as a predicted storm might fail to materialize, troubling results of prostate cancer screening tests often turn out to be false alarms.

PSA results are highly variable, with meaningless fluctuations of up to 30 percent from week to week.[1] A PSA of 3 one week could rise for no notable reason to 4.1 or sink to 1.9 by the next. An infection or inflammation in the gland can cause a rapid spike in your level that has nothing to do with cancer. A bigger prostate puts out more PSA, so benign enlargement of the gland alone, which happens in most men as they age, can cause your level to rise.[2]

The results of a digital rectal exam (DRE) are highly subjective. The same thing one doctor finds suspicious might be entirely overlooked or deemed insignificant by a different examiner. Tiny lumps or bulges may represent meaningless calcifications or benign enlargement of the gland. Fewer than 1 in 5 abnormal DREs turns out to be cancer.[3]

Recommending surgery or radiation on the basis of these uncertain tests would be irresponsible and overreaching. On the other hand, we don't want to miss the chance to identify and evaluate an early curable cancer or stop an aggressive tumor in its tracks. If your PSA or DRE raises a red flag that cancer may be present, a **biopsy** is the only way to determine whether or not you have the disease.

> NOTE: A biopsy is appropriate only if you would take action as a result of a cancer diagnosis. I would rarely recommend the test for a man so old or ill that his life expectancy is less than five years, unless he has symptoms of advanced prostate cancer, such as voiding problems or bone pain, and treatment would be useful to alleviate them.

MODERN BIOPSY TECHNIQUES AND HOW THEY DEVELOPED

Before the PSA test was developed, prostate cancers were typically suspected because of an abnormal DRE or symptoms of advanced disease, such as bone pain. As recently as 1985, the biopsies we did were targeted to suspicious thickenings or nodules we felt on the gland during a digital rectal exam. Guided by finger touch, we would insert a needle equipped with a pair of narrow cutting blades into the palpable lesion and remove one to three tissue cores, each about 1 inch long by $\frac{1}{14}$ inch wide. Because the needles were large, the procedure was done under general anesthesia.

The Development of
Ultrasound-Guided Biopsies

During World War I, very high frequency sound echoes in water (sonar) were used to detect enemy submarines and the sort of treacherous submerged iceberg that sank the Titanic. After the war, scientists began to investigate how this technology might be used in medical diagnostics. The first medical ultrasound device was developed by an Austrian physicist to visualize brain tumors. During the 1950s and 1960s, similar instruments were devised to detect breast, intestinal, and abdominal lesions and to monitor fetal development throughout pregnancy.

In the 1970s, Hiroke Watanabe, a Japanese urologist, designed a highly peculiar device to image the prostate. Patients sat on a chair fitted with a fingerlike ultrasound probe that was cranked into the rectum, allowing the examiner to visualize the gland.[4]

Danish scientists modified the Japanese probe in the 1980s, using a handheld wand that could be inserted into the rectum and manipulated to show the prostate from several angles. This **transrectal ultrasound (TRUS)** produced a clear, detailed picture of the prostate and surrounding tissues. (See page 164.)

Ultrasound probes had been used to guide needles into other organs, so once we had this flexible transrectal probe, a natural next step was the development of a long, thin, flexible needle that could be guided by ultrasound into the prostate. A further major breakthrough came in the early 1990s, with the production of the spring-loaded, handheld biopsy "gun." This device fires a hollow inner needle into the prostate, then instantly sends a sheath forward to slice off and retrieve a core of prostate tissue.[5]

Virtually all biopsies today are guided by ultrasound, which allows us to see precisely where a biopsy needle is placed into the prostate.

Once we've identified the target, the biopsy gun deploys an 18-gauge (18 would fit in an inch) or smaller "true cut" needle—which is sharp, disposable, and minimizes bleeding and pain—to obtain a core of tissue that measures 0.4 mm wide and 12 to 15 mm long.

Most prostate cancers are now discovered early, while they are too small to feel or to see on TRUS. Given the absence of palpable or visible nodules to target, our biopsy approach has shifted to sampling specified areas of the gland. Several studies have confirmed that these systematic segment biopsies are at least as effective at finding cancers as those targeted to suspicious areas. To maximize results, I also take an additional sample or two from any abnormal area that I see on ultrasound or feel on DRE.

It has become standard in the field to divide the prostate into sextants and take six samples (cores) from the left and right side of the apex, the middle, and the base of the outer peripheral zone, which is where most cancers arise. (See Chapter 1, The Prostate.) Needles are inserted at a 30- to 45-degree angle, running from the middle to the side of the prostate as they pass from the back toward the front.

Recent studies have found that the typical six-core biopsy may be inadequate. The more samples we get, the more likely we are to detect existing cancers.[6] Many doctors now advocate eight to fourteen, and some take many more. Unfortunately, more needles involve greater discomfort and increased side effects. About twelve cores appears to be an optimal number in most cases, ensuring a thorough biopsy that most men tolerate well.

NOTE: If a palpable abnormality was discovered on DRE but your ultrasound-guided biopsy is negative (no cancer), ask your doctor to add finger-guided biopsies directly into the abnormal area he can feel, along with the ultrasound-guided systematic biopsies. I have seen many cancers missed or seriously underestimated if the nodule is not deliberately targeted.

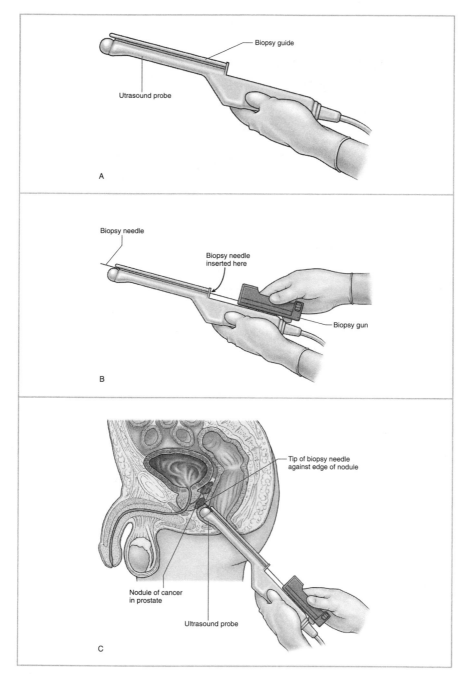

(a) Probe used to guide a biopsy by transrectal ultrasound.
(b) The needle is placed in a spring-loaded gun and inserted through the biopsy guide.
(c) The probe is placed in the rectum.

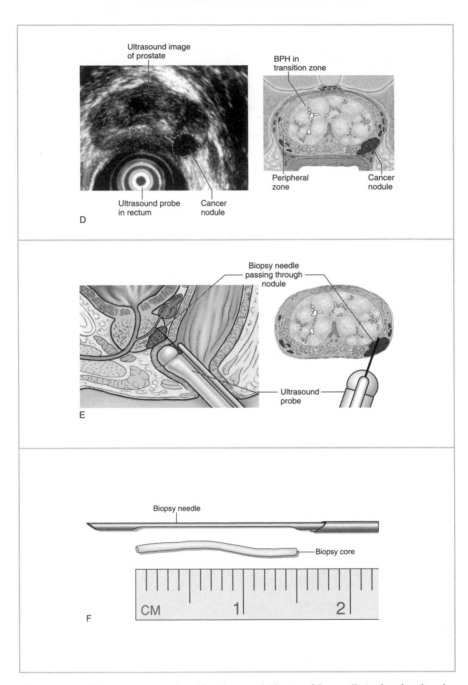

(d) An image of the prostate is produced by ultrasound. The tip of the needle is placed at the edge of the prostate or nodule.

(e) The needle is fired through the nodule.

(f) A core of tissues about 15 mm long is removed.

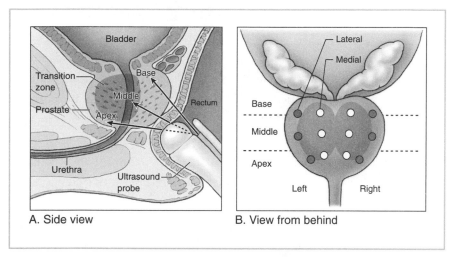

A. Side view | B. View from behind

The location of each biopsy core in systematic segment biopsy. A typical biopsy would sample twelve cores from the peripheral zone and perhaps two from the transition zone.

Saturation Biopsy

A twelve-core biopsy finds about 90 percent of existing cancers, leaving one of every ten cancers undetected. Because of that uncertainty, we tend to repeat the biopsy within three to six months if the first biopsy is negative, taking a total of twenty-six cores between the two biopsy sessions. In a deliberate effort to be sure no cancer is missed, no matter how small, some doctors perform "saturation" biopsies, taking 35 to 50 cores in a single biopsy session.[7]

Because saturation biopsies are painful, the procedure must be done under anesthesia, which carries its own risk of side effects. There is also a greater risk of bleeding than after an ordinary biopsy, as well as a greater risk of acute urinary retention, especially in men with a large prostate or obstructive voiding symptoms. While saturation biopsy does reduce the chance that we'll fail to find a cancer, it increases the likelihood that we'll overdetect tiny, indolent cancers that would pose little risk if left alone. (See Chapter 13, Watchful Waiting [Active Surveillance].)

Template-Guided Transperineal Biopsy

In a refinement of the saturation approach, we can use a template (the same one used to implant brachytherapy seeds for treatment) to guide needles through the perineum (area between the rectum and the scrotum) into the prostate at regularly spaced intervals. (See illustration on page 350 showing ultrasound guidance to place brachytherapy seeds.) An advantage of the template approach is that the precise location of each biopsy core can be mapped to its location within the prostate more accurately than is possible with the transrectal saturation biopsy. The probability of missing a cancer is reduced because the needles are spaced regularly with precision.[8] This approach has also received impetus from a budding interest in focal therapy to treat small, low-risk prostate cancers. Sometimes called a "male lumpectomy," focal therapy, which is now being studied, seeks to treat only the area of the gland containing a cancer. If trials of this approach go well, appropriate patients would be able to avoid the risks of radical therapy. (See Chapter 16, Focal and Other "Local" Therapies.)

The jury is still out on whether saturation or template-guided biopsies are a good idea, especially in anyone who might be a candidate for surgery if a significant cancer is found. The scarring from these biopsies can make the operation more difficult and nerve-sparing less effective.

WHAT DOES A BIOPSY ENTAIL?

PREPARATION

I don't recommend any special diet or bowel preparation such as an enema before the test.[9] If you're taking a blood thinner like warfarin (Coumadin), you'll have to stop it five days before the procedure and have your prothrombin time or INR (which is the ratio of your clotting time compared with a healthy norm) checked to be sure they are back near the normal range to prevent excess bleeding. Short-acting blood thinners, like heparin or its relatives, can be stopped about six hours before a biopsy. I've seen no evidence that eliminating aspirin, NSAIDs, or vitamin E is necessary, though some doctors routinely recommend doing so.[10] If stopping these drugs would cause you troubling symptoms of arthritis or other problems, you may want to question whether it's really necessary in your case.

Since prostate biopsy involves passing needles through the rectum, infection is a serious concern. Most doctors prescribe a broad-spectrum antibiotic, such as ciprofloxacin (Cipro) or levofloxacin (Levaquin). By starting antibiotics the night before the test, you'll build good protective levels in your bloodstream.

Special caution is in order if your immune system is compromised for any reason. This applies if you're taking immunosuppressive drugs because of a transplant or if you have an autoimmune disease or a low white blood count. Steroids, including hydrocortisone or prednisone, and chemotherapeutic drugs can also depress the immune system.

Be sure to discuss any of these situations thoroughly with your doctor before biopsy. The need for the test should be weighed against your increased risk of infection. For example, if an HIV-positive or AIDS patient has a mildly elevated PSA level, it might be preferable to follow the PSA over time and get a sense of the dynamics of change before exposing him to the risks of a biopsy.

Otherwise healthy patients who have artificial heart valves, heart murmurs, or a history of rheumatic fever may be at risk for **subacute bacterial endocarditis (SBE)**, an infection caused by bacteria that enter the bloodstream and settle in the heart valves or heart lining after invasive procedures. To prevent this, the American College of Cardiology recommends a powerful antibiotic regimen, including a high-dose oral ampicillin or amoxicillin along with intramuscular or intravenous antibiotics such as gentamicin or tobramycin. If you have to take antibiotics before dental work or any kind of surgery, or if you have had a joint replacement within the last two years, you should follow the special antibiotic regimen before a prostate biopsy.[11]

THE PROCEDURE

Typically, going through a biopsy takes only a bit longer than a standard checkup. You should allow time to visit with the doctor and nurse beforehand. The test itself involves about ten to fifteen minutes for the ultrasound, plus five to ten minutes to harvest the sample cores. If you're going to have a local anesthetic, plan on another ten minutes for the lidocaine to take effect.

Prostate biopsy (aside from saturation or mapping biopsies—see above) does not require general anesthesia, which carries a small but real risk of serious or even fatal complications. While no one likes having a prostate biopsy, only one man in one hundred refuses to have it again under local anesthesia because of pain or discomfort.

SIDE EFFECTS AND COMPLICATIONS

The degree of discomfort from a prostate biopsy tends to be directly related to the number of sample cores we take. Today, a local anesthetic, such as 1 percent lidocaine on each side to numb the gland before the test, has become standard, especially when we plan to take more than six samples.[12]

After the test, you may feel some soreness in your rectum or penis, but this should resolve within a matter of hours, and most men are able to return to work and resume most normal activities the same day.

About 50 percent of men notice blood in the urine and may pass small clots after a prostate biopsy. In most cases this clears up in about three days, though occasionally it continues for weeks. Rest and increased fluid intake to flush the system usually take care of the problem.

Bleeding from the rectum is common for the first day or two but rare after that. Occasionally, a biopsy needle hits a small artery in the rectal wall, causing more severe bleeding. About 1 in 1,000 patients needs to be admitted to the hospital for a blood transfusion or requires cauterization, fulguration (a radiofrequency that causes coagulation), or sutures to resolve rectal bleeding.

I advise patients to avoid vigorous exercise for a few days after the test until any rectal or urinary bleeding stops. For five to seven days, it's wise to be cautious about activities that might exert pressure on the prostate, such as riding a bicycle, a motorcycle, or a horse.

What you should or should not do depends on the specifics of the situation. For example, riding a very narrow bicycle seat on bumpy roads for several hours may be ill-advised, but sitting on a very well-padded seat on an exercise bicycle and peddling might not be a problem at all. The goal is to avoid trauma to the prostate until it heals.

It's a good idea to wait until rectal and urinary bleeding has stopped for at least twenty-four hours before you have a sexual climax after a biopsy. Orgasm causes the gland to contract, which can promote bleeding. Blood in the ejaculate is common for a month or more and should not be a cause for alarm, and it is not harmful to your partner.

If your bleeding has stopped but starts again after sex, it will almost always clear up uneventfully. Rest and increased fluid intake should help. Serious bleeding from sexual activity after a biopsy is very rare. Some men report a temporary problem with erections following a prostate biopsy. This should resolve on its own within a few months.

Be aware of rare but significant complications that can develop during the first week or two after the test. About 3 percent of men who take antibiotics—and 6 to 10 percent of those who don't—come down with a urinary tract infection or develop bacterial prostatitis, a serious infection of the gland.[11] During this time period, if you experience symptoms such as a fever of 101°F or higher, chills, muscle aches, or urinary problems (frequency, urgency, or burning), you should go to your doctor or emergency room *immediately* for a round of cultures. Be sure to tell the examining physician that you had a transrectal biopsy of the prostate and might need intravenous antibiotics. With appropriate treatment, the infection will be arrested promptly, and you can go home within a day or two. A wait-and-see approach is definitely unwise. If you allow an infection to build for even six to twelve hours, you can become overwhelmingly septic, which could result in a long hospitalization and serious health risks. Fortunately, this occurs in less than 1 of every 200 cases.

People who have an enlarged prostate or difficulty urinating before a biopsy are at risk of developing a sudden inability to urinate, **acute urinary retention**, because of swelling from the needles. As a preventive measure, your doctor may prescribe alpha-blocking drugs. (See Chapter 5,

BPH [Benign Prostatic Hyperplasia].) Still, if urinary symptoms worsen after the test or you are unable to urinate, let your doctor know.

Given the risk of infection or bleeding, I advise patients not to take any plane flight that lasts more than four to five hours until a week to ten days after the test. If you do travel, avoid remote or underdeveloped areas. You'll definitely want to have access to top-notch medical care if complications occur.

BIOPSY RESULTS: "POSITIVE" MEANS CANCER

While heart disease can be established by clinical means through an electrocardiogram (ECG), and we have chemical tests for diseases like diabetes, biopsy is the *only* currently available tool for diagnosing cancer. To make the call, a pathologist must examine tissue taken from the suspect organ under a microscope and decide whether cancer is present or not. There is no magical passing number, no blazing indicator light, no unequivocal reading on an electronic monitor.

A positive biopsy means the pathologist has found cancer. In one of the many ironies of medical terminology, "positive" in this case turns out to be what you don't want to hear, while a "negative" result is desirable. Still, knowing that you have a malignancy is far from the whole picture. Prostate cancers vary widely, and you have to understand the specifics of your particular disease to make a sound decision about whether, when, and how to treat it.

CAN BIOPSIES MISS A CANCER?

Because biopsies test a tiny fraction of prostate tissue, any given twelve-core biopsy will detect about 75 to 90 percent of existing cancers. If the result is negative, with no cancer found, a second biopsy session of twelve or more cores would pick up many of the remaining malignancies, bringing the total to 95 to 98 percent.[13] Biopsies can be scheduled six weeks to six months apart, allowing time for swelling and bleeding from the previous test to resolve, so the prostate can be examined anew.

Occasionally, it can take three or even more attempts to find a prostate cancer. Still, in the overwhelming majority of cases, two good sets of biopsies using modern techniques and taking at least twelve cores are sufficient. On the second set, I'd add two anterior, transition-zone biopsies and a targeted biopsy to any suspicious areas I felt on DRE. If two twelve-core biopsies failed to find cancer and I'm still highly suspicious that a man has cancer (i.e. the PSA level continues to rise, the free PSA level falls, or a DRE abnormal), I would image the prostate before biopsy with an **endorectal MRI with spectroscopy** or color duplex Doppler ultrasound,[14] with or without contrast. These highly sophisticated studies may yield better information about where a cancer might be. I'd be especially inclined to use these tests if a patient has a high PSA level given the size of his prostate (PSA density over 0.15), or a low free PSA level (less than 10 percent) in combination with an elevated PSA, both of which point to a higher likelihood that a cancer exists. (See Chapter 8, Detecting Prostate Cancer with PSA and Other Tests.)

After a third such biopsy, where despite imaging and finger guidance no cancer has been found, I would recommend no further biopsies, but would follow the patient, testing the PSA and free PSA every six months and doing a digital rectal exam annually. I would suggest another biopsy only if these test results became substantially more abnormal.

NOTE: Though some people worry that a biopsy might spread cancer, there is no real evidence that this is true with modern transrectal biopsy techniques.[15] With the old technique, using large needles placed through the perineum, cancer was sometimes spread along the needle track. So far, that has not been reported with the modern transperineal template biopsy techniques, but it's too soon to be sure.

THE PATHOLOGY REPORT AND GLEASON GRADING

The standard pathology report will include your diagnosis, a description of what was found on gross and microscopic inspection, and a summary comment about the findings.

Adenocarcinoma

Ninety-eight percent of prostate cancers are **adenocarcinomas**, from the Greek root *adeno,* referring to a gland, and *carcinoma,* which describes a cancer that arises in epithelial cells, the lining cells of the ducts and glands that secrete seminal fluid. When these malignant cells are contained within the individual ducts and glands, they are called **high-grade prostatic intraepithelial neoplasia (PIN)**.[16] Once they invade through the surrounding "basement" membranes, internal fences that separate the ducts and glands, they are considered to be invasive adenocarcinomas, commonly known as prostate cancers.

Grade

The term **grade** refers to the degree to which cancer cells resemble the normal cells from which they arose. Low-grade cancers are well-differentiated. Under the microscope, they look very much like their normal counterparts with many features of the normal cell still recognizable. Moderately differentiated, also known as intermediate-grade cancers, still have some identifiable features, but they are more disrupted and disorganized than low-grade cells. High-grade, poorly differentiated cancers are wild and bear little, if any, semblance of their original form.[17] Compared with a box of berries, low-grade cells would be pretty regular with some minor variations in shape and size, intermediate-grade cells

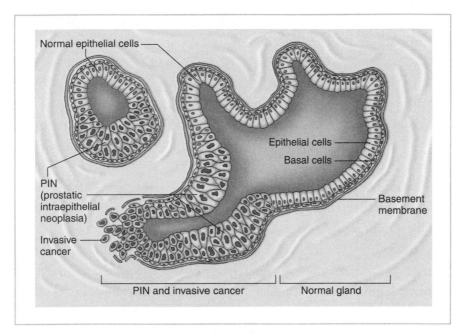

Microscopic view of a prostate gland showing normal cells and premalignant changes seen in high-grade PIN, and cancer cells invading through the basement membrane.

would have some fairly normal-looking elements and some that were crushed or distorted, and high-grade cancer would be very irregular with some unusually large cells, some abnormally small, and many distorted by lumps or otherwise misshapen.

The concept of grade arose from looking at cancers under a microscope and recognizing that the more normal a cancer cell looks, the slower it grows and the better it's likely to behave. Cancer cells with close to normal architecture pose less of a risk and are less likely to spread beyond the original organ than are higher grade cells. Wilder, stranger-looking cells are more likely to escape their local confines, set up camp in distant sites (metastasize), and prove lethal.

GLEASON GRADING

In prostate cancer we use the Gleason grading system as a simple means to characterize the seriousness of the cancer. The system is named after its inventor, a pathologist named Donald Gleason. After studying count-less prostate cancers under a microscope, he devised a scale of patterns ranked from 1 to 5, where 1 is closest to normal glandular architecture and 5 is the wildest, most poorly differentiated, and highest grade.[18]

Gleason observed that the same man frequently had more than one malignant pattern within his biopsy sample. To reflect this, his grad-ing system reports on the primary pattern plus a secondary pattern if it represents at least 5 percent of the cancer. The grades of the dominant and secondary patterns are added together to yield the **Gleason sum**, **score**, or **grade**, which can range from 2 to 10. If there is no secondary pattern, the primary pattern is added to itself (e.g., 3 + 3 = 6).

Gleason grouped his grades into 2 to 4 (well differentiated and with little or no risk), 5 and 6 (moderately differentiated, with a low risk and a favorable prognosis), 7 (moderately to poorly differentiated and with intermediate risk), and 8 to 10 (poorly differentiated, with high risk, and most aggressive). It is best to note the primary and secondary **Gleason pat-terns** separately, since the presence and amount of poorly differentiated

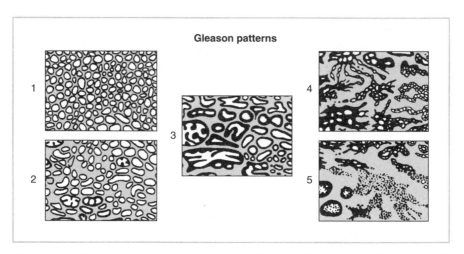

Gleason patterns

The microscopic appearance of prostate cancer typical of each Gleason pattern. Patterns 1 and 2 are well differentiated and closest to normal; pattern 3 (the most common) is moderately differen-tiated; and patterns 4 (the next most common) and 5 are poorly differentiated.*

*Source: Modified from Myron Tannenbaum, *Urologic Pathology: The Prostate*. Philadelphia: Lea & Febiger, 1977. © 1977 Myron Tannenbaum. Reprinted with permission from Lippincott Williams & Wilkins.

pattern 4 or 5 cells tend to drive the behavior of the cancer. A Gleason 2 + 4 would cause more concern than a 3 + 3, even though both patients would have a Gleason score of 6. And a 4 + 2 where the predominant finding is poorly differentiated cancer would be far more worrisome than a 2 + 4, with a smaller amount of high-risk cancer. Cancers tend to behave according to their worst components. The presence of poorly differentiated cells suggests that a cancer is growing quickly. The more high-grade cancer there is, the faster the tumor is likely to grow.[19]

NOTE: Many experts today believe that patterns 1 and 2 may not be cancer at all, so it's rare to have a Gleason sum of less than 3 + 3 = 6. If your biopsy report indicates that you have a Gleason 5 or lower, be very wary. A review of your slides by a highly skilled pathologist may find that you don't have cancer at all. Another possibility is that the first pathologist underestimated your Gleason sum, and a review will find that you have a higher-grade, more serious cancer.

NOTE: Analyzing biopsy slides is highly subjective. What appears to one pathologist to be a Gleason pattern 3 may strike another as a pattern 2 or 4. What one doctor considers normal tissue may be deemed cancer by a different pathologist. Sometimes a biopsy finding of cancer is reversed by a reviewing expert. Often, the doctor who first reviews the slides is not a prostate specialist at all.

For all these reasons, *I strongly urge you to have a second pathologist review your biopsy slides!* I advise against having this done by a different practitioner in the same office or department, because there may be pressure—no matter how subtle or subconscious—for colleagues to agree. To get the most valid second opinion, ask your diagnosing physician to send the slides to a recognized expert in the field. So-called referee centers, such as the Armed Forces Institute of Pathology, Memorial Sloan-Kettering Cancer Center, or Johns Hopkins, have pathologists whose sole job is analyzing prostate tissue.[20] Make sure that all of your slides are sent and that you get a complete report of all findings.

TIPS ON INTERPRETING YOUR BIOPSY RESULTS

After you've had your slides reviewed, be sure to ask whether there was any poorly differentiated component to your cancer. Generally, that would mean you have been assigned a Gleason score of 7, 8, 9, or 10, but sometimes there's a third component, less than 5 percent of what the pathologist sees is poorly differentiated, and that would not normally be included in your Gleason score, but it could have an effect on your prognosis. For example, if your tumor was 3 + 3, but 4 percent was composed of Gleason pattern 4, the cancer would behave worse than a 3 + 3 with no minor area of poorly differentiated cells.

If your cancer shows any pattern 4 or 5 cells, the prognosis is more serious. If your cancer is a Gleason 7, you'll want to know whether your biopsy findings were 4 + 3, which means that the dominant pattern was poorly differentiated, or 3 + 4, with a majority of more moderately differentiated cells.[21] This also makes a difference in prognosis. A 3 + 4 tumor poses less threat than does a Gleason sum of 4 + 3.

If all this seems unreasonably confusing, try to focus on the two critical issues in grading: *Was there any poorly differentiated cancer in your biopsy, and if so, how much?* A poorly differentiated cancer should be treated with all deliberate speed, not watched. While you should wait for the prostate to heal following a biopsy, aim to begin treatment within six to eight weeks after diagnosis.

At the time of your biopsy, the doctor probably took at least six and more likely as many as twelve or more sample cores from your prostate. The pathologist who read the slides reported on every core, whether it contained cancer, and if so, the Gleason primary and secondary pattern in each core. The conventional approach is to assign the overall Gleason grade of your cancer the single core with the highest Gleason core. For example, if one of your cores contains pattern 4 + 4, you would be assigned an overall Gleason sum of 8. It is important to know the amount and proportion of poorly differentiated cancer in all the cores. This is more reflective of your prognosis and a better basis on which to make a treatment decision.

NOTE: Criteria for assigning Gleason grades have changed over the last 15 years, but the studies we use to predict prognosis were based on samples collected 10 to 15 years ago. Since prostate cancer is slow-growing, we don't know the results of treatment for many years. In the modern era, pathologists assign many tumors a 3 + 4 that would have been 3 + 3 a decade ago. Prostate pathology has seen the equivalent of grade inflation.[21] Consequently, a man diagnosed with a Gleason 7 cancer today generally has a more favorable prognosis than someone assigned a Gleason sum of 7 fifteen years ago. A high Gleason sum should not be cause for panic or undue pessimism. Many of the highest Gleason score cancers today are curable (even so-called high-risk Gleason 8 through 10).

HOW RELIABLE IS THE PATHOLOGY REPORT?

Most often, the Gleason grade of the cancer found in the biopsy cores accurately reflects the grade of all the cancer in the prostate. Nevertheless, in 30 percent of cases the tumor will turn out to be higher grade than it appeared to be in the biopsy, and 5 percent of the time the grade will be lower.[22] A biopsy session, even one where twelve or more cores are taken, randomly samples only a tiny fraction of prostate tissue, so complete accuracy can't be guaranteed. Sometimes we repeat a biopsy to learn more about the nature of the tumor. In about a fourth of cases, we find no cancer the second time, not because the cancer has disappeared but because the needle cores missed a small malignancy that was hit the first time. On the other hand, about a fourth of the time we also find that there is substantially more cancer present or a higher Gleason grade.[23]

Think of a biopsy as a good approximation, but not an exact replica, of what is actually in the prostate gland.

RARE TYPES OF PROSTATE CANCER

NEUROENDOCRINE (SMALL-CELL) CARCINOMA

These extremely rare tumors are very aggressive. They grow rapidly and metastasize early. Small areas of neuroendocrine carcinoma can be found in many prostate cancers, especially large, poorly differentiated tumors with a high Gleason sum (8 or more), but these tiny findings do not have any special significance. However, when the predominant element is neuroendocrine, the prognosis is poor, and chemotherapy to shrink the tumor is generally the treatment of first choice.[24] Patients with a neuroendocrine tumor can have an elevated level of a chemical called **chromogranin** their blood.

TRANSITIONAL CELL CARCINOMA

The prostatic ducts and the urethra running through the prostate are lined by the same transitional cells as the bladder. A cancer arising in these lining cells can spread into the prostate. If you have this rare carcinoma, you'll need a thorough evaluation to determine where the cancer arose, whether the urinary bladder or the ureters are involved, and whether it should be treated as a prostate cancer or a bladder cancer.

DUCTAL OR ENDOMETRIAL CARCINOMA

Adenocarcinomas that arise in or invade the ducts of the prostate have a characteristic appearance, are usually high-grade, and have a worse prognosis, but are otherwise typical prostate cancers.[25] Some of these make an unusual appearance by growing through the prostatic ducts into the urethra, creating the characteristic appearance of what was once called "endometrial" carcinoma. We now know that these are a particular manifestation of ductal carcinoma.

OTHER RARE CANCERS OF THE PROSTATE

In a tiny fraction of cases, a biopsy of the prostate finds sarcomas, melanomas, or cancers that have spread from the kidney, bowel, stomach, or lung. Each case must be evaluated thoroughly to determine the appropriate treatment.

ASIDE FROM CANCER, WHAT OTHER IMPORTANT FINDINGS MIGHT THE PATHOLOGY REPORT CONTAIN?

PROSTATITIS

If the pathologist sees many white blood cells within the prostate tissue, he or she may report the diagnosis of "prostatitis." **Chronic prostatitis** indicates that the type of white blood cells found are typical of lasting inflammation, while **acute prostatitis** means the white cells are more likely due to recent inflammation. Such a finding does not necessarily mean that you have an infection. There seems to be little relationship between these microscopic observations and the troublesome symptoms of clinical prostatitis or chronic pelvic pain syndrome that lead men to seek medical treatment. (See Chapter 4, Prostatitis.) Some men simply have higher levels of white blood cells in their prostates, which tends to mean higher PSA levels, and thus these men are more likely to be referred for biopsy.[26]

> NOTE: Though prostatitis may cause an alarming increase in PSA, men with an active infection in the gland *should not* undergo a biopsy. Wait until your infection disappears, your urine cultures are normal, you complete the course of antibiotics, and your prostate has had time to heal.

PROSTATIC INTRAEPITHELIAL NEOPLASIA (PIN)

High-grade **PIN** is not cancer, but it is probably the main precursor. This common lesion can be recognized because the cells resemble cancers, except that the basement membrane, which functions like the skin around a grape, remains intact. (See page 172.)[27]

Since these cancerous-appearing cells do not invade surrounding tissues, we refer to high-grade PIN as carcinoma in situ (cancer cells that remain in their site of origin). In other organs, fairly aggressive treatment of carcinoma in situ is common, but current thinking in the prostate field is that treatment would be overkill. Having high-grade PIN *does not mean* you'll inevitably develop prostate cancer. We view it as an early-warning sign, similar to an elevated PSA. Early studies found that 50 percent of men with high-grade PIN had prostate cancer on a subsequent biopsy over the next five years. Eighty-five percent of patients diagnosed with prostate cancer also have areas of high-grade PIN. Most malignant lesions in the prostate start out as high-grade PIN. Still, recent studies stress that while having high-grade PIN increases your prostate cancer risk, the level of that risk depends on a host of risk factors, including age, PSA level, size of prostate, the findings on DRE, and family history.[28]

High-grade PIN is a cancer precursor and calls for vigilant monitoring, but it is not a disease or pressing emergency. The condition *will not* suddenly develop into an aggressive cancer or metastasize. If your pathology report shows areas of high-grade PIN but no cancer, your doctor may recommend a repeat systematic biopsy within six to twelve months, depending on your particular situation. Your chances of eventually being diagnosed with cancer depend on your age, your family history of prostate cancer, your PSA level, and many other factors, and can best be measured on a recently published nomogram. (For more information about nomograms, see the Resources section at the end of this book or visit www.nomograms.org.)[29]

ATYPICAL SMALL ACINAR PROLIFERATION (ASAP, ATYPIA)

The pathologist sees a cluster of cells with malignant features, but the suspect sample is too tiny or uncertain to warrant a cancer diagnosis. A finding of ASAP means you are at increased risk of having a cancer. A second pathologist's opinion is particularly important in these cases, and a repeat biopsy is in order if both doctors agree that the cells are atypical and suspicious. You should wait six weeks to three months until the effects of the previous biopsy have resolved. The repeat biopsy should

Special Stains

When viewing biopsy specimens, pathologists sometimes find cells that lack the typical distinguishing features of prostate cancer or high-grade PIN. Special stains can help identify the cell types in this situation. These stains contain antibodies that pick up the signals or markers that characterize different cell types within the prostate. The most commonly used stains identify the basal cell layer beneath the epithelial cells. In high-grade PIN, the basal cell layer remains intact. With invasive cancer, the malignant cells displace the basal cell layer and invade through the basement membrane.

Another commonly used stain is for racemase, a marker that is almost inevitably found within cancer cells and rarely in any other (benign) cells. These special stains can help the pathologist determine whether small abnormal lesions are truly malignant or just cancer look-alikes.

pay special attention to the region of the prostate where the abnormal glands were found.

ADENOSIS (ATYPICAL ADENOMATOUS HYPERPLASIA, AAH)

Adenosis is not cancer and does not suggest an increased cancer risk, but an inexperience pathologist might mistake this overgrowth of benign abnormal cells for a low Gleason score cancer of 3 + 3 or less.

THE FUTURE

A needle biopsy of the prostate is nobody's idea of fun, and the procedure can seem even more onerous for men who need to go through it several times. You may be wondering why we can't find a kinder, gentler way to diagnose prostate cancer without having to pierce the gland with needles. In fact, researchers are exploring possible alternatives to traditional biopsy that would enable us to do just that.

Prostatic fluid, whether collected as a semen sample or in a urine specimen passed after prostatic massage, contains thousands of prostate cells as well as a number of distinctive proteins that are secreted by the gland. A particularly promising approach would be to examine prostatic fluid for the presence of malignant cells or specific genes or proteins that might prove as useful in diagnosing cancer as a biopsy specimen. The PCA3 test is commercially available and is being actively studied as a way to detect the likelihood of cancer, and researchers are beginning to develop tests to identify the TMPRSS-2 fusion gene, which is found in prostate cancers but not in normal cells or cancers from other organs. Another promising molecular test would identify a gene called GST, the earliest known molecular change leading to prostate cancer. We are also seeking ways to measure telomerase, which increases markedly in the presence of cancer. If we can develop reliable ways to test for these substances in a clinical laboratory, we might be able to use them in lieu of a biopsy.

Though PSA is not reliable enough to use in diagnosing cancer, we may be able to use sophisticated technology to isolate and identify small numbers of prostate cancer cells in the bloodstream. These **circulating tumor cells (CTCs)** are regularly found in the blood we draw from men with metastatic cancer. These tests are becoming exquisitely sensitive, with the ability to identify a single cell in 10 million in the bloodstream. As the technology continues to evolve, tests for CTCs may one day be used to detect prostate cancer. The CTC test could prove to be the discriminator we've long been hoping for, capable of finding serious cancers while avoiding the overdetection of trivial cancers that don't pose any significant threat and do not need to be treated.

IN SUMMARY

A biopsy is the only means we currently have to diagnose prostate cancer, but the test is far from foolproof. Be sure to have a second, independent expert pathologist review your results. Always request a complete pathology report, including information on what was found in every sample core and whether there was any finding of high-grade, poorly differentiated cancer.

10

■

Understanding Your Cancer

READ THIS CHAPTER TO LEARN:

- How do we determine the clinical stage of a cancer, and what does it mean?
- How can you better understand how serious your cancer is by factoring in all the diagnostic information?
- What are nomograms, and how can they help you decide what to do about your prostate cancer?

often wish that we could find a name other than *cancer* for a malignant tumor in the prostate. Few words carry a more explosive emotional charge, and few medical conditions provoke such overwhelming distress and anxiety. In the minds of many people, cancer spells doom—end of story. But that's far from the actual fact.

While it is true that all cancers share risky features, including the potential to spread to surrounding tissues and distant sites, the course of the disease varies tremendously from organ to organ and from case to case. Some malignancies, including certain forms of leukemia and pancreatic cancers, are overwhelmingly destructive, often causing death within a few years. Fortunately, we can diagnose, treat, and arrest many other cancers before they have the chance to do any serious or lasting harm. Some slow-growing tumors, especially in older patients, may not warrant any treatment at all.

Given current diagnostic and therapeutic tools, a huge and growing number of people get through a bout with cancer and go on to live out a normal life span. In fact, there are currently over 11 million cancer survivors in the United States alone, and over 2 million of them have survived prostate cancer.[1]

The outlook for prostate cancer patients has improved dramatically in the past twenty-five years. Before the advent of PSA testing, many of these tumors went undiscovered until they were well beyond any hope of a cure. Today, thanks to greater awareness and widespread screening, the vast majority of cases are diagnosed while the tumor is still small, contained, and curable. Most prostate cancers grow slowly and aren't likely to cause any problems or symptoms for many years. Still, if you have a serious cancer, having treatment now may prove to be an important investment in your future. I think of it as similar to a retirement fund. If you don't plan ahead, you could find yourself with a serious, irremediable problem down the road.

That said, prostate cancer *is not* a medical crisis that requires immediate or emergency intervention. The wisest approach is to weigh your options

NOTE: Men commonly believe that if they are diagnosed with prostate cancer, it just appeared and must be removed immediately. But unlike some cancers, prostate cancer is slow-growing. The usual time it takes for the cancer to double in size is two to four years. Even if the cancer is more advanced, with a doubling time as short as three or six months, the tumor has been there for many months or years, perhaps even decades, and it is not an emergency. Making the right treatment decision is more important than making a quick decision. Be sure any treatment you require is done well and safely.

carefully and commit to a therapeutic strategy within about three to six months after you're diagnosed. (The exception is men whose tumors are large and high-grade. They should aim to begin treatment as soon as the cancer has been thoroughly evaluated.) That should give you ample time to gather the information you'll need to make an informed decision about what course of action would be best in your particular case.

HOW SERIOUS IS YOUR CANCER?

Suppose you were awakened by a sound in the middle of the night. Before you leapt into full combat mode, you would be wise to take a moment to consider the source of the noise. It might be perfectly innocent: the dog knocking something over or a child padding into the kitchen for a midnight refrigerator raid. Maybe you come fully awake and remember that you have a friend visiting or that one of the kids was expected home late. Waiting a beat to figure out what's really going on can help you to respond rationally and avoid doing something you might regret.

The same holds true when the diagnosis is prostate cancer. To arrive at a sensible plan of action, you need to learn as much as possible about your disease. How large and extensive is your cancer? How dangerous and aggressive is it? What risk, if any, does it pose to your life and health?

The "Stage" or Extent of the Cancer

Clinical **stage** refers to the size and extent of your tumor. How big is it, how much of the gland does it occupy, and does it extend into surrounding tissues. In most cases, the estimate is based on the results of the **digital rectal exam (DRE)**.

Digital Rectal Exam (DRE)

While it's standard practice to base clinical stage on the DRE alone, the test has serious limitations. A doctor can only examine the rear portion of the prostate that rests against the front rectal wall. Tumors in other areas of the gland will not be detected, nor will cancers that are too small to feel.

Still, it's important to know whether your doctor detected any suspicious lumps or nodules during your DRE. If so, request a written report including significant details. How large was the affected area? In what part of the prostate was it located? Does the doctor believe that the lump or nodule he felt was confined within the gland, or is there any reason to suspect that it has eroded through the capsule or invaded nearby structures?

It's useful to collect the results of all the DREs you've ever had. If you have been examined regularly, especially by the same physician, an abrupt change could signal that your tumor has suddenly become aggressive. On the other hand, if your last exam was a decade ago and your doctor finds a nodule now, it's impossible to know whether the tumor has been slowly, steadily increasing in size or has accelerated recently.

If more than one doctor examines you, be sure to note whether or not the DRE findings are consistent. It can happen that one physician feels a nodular thickening on the right base (top) of the prostate, while another reports an abnormality on the upper left. The DRE is a difficult test to learn, and accuracy depends on the doctor's sensitivity and training. Family doctors or internists who don't do these exams routinely often fail to pick up subtle abnormalities that an experienced urologist might detect. Findings are highly subjective, and even experts may disagree. Where results are discordant, I would rely on the opinion of the doctor who has the most experience in the field.

What is found on DRE should conform to what was seen on ultrasound during your biopsy. If the doctor felt something on the right base and that area appears abnormal on the ultrasound as well, I would have far more confidence that the results really reflect the cancer. I am less confident when the doctor feels something in the right base and that area appears normal on an MRI. In that case, I'd turn to the map of the cancer I can get from systematic biopsies to resolve the question (see page 162). If that still doesn't clear things up, a repeat biopsy may be required to determine exactly where the cancer is located and how large and serious it is.

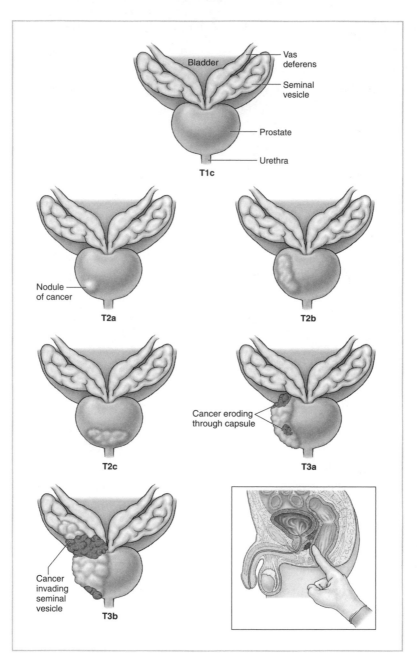

The TNM classification of prostate cancers is used to indicate the size and extent, or stage of the cancer. T stands for "tumor," or the extent of the primary cancer in the prostate. Cancers are designated T1 if they cannot be felt by DRE. T2 cancers are palpable but confined within the capsule of the prostate. T3 cancers extend through the capsule. Biopsy results play no role in assigning the T stage. The stage is based on DRE results alone. (See page 193 for more on TNM staging.)

What Other Tests Can Help to Confirm Tumor Stage?

PSA   Generally speaking, your PSA reflects the volume of the tumor: larger cancer equals higher PSA. Since tumor size typically correlates with the seriousness of the disease, PSA provides a useful piece of the diagnostic puzzle.

As a rule, PSA levels lower than 2 are associated with a highly favorable outlook and a high probability that a cancer is contained in the prostate and curable with surgery or radiation if it even needs to be treated. PSAs over 10 are progressively less favorable. The more elevated the level, the more likely the tumor is to have spread.[2]

Interpreting PSA levels between 2 and 10 is tricky. Elevations in this range may stem from benign enlargement of the prostate, or from cancer. To accurately interpret your PSA, you have to factor in the size of your prostate. A larger gland naturally produces more PSA, which registers as a higher number on the test. This does not suggest that any tumor present is likely to be large and aggressive. In fact, precisely the opposite is true. Our research has confirmed that the bigger the gland, the smaller and more favorable any cancers we find tend to be.[3]

A favorable ratio of PSA to prostate size is anything less than 1 to 10.[4] A 20-gram prostate can be expected to account for a PSA of up to 2. For a 100-gram prostate, the PSA would ideally be less than 10. Since most prostates in adult men weigh between 20 and 100 grams, much of the PSA between 2 and 10 may be due to benign enlargement of the gland (BPH). As a result, numbers in this range are less reliable in measuring the seriousness of a cancer than are numbers below 2 or above 10.

SYSTEMATIC BIOPSY RESULTS   We can use systematic biopsy results to create a virtual map of the tumor. If one core out of twelve or fourteen contains only a tiny amount of cancer, it's probable that we're dealing with a small, early-stage tumor. On the other hand, if many of the biopsy samples turn up large amounts of cancer, the malignancy has obviously progressed further, involving more of the gland and a greater risk of spread beyond its confines.

Interpreting biopsy results is a simple matter of connecting the diagnostic dots. When a large percentage of several adjacent cores are positive

Diagram of the amount of cancer in systematic needle biopsy cores

Patient: Joe Smith (single, small cancer)

Part of the prostate	Left	Right
Apex	1 mm	
Middle		
Base		
Ruler 15mm	0 5 10 15	0 5 10 15

Patient: Bill Jones (large, multifocal cancer)

Part of the prostate	Left	Right
Apex	7 mm	5 mm
Middle	12 mm	
Base	9 mm	

Normal tissue   Cancer

Diagram used to represent the amount and location of cancer in systematic needle biopsy cores.

for cancer, the tumor is likely to be large, bulky, and more serious. In contrast, if tiny clusters of malignant cells are scattered randomly throughout the gland, we're probably dealing with a number of smaller, less advanced, and lower–risk tumors.[5]

Ultrasound and MRI of the Prostate

Sophisticated imaging studies, along with a careful analysis of other test results, can shed additional light on the tumor's size and location. Though the prostate's particular anatomy and its obscure location deep in the pelvis make it difficult to visualize as clearly as we can a kidney or lung, dedicated prostate imaging specialists using state-of-the-art technology can make a valuable contribution to our understanding of a patient's particular disease.

TRANSRECTAL ULTRASOUND (TRUS) Cancerous tissue responds differently from normal tissue to ultrasound waves.[6] An expert can evaluate these visible areas of low sound reflection to calculate where in the gland cancers lie and how big they are. (See figure on page 163 for an image of the prostate produced by ultrasound.) While ultrasound provides a very good picture of the prostate gland and allows us to measure its size and configuration accurately (making it useful for guiding needles into the prostate for biopsy) and for calculating PSA density, it has serious limitations for detecting cancers. Ultrasound is fairly accurate at imaging large cancers, which, given widespread prostate cancer screening, are uncommon in the United States today. The test is not very good at picking up cancers smaller than 7 mm in diameter, or those that are Gleason 6 or less. I am often surprised that I can feel on DRE a cancer that I am unable to see on the ultrasound during an ultrasound-guided biopsy.

Adding futuristic technology such as color Doppler effects (a name you may recognize from those vibrant weather maps on the Internet and TV) may enhance the diagnostic accuracy by allowing the imaging specialist to visualize the complex blood vessels that cancers require to grow.[7] Researchers are investigating the value of contrast agents such as micro-bubbles to further increase the ability of ultrasound to detect small cancers.

MAGNETIC RESONANCE IMAGING (MRI) This procedure creates a magnetic field that causes protons in the atoms that comprise the prostatic tissue to align and emit radio waves that can be recorded and interpreted. It has proven to be the best means we have today for seeing a cancer in the prostate.[8] Prostate imaging with MRI requires state of the art technology and expert interpretation. MRI experts such as Dr. Hedvig Hricak at Memorial Sloan-Kettering Cancer Center, a radiologist specializing in prostate imaging, can examine areas of the prostate that cannot be felt on DRE or seen on conventional imaging studies and

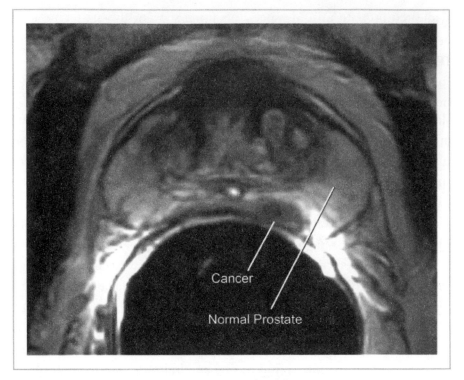

MRI scan of the prostate in a man with an early-stage prostate cancer. The normal prostate appears gray and uniform. The cancer at the edge of the prostate is dark and nodular. (T2-weighted endorectal MRI of the prostate. Courtesy Dr. Hedvig Hricak, Memorial Sloan-Kettering Cancer Center, New York.)

provide far greater anatomical detail than conventional imaging studies, including CT scans. MRI can help to determine extracapsular extension and seminal vesicle invasion. MRI is as good as CT scanning at detecting lymph node metastases and better at finding spread to bones in the pelvis. The test also provides detail about the size and anatomy of the gland, which is useful in treatment planning. (See illustration above.)

A number of techniques can improve the accuracy of MRI. Diffusion-weighted imaging (DWI) can enhance the distinction between cancer and normal tissue. At MSKCC, we use an endorectal coil, which places the MRI detectors in the rectum right next to the prostate, markedly magnifying the view. The coil also allows us to analyze the chemical composition of prostatic tissue, enhancing our ability to distinguish cancer from benign tissue. Other centers use **dynamic contrast enhanced (DCE) MRI**, which highlights vascular areas of cancer that are not found in normal tissue. Nevertheless, even this powerful technique can be stymied by prostate cancer's ability to mimic normal tissue. Cancers smaller than 5 mm, those located in the transition zone, and those of low Gleason grade (6 or lower) are almost always missed by MRI.

With prostate MRIs, false positives can also be an issue. Changes in the gland such as BPH or the effects of previous biopsies can emit a signal similar to cancer, though no malignancy exists.

> NOTE: Unless you have a high-risk or locally advanced cancer, an MRI is probably not useful. To get the best information from a prostate MRI, you should have it performed in a center with special interest and expertise in this test.[9]

TNM STAGING

TNM Staging is the system most commonly used to stage all cancers. (See the table on page 195.) In addition to describing the extent of the primary or largest tumor (T stage), this approach notes whether a cancer has spread to lymph nodes (N stage) or if it has metastasized to distant organs (M stage).[10]

Stage T1 describes cancers that are either too small for the doctor to feel or located in the front (anterior) part of the gland, which cannot be reached during the digital rectal exam. Given early detection with PSA, this stage describes the majority of cases we diagnose today. Some prostate tumors are discovered incidentally when a pathologist examines tissue that has been removed to treat the urinary obstruction caused by BPH. If less than 5 percent of the specimen is found to contain cancer, the clinical stage is set at T1a. When the cancer involves more than 5 percent of the excised overgrowth, the stage is reported as T1b. Clinical stage

T1c describes a tumor that cannot be felt on DRE but is discovered during a biopsy that was triggered by an elevated PSA.

If we feel a tumor on only one side of the gland, occupying less than one half of the lobe, and it appears confined to the prostate, the clinical stage is T2a. A larger cancer involving one lobe is designated stage T2b. If the cancer involves both lobes, it is T2c. T3a cancers extend beyond the prostate's outer covering (capsule) on one or both sides, while T3b refers to tumors that have invaded the neighboring seminal vesicles. If the cancer has spread to other nearby structures such as the bladder neck, the external urinary sphincter, the rectum, or the pelvic wall, we classify it as stage T4.

Where there is no evidence of lymph node involvement, the node stage is recorded as N0. N1 refers to a cancer that has spread to pelvic lymph nodes. The presence of cancer in lymph nodes can be determined by imaging studies such as CT scans or MRIs, but only if the nodes are enlarged. A negative CT scan or MRI is no guarantee that the nodes are free of microscopic metastases. These scans are not sensitive enough to detect tiny clusters of malignant cells in lymph nodes.

Stage M0 means there is no evidence of spread beyond the local area. If cancer is evident in lymph nodes beyond the pelvic region, we assign a stage of M1a. Where metastases to skeletal bones have been detected on a **bone scan or other imaging studies**, the M stage is M1b. M1c describes spread to other distant sites such as the liver, lungs, or brain.

NOTE: If your cancer is found in tissue removed during a TURP to treat the symptoms of prostate enlargement (BPH), further testing is usually needed to determine whether you need treatment. If the cancer is high-grade (Gleason 7 through 10), further treatment is usually warranted. Otherwise, I recommend waiting six to eight weeks after the TURP until the prostate is healed, and then reassessing the extent of the cancer with a DRE, PSA, MRI imaging if available, and a repeat needle biopsy. The decision about whether to have further treatment depends on the amount of cancer found after this restaging, not on the initial evaluation.

TNM STAGING SYSTEM FOR PROSTATE CANCER*	
STAGE	CHARACTERISTIC
T1 T1a T1b T1c	Can't be felt on DRE or seen by imaging Incidental finding in <5% of tissue removed to treat BPH or bladder cancer Incidental finding in >5% of tissue removed to treat BPH or bladder cancer Tumor identified by needle biopsy, for any reason (e.g., elevated PSA level)
T2 T2a T2b T2c	Palpable or visible tumor, confined within the prostate Less than half of one lobe One lobe Both lobes
T3 T3a T3b	Tumor extends through the capsule ECE, unilateral or bilateral Seminal vesicle invasion
T4 T4a T4b	Tumor is fixed or invades adjacent structures Invades bladder neck, external sphincter, or rectum Invades levator muscles or fixed to pelvic sidewalls
N0	No spread to regional lymph nodes
N1	Metastasis (spread) in a single lymph node, <2 cm in greatest dimension
N2	Metastasis in a single lymph node >2 cm but <5 cm, or in multiple lymph nodes, none >5 cm in greatest dimension
N3	Metastasis in a lymph node >5 cm in greatest dimension
M0	No distant metastasis
M1 M1a M1b M1c	Distant metastasis exists Metastasis to lymph nodes beyond the prostate region Bone metastasis Metastasis to other sites

Extracapsular extension (ECE) of a prostate cancer refers to microscopic penetration through the capsule into the surrounding tissue. In most cases the cancer has not spread to distant sites and is still curable with surgery or radiation. While ECE indicates that the cancer is capable

*Source: Modified from M. Ohori, T. M. Wheeler, and P. T. Scardino, "The New American Joint Committee on Cancer and International Union Against Cancer TNM Classification of Prostate Cancer: Clinicopathologic Correlations," *Cancer* 74 (1994): 104–114. © 1994 M. Ohori, T. M. Wheeler, and P. T. Scardino. Reprinted with permission from Wiley-Liss, Inc., a subsidiary of John Wiley & Sons, Inc.

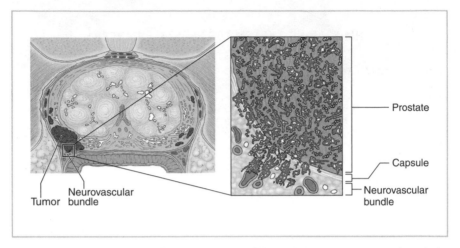

Extracapsular extension (ECE) of a prostate cancer refers to microscopic penetration through the capsule into the surrounding tissue. In most cases the cancer has not spread to distant sites and is still curable with surgery or radiation.

of invading through normal tissue boundaries, cancers within the prostate can metastasize by invading into blood vessels or lymphatics within the gland. ECE is not the normal route of distant dissemination of prostate cancer.

STAGE AND TREATMENT

Traditionally, clinical stage has dictated the kind of treatment we advise. Men with small, early-stage T1 or T2 cancers are seen as good candidates for curative radiation or surgery to remove the gland. Large, extensive T3b or T4 tumors are usually not curable with local therapy alone, so systemic treatments such as hormone therapy in combination with local therapy would be more appropriate.

A major area of confusion and misunderstanding is what to do about T3a tumors, where the cancer has penetrated the capsule of the gland. **Extracapsular extension (ECE)** means the disease is no longer organ-confined, but that *does not mean* it has spread to other organs. Sticking your head out the window is not the same as leaving the house. You'd still be able to feel the air-conditioning and hear the radio, though you might have to turn both up to maintain the same effects.

In similar fashion, surgery or radiation can cure a tumor that has broken through the capsule of the gland, as long as it's contained in the local area. Radical prostatectomy can succeed as long as the surgeon operates widely enough to ensure that no cancer cells are left behind. Where there is extracapsular extension, we have to take extra care to remove sufficient tissue. If we leave cancer at the edge of what's removed (**positive surgical margins**), the risk of recurrence is far greater. Sometimes, getting safely around an area of ECE risks damaging one or both erectile nerves, These nerves generally recover if they are not completely resected, in which case one or both can be replaced with nerve grafts by a surgeon skilled in this procedure.

If radiation is the treatment choice, the area of ECE must be included in the target field. A careful assessment should be made of whether seed implants, which are normally recommended for favorable cancers, are appropriate in this setting.

THE STAGING (PARTIN) TABLES

The **Partin tables** are mathematical models that predict what a pathologist would find if the prostate were surgically removed and examined under the microscope.[11] Pathological stage—the actual size and scope of the cancer—may turn out to be very different from the clinical stage we estimate from the DRE and other studies.

The Partin tables combine the Gleason grade, PSA, and T stage (based on the DRE) to estimate pathological stage. Partin 1 indicates the probability that the cancer is confined to the prostate. Partin 2 is the likelihood of extension through the capsule without seminal vesicle invasion or lymph node involvement. Partin 3 is the chance that the cancer involves the seminal vesicles but has not spread to the lymph nodes, and Partin 4 is the probability of metastasis to the lymph nodes. Because they take the three most important diagnostic factors into account, the Partin tables were a major advance and provide a more accurate estimate of the extent of the cancer than we can get from any one of these factors alone.

But Partin tables can overgeneralize. For example, by clustering patients with a broad range of PSA levels, the Partin tables suggest that a man with a PSA of 10.1 would have an equal risk that his cancer has spread to lymph nodes as would a man with a PSA of 19.9. This is similar to suggesting that boxing any middleweight is the same, no matter if your opponent is at the very bottom or at the maximum for the weight class. In fact, higher PSA levels indicate an increased risk that cancer has spread beyond the prostate.[12]

Another limitation of the Partin tables is that they predict mutually exclusive **disease states**. A patient expected to have extracapsular extension is placed in a different group from a man predicted to have seminal vesicle invasion, even though the latter would typically have ECE as well. Consequently, the risk of having extracapsular extension, which has important implications for treatment planning, can be underestimated by this system.

The Partin tables do not help us localize the area of presumed abnormality. For example, estimating the likelihood of extracapsular extension gives no information about where cells likely penetrate through the capsule. This is crucial data for a surgeon attempting to remove all the cancer while minimizing damage to the neurovascular bundles, which contain the nerves responsible for penile erections.

As valuable as they are, the Partin tables are often misused to try to estimate a patient's chance of cure (prognosis) rather than their intended use, which is to predict the extent (stage) of the cancer. Many patients and physicians assume that only cancers confined to the prostate can be cured with surgery. If the Partin tables suggest that there is only a 50 percent chance the cancer is confined, some users erroneously conclude that there is only a 50 percent chance of a cure. In fact, most men with extracapsular extension and many with seminal vesicle invasion or lymph node metastases can be cured with surgery or radiation alone.

HOW IS STAGE DIFFERENT FROM PROGNOSIS?

Stage describes the size and extent of the cancer. But knowing the size of the enemy army, where the troops are encamped, and how much of your land they have infiltrated does not fully inform you about how fiercely they are going to fight or how likely they are to win the war. As a general rule, a larger, more extensive tumor poses a greater threat (as does a larger opposing army), but this is not universally true. What happens on the battlefield will ultimately depend on how well-armed, well-trained, deft, and determined the enemy forces prove to be, and how successful they are at defeating your efforts to thwart them. On the cancer front, some small prostate cancers are fiercely aggressive, while some large tumors, like slow, lumbering beasts, are not.

With cancer and other diseases, **prognosis** is an estimate of your outlook. How big a threat, if any, does the cancer pose to your long-term health and survival? Do you have a tumor that needs to be treated now, or can treatment be postponed until the cancer shows convincing signs of progression? How urgently should you begin therapy, and how force-ful does your treatment need to be? What is the likelihood that any given treatment will cure or arrest the disease?

HOW AGGRESSIVE IS THE CANCER? THE GLEASON GRADE

The Gleason grade measures the cancer's aggressiveness and predicts how serious and dangerous it's likely to be. After your biopsy, a pathologist examines the sample cores that were taken under a microscope. Based on how closely the cancer cells resemble normal cells, each core is assigned a primary and secondary **Gleason pattern or grade**. Those two pat-terns are then added together to arrive at your **Gleason score** (sum, or simply, Gleason). (For a full discussion of the Gleason grading system, see Chapter 9, Biopsy.)

The more normal cancer cells appear to be, the more predictably and reasonably they behave. Poorly differentiated cancers with few remaining normal features are like wild animals that must be considered dangerous and erratic.

To gauge your prognosis, it's important to know the details of your Gleason grade. Like a rioting crowd, cancers tend to be driven by their worst elements. If your tumor has any poorly differentiated Gleason 4 or 5 components, it will be more aggressive, grow more rapidly, and is more likely to spread.

If the pathologist reports any high-grade cancer, be sure to find out how much. One tiny focus of poorly differentiated cells is far less ominous than biopsy results in which the predominant finding is high-risk Gleason pattern 4 or 5. Be sure to request a report of the Gleason grade of each biopsy core that was found to contain malignant disease. Having one core with a small amount of Gleason 3 + 4 cancer is far less worrisome than having multiple cores filled with Gleason 4 + 3, even though the overall Gleason score would be 7 in both cases.

PSA LEVEL AND PROGNOSIS

Along with Gleason score, the best predictor of prostate cancer is your PSA level. In addition to reflecting tumor size, PSA can help us to understand how a cancer is likely to progress. In general, a higher level carries a worse prognosis, but there are many exceptions to this rule. I have seen men with a PSA of 50 with a large cancer in the transition zone that was completely confined to the prostate and cured with surgery alone. At the same time, poorly differentiated cancers, which can be the most aggressive, typically produce little PSA per gram of cancerous tissue, so a cancer can spread to the lymph nodes despite a low PSA (e.g., below 2).

While it can provide useful information, PSA is not a sure thing. It behaves more like a barometer reading that may correlate strongly with the weather but certainly does not guarantee clear skies or rain.

It is not an absolute indicator of how cancers are going to behave. Every little increase doesn't necessarily mean the cancer is growing, and every decrease does not guarantee that the tumor is shrinking. While the cancer is in place, changes in PSA can reflect changes in the gland that are unrelated to the tumor. PSA is an important, but imperfect, measure.

It is sensible to assume that if PSA is so important and so clearly reflects the extent of the cancer, the changes in PSA level absolutely indicate change in the cancer. Many studies argue that rapid rises in PSA, for example, greater than 2 ng/ml/year, indicate an unusually aggressive cancer highly likely to metastasize.[13] High PSA velocity and short PSA doubling time (see Chapter 8, Detecting Prostate Cancer with PSA and Other Tests, for more discussion of PSA kinetics) have repeatedly been associated with a more serious cancer. The trouble is, few of these studies take into account the PSA at the same time. When rigorously analyzed, the absolute level of PSA means more than the rate of rise.[14] The problem with changes in PSA is that they are highly variable in a man whose prostate is in place and untreated.[15] The normal variations in PSA over time, and the difference between assays, swamp any real change in PSA that could be meaningfully used to compute PSA velocity. I recommend repeating the PSA after a few weeks in any man diagnosed with prostate cancer. Often the repeat level is lower and the velocity less. Nevertheless, doctors appropriately worry when a man's PSA rises rapidly. Occasionally, the rise is real and the prognosis truly ominous.

NOTE: The phenomenon of the sophomore jinx in baseball has long been used to explain the frustrating drop in batting averages of last year's leading sluggers. Such regression to the mean also affects PSA levels, which often fall after a biopsy triggered by a rising PSA. When the PSA is checked again six weeks later, it is usually lower. Consider the sophomore jinx phenomenon before becoming too concerned about a PSA that rises rapidly right before a biopsy and then falls. To assess true PSA levels, keep checking over the months following biopsy.

Try to assemble every PSA you've had, going back to the very first time you were screened for prostate cancer. Given the long, slow evolution of this disease, we can learn far more from a historical time-lapse perspective than we can from a current snapshot. Even changes within so-called "normal" limits may be significant. Recent studies have shown that it's possible to observe telling changes in PSA ten, fifteen, or even twenty years before a man is diagnosed with prostate cancer.[16]

In evaluating PSA, it's important to focus on trends. Just as a one-day boost in the Dow Jones Industrial Average does not necessarily mean a bull market, a sudden spike in your PSA does not automatically spell serious trouble. Inflammation or any manipulation of the prostate, including a biopsy, can cause your level to soar. If your number has hovered in the 1 to 2 range over many years and it suddenly jumps to 6 or 26, something other than cancer is probably the cause. Retesting after a few weeks or months is certainly in order. This is true even after a biopsy has determined that you have prostate cancer. A follow-up test might confirm a lower PSA that is far more representative of the state of your disease.

A recent study suggested that men whose PSA rose by more than 2 ng/ml per year in the year before radical prostatectomy had a 28 percent chance of dying of prostate cancer within seven years. This alarmed many men who had a rapidly rising PSA before surgery.[17] Our group tried to duplicate this research, but we found no such alarming results associated with a steep PSA rise. In fact, men whose PSA rose more than 2 in a year did no worse than those with a slower rate of increase. For both groups, the chances of dying of prostate cancer within seven years was only 3 percent, not 28 percent. A rapidly rising PSA may reflect a serious cancer, but more often, it is caused by normal variation in PSA levels.[18]

To get the most accurate picture, you should continue monitoring your PSA until you begin treatment. Wait three to six weeks after the biopsy to be sure the inflammation has resolved, and then have your PSA tested periodically. Every six weeks is a reasonable interval to track changes, determine the true baseline, observe whether the cancer is growing slowly or quickly, and judge how great a risk there is of local or distant spread.

SHOULD YOU HAVE FURTHER TESTS TO TELL IF THE CANCER HAS SPREAD?

A prime worry with any cancer is whether the disease has spread to distant sites (metastasized). Many patients seek further testing in a quest for reassurance. It seems logical, in this age of futuristic scanning and imaging techniques, that there should be a way to determine the precise extent of your disease and predict its course with absolute certainty.

Unfortunately, there is no such crystal ball for prostate cancer. Scans that work well for other organs are unreliable in looking at the prostate. Results can be uncertain or yield false positives. The net effect may be to multiply your concerns unnecessarily. Worse, unclear findings might lead you down a treacherous path of ever more invasive and riskier diagnostic procedures.

To resolve this problem, the National Comprehensive Cancer Network (NCCN) has developed guidelines that patients and physicians can follow in deciding whether such tests are warranted.[19] These experts state that bone scans are not necessary for men with stage T1 or T2 cancer, who have a PSA less than 10 and a Gleason score of 7 or below. Bone scans are recommended for men with stage T3 or T4 cancer, and for patients who have symptoms of advanced prostate cancer, such as bone pain. CT or MRI scans of the pelvis are seen as appropriate for all men with T3 or T4 cancer, and for patients whose clinical stage is T1 or T2 if an analysis of their test results suggests at least a 20 percent probability of lymph node involvement. To be absolutely safe, I'd advise that you have a CT scan or MRI to check your pelvic lymph nodes if a nomogram (see below) or Partin tables calculate that your risk of spread to the nodes is 5 percent or greater.

> NOTE: At Memorial Sloan-Kettering Cancer Center we've developed special mathematical models called **nomograms** to assess the risk that your disease would spread to lymph nodes.[20] Our entire suite of prostate nomograms is available at no charge. They're easy to use online at www.MSKCC.org (search the site for "prostate nomograms"). If you prefer, you can download them to your computer or you can work them out in paper form. Input a few simple test results and you can get a much better notion of how serious your cancer appears to be. (See page 208 for more on nomograms.)

BONE SCAN

Since PSA screening came into wide use in the late 1980s and we began to detect prostate cancer earlier and earlier, the value of a bone scan in most cases is highly questionable.

While it is common for advanced prostate cancer to spread to bones, it's very uncommon for cancer to register on a bone scan if the PSA is less than 20 and extremely rare with a PSA under 8.[21] Having a bone scan makes little sense unless you have a high-stage or very aggressive cancer. Otherwise, you'd run a serious risk of false positives. Many things, including arthritis and old injuries, can register as suspicious on bone scans. Making sure that such findings are benign requires further tests. While the bone scan itself is largely harmless and not invasive, follow-up studies to rule out metastases can be risky and more involved. Simple X-rays or even an MRI may not provide sufficient information. Even a bone biopsy, which can be difficult and painful, may not provide conclusive evidence of the presence or absence of cancer in the bone.

If your cancer puts you in the high-risk category for metastases

(Gleason 8–10, PSA over 20, and stage T3 or greater), the test may provide some useful information for treatment planning and gives a baseline for comparison with future studies, but if that doesn't describe your situation, a bone scan offers little of value and has considerable potential to cause unnecessary problems.

NOTE: Unless a patient has symptoms of bone pain, I would rarely recommend a bone scan, as long as the pretreatment nomogram predicts a 70 percent or greater chance that his cancer can be cured with radiation or surgery (for more on nomograms, see page 208 or www.MSKCC .org. Search for "prostate nomograms"). If a bone scan shows a "hot" area that might indicate a site of spread of the cancer, doctors will often order a plain X-ray of the bone. The purpose of the X-ray is not to confirm the presence of cancer, but to find an alternative explanation for the hot spot, such as an old fracture or an area of arthritis. A hot spot on bone scan combined with a normal X-ray strongly suggests cancer. Today, we have sophisticated diagnostic tests that are much more sensitive than plain X-rays. The best is a bone marrow MRI.[22]

CT SCAN

The CT scan is not very good at detecting metastases or the presence of cancer in bone. Lymph nodes can only be seen on the scan if they are enlarged. Microscopic deposits of cancer cells won't show up at all.

Because of this general lack of sensitivity, CT scans have little use in the evaluation of prostate cancer, except for patients with aggressive disease and a high suspicion of lymph node involvement (see note above).

Unless you are at high risk of having metastases, it's not worthwhile to have a CT scan to look for them.[23] The test is not totally harmless. It exposes you to radiation and to contrast agents, which, in rare cases, can cause serious allergic reactions or kidney damage. In general I find that a prostate MRI provides as good an evaluation of pelvic lymph nodes as does a CT scan, and gives us much more information about cancer within the prostate.

PELVIC LYMPH NODE DISSECTION FOR STAGING

If your cancer is going to be treated with radical prostatectomy, a **pelvic lymph node dissection** is normally included in the surgery for all but patients with low-risk cancers. Even when enlarged pelvic lymph nodes are found on pelvic CT or MRI, many doctors would proceed with surgery and remove the enlarged nodes, as long as they are in the normal operative field and are not so enlarged as to make complete removal problematic. Some men who are going to be treated with radiation ask whether it's reasonable to do an operation to remove and examine pelvic lymph nodes to determine the size and extent of the cancer. The answer is generally no, with few exceptions. The risks of such an operation are not trivial and scar tissue could make subsequent surgery to remove the prostate more difficult and complicated, should the cancer recur. If radiation is the chosen treatment, previous lymph node surgery could also increase the risk of bowel damage from radiation.

If enlarged lymph nodes are found on MRI or CT scan, the best way to evaluate them further is to have a needle placed in the lymph node under CT guidance by an interventional radiologist. The doctor can draw cells from the lymph node and send them for microscopic examination by a pathologist to determine if they are malignant. Another way to determine if enlarged lymph nodes are cancerous is to administer a three-month course of LHRH agonists, such as leuprolide or goserelin. If the nodes decrease in size back to normal, a reasonable presumption is that they were malignant.

NOTE: Prostate cancer can spread without affecting the lymph nodes, so a negative pelvic lymph biopsy does not rule out the presence of microscopic metastases elsewhere.

TIPS ON INTERPRETING YOUR TEST RESULTS

In medical practice it's common to invoke general rules. Call the doctor if your fever hits 101 degrees. Have a flu shot if you're over 55. Start screening for colon cancer at age 50.

In similar fashion, it's neat, simple, and convenient to divide men with prostate cancer into risk groups. Low-risk cancer is defined as a PSA under 10, a Gleason score of 6 or less, and a stage T1 or T2a tumor. Intermediate-risk cancers are those with a PSA between 10 and 20, Gleason 7, and tumor stage T2b. A PSA over 20, Gleason grade of 8 to 10, or stage T2C or higher places a man in the high-risk group.[24]

Unfortunately, risk grouping carries risks of its own. Dealing with low-risk tumors is fairly straightforward. Very tiny cancers, which we refer to as indolent, might never cause any problems, especially in older men. The same is true for small, localized tumors with favorable characteristics (Gleason 6, PSA < 10). Depending on a man's remaining life expectancy, it may be appropriate to monitor rather than treat the disease. If treatment is indicated, surgery or radiation would offer a high probability of cure. Seed implants, which are appropriate only for favorable cancers, might be a reasonable treatment choice as well.

For men in the intermediate- and high-risk groups, the situation is much murkier. Someone with a small focus of Gleason 3 + 4 = 7 cancer could be lumped as intermediate risk with patients who have extensive areas of pattern 4 + 3 = 7. Some patients whose numbers suggest high-risk cancer actually have a far more favorable prognosis when all of their diagnostic factors are considered.[25] Risk groups do not provide us with the tools we need to make sound treatment decisions for an individual patient. What's right for men with similar test results might be completely the wrong approach for you when all relevant factors are considered.

Nomograms:
The Key to Understanding Your Risk

Mathematical models that factor in all the relevant data are a much better way to gauge the current extent of your disease and what's likely to happen in the future. (See Chapter 12, Deciding How to Treat Localized Prostate Cancer.) The Partin tables are staging nomograms. They use a mathematical formula that combines your stage, grade, and PSA to compute how extensive your cancer would prove to be if the gland were removed and examined. At Memorial Sloan-Kettering Cancer Center we have refined these staging nomograms and added many others that predict the chances of successfully curing the cancer with each treatment: surgery, external beam therapy, or seed implants. You can find these online (visit www.MSKCC.org and search for "prostate nomograms").[26]

Beware of being brushed off as "incurable" if your cancer is deemed "high-risk." One of my patients with a clinical stage T2b, Gleason 8 cancer in 3 of 12 biopsy cores was told that such an aggressive tumor could not be cured with surgery, but his PSA was only 4, and there was no clinical indication that the cancer had spread beyond the gland. The presence of poorly differentiated cancer cells was troubling, and the Partin tables predicted that he had only a 39 percent chance of having an organ-confined cancer.[27] When we calculated his chance of being cured of cancer ten years after surgery using the pretreatment nomogram, his overall picture looked much brighter. I was pleased to tell him that his chance of being cured at ten years was 81 percent with surgery alone.[28]

When all the diagnostic information is considered and a nomogram is used to estimate the chances of treatment success, the outlook is often much brighter. With good modern surgery or radiation, many "high-risk" cancers stand an excellent chance of being cured.[29]

THE FUTURE

The critical issue in modern treatment of men with prostate cancer is to determine which cancers need to be treated with surgery or radiation therapy, which can be left alone and monitored in a watchful waiting program, and which need intensive combinations of systemic and local therapy. For men with advanced cancers, the central question is which targeted therapy is right for which patient.

We have long relied on Gleason grade to characterize prostate cancers. But Gleason grading has limitations. Two thirds of the prostate cancers we diagnose today are Gleason $3 + 3 = 6$ on biopsy. Even when the Gleason score, clinical stage, and PSA are incorporated into nomograms, our ability to predict the course of a cancer is limited. Understanding their genetic bases has led to breakthroughs in the treatment of lung cancer, breast cancer, and leukemia. As we begin to crack the genetic code of prostate cancer, I'm confident that we will develop similar tools to characterize this common malignancy more accurately.

IN SUMMARY

Prostate cancer is not a medical emergency. You can and should take time to size up your particular disease so you can make a sound choice about treatment. To get the most accurate picture of what you're up against, consider all the relevant diagnostic factors. Mathematical models called nomograms can help you evaluate the odds that you'll be cured with any given approach and whether you need treatment immediately or it is safe to wait.

11

■

Understanding Yourself

READ THIS CHAPTER TO LEARN:

- Which emotional responses are common in prostate cancer patients and their partners?
- What can you do to cope with this disease effectively?

Few pieces of news are harder to hear than a cancer diagnosis. It's perfectly normal to feel angry, overwhelmed, disbelieving, horrified, or scared. People commonly equate cancer with a death sentence. On learning they have prostate cancer, many patients presume that what they need to do is get their affairs in order and await the worst. Even men who understand intellectually that prostate cancer is typically slow-growing and never an imminent threat often fear for their immediate survival. One patient described his initial shock and panic with poignant clarity: "Normally, I'm an optimist, but when I found out I had prostate cancer, I couldn't shake this image of an awful, gruesome death. I kept picturing crazy things like my bladder exploding. All I wanted to do was get this thing out—fast!" Another man recounted a similar sense of impending doom: "I started imagining that I might die of a heart attack or an accident first. I almost wanted those things to happen, so I wouldn't have to deal with this."

NORMAL STRESS
OR SERIOUS DISTRESS?

Denial is a protective response to highly disturbing news. Until we are psychologically prepared to confront an overwhelming reality, our minds try to blunt the situation with soothing doubts. How could I possibly be sick when I feel so well? Couldn't the pathologist be mistaken? What if my results were mixed up with someone else's? I bet I'll wake up tomorrow and find out this was all a bad dream.

Such thoughts help you to cope in the short run, but persistent denial poses a serious roadblock to rational decision-making. Joe F., a 62-year-old commercial realtor, suffered from prolonged, paralyzing denial: "For almost a year, I honestly couldn't hear what the doctors were telling me. After every consultation, my wife would want to discuss whether I should choose surgery or radiation, and I'd argue that I didn't need treatment. I was fine. Nobody and nothing could get through to me. I was living in some sort of a bubble that protected me from what I couldn't face."

As denial yields to acceptance, men with prostate cancer must confront several disturbing unknowns. How serious is the tumor? What's the best way to treat it? What will it be like to go through surgery, radiation, or combination therapies? What's the chance that I'll have to deal with side effects like incontinence, impotence, or bowel problems? What, if anything, can be done about such things if they happen to me? How likely is my cancer to recur? What impact is all of this going to have on my life and my loved ones? "When I finally accepted that this was real, it was like opening Pandora's Box," Joe recalls. "I was so overwhelmed with the awful possibilities. I felt totally out of control."

This particular disease hits men right where they live. All approaches to treating prostate cancer, including watchful waiting, carry a risk of sexual dysfunction, urinary disturbances, and bowel problems. To some men this feels like a Hobson's choice—in other words, no real choice at all. Henry Ford famously declared that his 1914 Model T was available in any color, as long as it was black. As a prostate cancer patient, you can elect surgery, brachytherapy, external beam radiation, combination treatments, or watchful waiting, as long as you accept that all of these involve some risk of harm to normal bodily functions.

Venturing into such alien, uncertain territory is bound to provoke anxiety, but the level of apprehension is highly individual. Your feelings might range from a mild undercurrent of edginess to unbearable, screaming-neon alarm. Anxiety can announce itself with physical symptoms, such as rapid heartbeat, tightness in the chest, shortness of breath, dizziness, stomachache, or the need to urinate with unusual frequency. Psychologically, extreme worry can leave you irritable, angry, or distractible. In severe cases of panic, you might feel as if you're losing touch with reality, having an out-of-body experience, going crazy, or even about to die. "I couldn't sleep, couldn't focus, couldn't function," Joe says. "I can't remember ever being so utterly lost and overwhelmed."

When you have a serious disease, some measure of anxiety is normal and possibly useful. There is some evidence that the accompanying jolt of extra adrenaline might enhance your mental or physical performance. But crushing or paralyzing anxiety is quite another story. If you suffer from overpowering fear, dwell obsessively on your disease, or feel the need to cling to others compulsively for reassurance, the problem is out of control and you should seek help. (See Ways to Cope, page 217.)

The same is true of depression. While sadness about being ill or grief over a possible loss of function is perfectly normal, having a disease should not throw your entire existence into total eclipse. Signs that your blue mood has crossed the line into major depression include severe lethargy, apathy, sudden changes in appetite or sleep patterns, or a loss of interest in things you previously found pleasurable. You might find it difficult to think, concentrate, or go about your normal routines. Severe depression can lead to suicidal thoughts or a preoccupation with death. "I had trouble with anxiety *and* depression," one patient explained. "When I first got the diagnosis, I honestly thought I'd sail through this thing with no problems at all. Instead, everything seemed worse than I expected. The slightest thing would set me off. I'd sink into a tailspin or fly off in a rage."

The stress of deciding what to do about your cancer can leave you feeling hopelessly ambivalent or utterly confused. Often there's no obvious best treatment choice with this disease. Experts and others may offer conflicting opinions, increasing your unease. Many men, in a quest to learn all they can and make the best decision, wind up suffering from information overload. They read everything they can find on the Internet, consult with everyone they can think of who might have any knowledge of this disease, and, unfortunately, wind up more uncertain than they were at the outset.

In times of extreme stress, some patients resort to self-medication with drugs or alcohol or become more deeply dependent on substances they already abuse. Such chemical coping can interfere with the clear thinking required to make a sensible treatment choice, alter the effectiveness of anesthetics and other medications, and stand in the way of an optimal recovery. If this applies to you, I urge you to seek help so you can develop other, healthier coping strategies.

Many men find it difficult to discuss personal issues or admit to having emotional distress. Instead, they withdraw and let their feelings fester. If that describes your response to stressful situations, you might suffer a sense of isolation, and your close relationships may be placed under extra strain. "He keeps everything bottled up," one patient's wife said. "How can I help if he won't tell me what's going on?" Often, it's the partner who tells the physician that a patient is not coping well.

Men who are able to express what they're going through don't always get the desired response of support and understanding. Though we've come a long way, cancer still carries a degree of social stigma. Many people feel awkward around illness or are unclear about how to react. Such discomfort may be magnified when a patient expresses his own emotional problems in coping with the disease. At times, even the most well-intentioned comment can miss the mark and strike a raw sensitivity: "I love my sister, but she can drive me nuts," one patient told me. "In the car on the way to the hospital for my operation, she was still questioning why I wasn't getting seed implants. If seeds plus external radiation and hormones were good enough for Mayor Giuliani, why weren't they right for me? Though I was definitely not in the mood, I tried joking in the hopes that she'd give it up. I told her that particular combination therapy has only been proven effective on big-city politicians, but she just wouldn't stop. She had no idea how much I'd put into making this choice, how important it was for me to have my family's support."

Dr. Andrew Roth, a psychiatrist at Memorial Sloan-Kettering Cancer Center who specializes in treating patients with prostate cancer, says that many men he sees feel angry and betrayed. They've done everything right, watched their diet, exercised regularly, been religious about checking their PSA, and still their bodies had the audacity to develop this frightening disease.

Roth notes that for many men, the hardest part of having prostate cancer is a real or perceived loss of control. In dealing with the medical system, you may feel as if you're being forced to cede some of your power and autonomy to others. Specialists define what tests you should have and which therapeutic options are available to you. Those tests and treatments can involve embarrassing incursions into your intimate space. Prostate cancer therapies can also make unwelcome demands on your time, not to mention your physical, financial, and emotional resources. "To me, having this disease was a major kick in the pants," one man confessed. "At work, I was accustomed to taking charge, putting my finger on a problem and finding the right solution. Suddenly, this cancer was at the very center of my world. Everything seemed to revolve around it, and I was stuck on the outside, looking in."

NOTE: It's very important to be honest with your doctor about any and all drugs you're taking, including the amount of alcohol you're drinking and any "recreational" drugs you use.

WHY IS PROSTATE CANCER PARTICULARLY STRESSFUL?

Many cultures prize stoicism, strength, and independence as the masculine ideal. From early childhood, boys are urged to avoid appearing needy or vulnerable. Those ingrained imperatives can be powerful enough to keep some men from seeking medical care, including potentially lifesaving checkups and tests.

The same masculine mystique can throw men diagnosed with an illness into serious conflict. They fear that being sick will mark them as weak. This can be especially true with a disease like prostate cancer that poses a threat to sexual potency and urinary continence. It's not unusual for prostate cancer patients to expend a great deal of emotional capital on keeping their disease under wraps or agonizing over what might happen if they decided to disclose it. As one patient explained, "I couldn't stand the thought of people looking at me differently, feeling sorry for me. When I went for my radiation treatments, I'd put the newspaper over my face. I didn't want to see other patients or to have them see me."

Men often see prostate cancer as a direct assault on their virility. They worry about being able to perform sexually and satisfy their partner. They fear that they'll be diminished in the eyes of friends or colleagues. They are concerned about the effect this disease will have on their relationships, their earning capacity, their future plans. Men who are single or dating may feel particularly threatened by the potential loss of sexual function or fertility, and uncertain about whether, when, and how to discuss these issues with a potential new partner.

Prostate cancer often adds to the stress for older men, who are already burdened by ageist stereotypes and our society's obsession with eternal youth. The situation can seem even more intolerable if this is your first major run-in with illness. Living for many years without a serious disease can lull you into believing that you're going to dodge that bullet indefinitely. As one patient put it, "When the doctor said I had prostate cancer, I couldn't believe my ears. Suddenly, I felt like my own body—old faithful—was turning on me. It was as if all bets were off, and I couldn't count on anything anymore."

The average age at prostate cancer diagnosis is 68, a time when many men are grappling with major lifestyle changes such as retirement or the mounting independence of their grown children. Having this disease forces them to confront a possible reduction in sexual, urinary, and bowel functions as well. With advancing age, the risk of sexual and urinary side effects from prostate cancer treatments increases. Though it's commonly believed, even among some health professionals, that older men are unconcerned about sexual decline, in fact, for many men it continues to matter a great deal.

Race can also pose a particular challenge. African-American men, who have the highest prostate cancer incidence in the world, are far less likely than whites to undergo routine screening for this disease. For some of these men, cultural male values of strength and stoicism can be compounded by limited access to health care and inadequate awareness of their heightened vulnerability to this disease.

Sexual orientation may also increase the psychological burden. Many physicians lack awareness of the special sexual concerns of gay men with prostate cancer or feel uneasy addressing them. Some gay men find it difficult to be frank and open with their physicians as well. To make matters worse, prostate cancer resources, including support groups, websites, articles, and books are overwhelmingly geared toward men in heterosexual relationships. Understandably, homosexual patients and their partners can feel excluded or poorly served. As one man put it, "The doctors simply had no idea about how all of this applied to me as a gay man. Here I was, struggling with what to do, and I had to explain things to them."

Being in a loving, supportive relationship can lessen the distress, but if the bond with your significant other is already frayed or tenuous, having a disease can make matters worse. Some shaky marriages crack under the strain of prostate cancer diagnosis or treatment.

For many men with prostate cancer, PSA anxiety is the number one source of emotional anguish.[1] They worry obsessively about their blood-test results, even to the point of needing sleeping aids or anti-anxiety medications. The slightest elevation in PSA level sends some patients spiraling into serious depression, though the result might be nothing more than normal variation or a laboratory error. Even in cases where a rising PSA signals that local treatment has failed to cure the disease, salvage treatments are often effective, and therapies to control the cancer can keep most men active and symptom-free for many years, if not decades. Still, a morbid preoccupation with PSA can reduce a man's capacity to enjoy those years. "To me, waiting for PSA results is like hearing bullets flying overhead. You're constantly aware that the threat is out there, and you never know when you might get hit," one patient observed.

WAYS TO COPE

The National Comprehensive Cancer Network (NCCN) defines psychological distress as "an unpleasant experience of an emotional, psychological, social, or spiritual nature that interferes with the ability to cope with cancer treatment. It extends along a continuum, from common, normal feelings of vulnerability, sadness, and fears to problems that are disabling, such as true depression, anxiety, panic, and feeling isolated or in a spiritual crisis."[2]

If having prostate cancer has tossed you into serious emotional turmoil, you're far from alone. Experts estimate that 25 percent of all cancer patients experience distress severe enough to interfere with their treatment, heighten the focus on physical symptoms, or hamper their recovery, and men with prostate cancer are no exception. In fact, at some prostate cancer clinics, up to 31 percent of patients suffer sufficient psychological distress to warrant psychiatric evaluation. Anxiety accounts for the majority of these cases, with depression a close runner-up.

To manage the problem, the NCCN recommends that all cancer patients be screened to gauge their level of distress, followed by evaluation and treatment where appropriate. The call for universal screening acknowledges that doctors often believe that patients are faring better psychologically than they actually are. One study found that only 2 percent of cancer patients with serious psychological problems were referred for psychiatric evaluation. Other researchers found that oncologists missed signs of clinical depression in their patients more than half the time. Simple screening tests, readily available to medical personnel, such as the Hospital Anxiety and Depression Scale, the Distress Thermometer, or the Brief Symptom Inventory can signal that you might be in need of additional emotional support or the help of a mental health professional.

If screening suggests that you're having significant coping problems, you should have a thorough evaluation to pinpoint the reason. The issue may be highly specific, like anxiety over losing time from work or difficulty arranging transportation to radiation treatments. In some instances, you might find that appropriate help is available within the cancer-treatment setting. Still, many patients, even those who are not having serious psychological problems, benefit from counseling or other forms of emotional support. Certainly, if you're having serious symptoms, such as disorientation or suicidal thoughts, you should seek psychiatric help without delay.

Depending on your individual needs and preferences, treatment might take the form of individual psychotherapy, group therapy, participation in support groups, complementary strategies to reduce mild to moderate anxiety, such as meditation, exercise, or massage, and/or medications to control psychiatric symptoms. Getting the right help can make all the difference in how well you'll fare in dealing with this disease.

For Joe, joining a local support group made all the difference. "It was such a relief to meet other men who'd been through this. Looking at them, I realized it was possible to have treatment and come out okay. Finally, I was able to face this thing with a clear head."[3]

MAKING WISE DECISIONS
ABOUT TREATMENT

Try to identify and analyze emotional issues that may be driving your decision off the best possible course. Many men focus on one or two frightening things they've heard about treatment for prostate cancer. It may be impotence or incontinence or rectal bleeding or wound infection. Some patients are terrified of operations because someone close died unexpectedly after routine surgery, or they themselves had a difficult experience in the past. Others fear radiation because they heard a horror tale about a serious burn or saw something disturbing in a film.

There is an old dictum in psychiatry that the very thing you're most afraid to talk about may be the most crucial matter to discuss. This certainly holds true when deciding about prostate cancer treatment, where your biggest fear might be a nonissue in your case or represent only a small, relatively insignificant piece of the puzzle. Perhaps in your mind "incontinence" evokes the specter of adult diapers or having to wear a catheter and leg bag, while the physician is actually referring to a slim possibility that you'll have some temporary, minor leakage that may require the use of a couple of small pads a day. Serious lasting incontinence is rare after prostate cancer treatment, and even when problems persist, pelvic floor (Kegel) exercises or an artificial sphincter can typically restore urinary control. (See Chapter 17, Urinary Side Effects.)

While fear of erectile dysfunction is completely understandable, most men, given time, can enjoy a satisfying sex life following treatment. After nerve-sparing surgery, impotence is often transient. In many patients erections return after a few months, though others can take as long as three years to recover fully from the trauma radical prostatectomy inflicts on erectile nerves. Some men regain partial erections, which can be made fully functional with the aid of a pill like sildenafil (Viagra) or with penile injections or suppositories. Those who can't tolerate medications may achieve satisfactory erections using vacuum devices and penile rings that maintain rigidity. Where other methods fail, penile prostheses can restore function.

Unfortunately, some men reject such treatments, feeling that any erection that is not induced in the natural way is not okay with them. Worried about not being able to achieve satisfactory erections, they may avoid physical intimacy with their partners. This can place unnecessary strain on relationships.

"I realized that what I was terrified about, above all, was impotence," Joe said. "I thought having this cancer meant I'd never be able to have sex again. But then I talked to my doctor about what was likely to happen if I had my prostate removed. My tumor was small and nowhere near the erectile nerves, so they could almost certainly be spared. Since I was functioning well in that department before the operation, chances were I'd regain full or near normal function eventually. Regular arousal would help, and I certainly had no objection to that. Also, I found out that I'd have normal sensation in my penis and still be able to have orgasms, even though I wouldn't ejaculate. Suddenly, this didn't seem like such a major catastrophe after all."

Making a treatment choice for prostate cancer can resemble a game of chance. There is no crystal ball or absolute correct answer. You have to calculate probabilities, weigh risks against rewards, examine your risk tolerance, and, ultimately, go with your best instincts. However you decide to proceed involves some gamble. If you monitor the disease, you might miss the chance for a cure. If you treat it, you could suffer troubling side effects and require further treatment. You might choose surgery and afterward feel that radiation might have served you better, or vice versa. If you decide to start hormones early, you might later wish you'd waited. You might refuse systemic treatment and later wish you had not.

The fledgling field of **medical informatics** develops tools that are designed to optimize decision-making and minimize regret. Instead of flying by the seat of your pants, you can use these tools to gauge the risks and benefits of treatment choices and get a clearer idea of your personal preferences.

An interesting and potentially illuminating informatics exercise challenges you to consider how large a risk you'd be willing to take to cure your disease, delay its progression, or avoid a certain side effect. The standard gamble asks the following: Suppose there was a pill you could take tonight at bedtime that would make your prostate cancer disappear (or guarantee you would live an extra five years or that you would not be impotent), but there was a possibility that instead you would gently die in your sleep before morning.[4] Would you take that risk if your chance of death was 10 percent? How about 5 percent or 1 percent? Would you risk treatment if, instead of death, there was a chance you might go

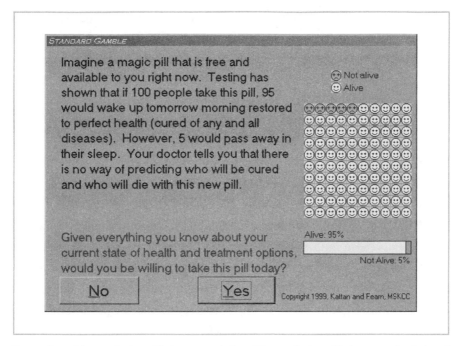

Screen shot of the standard gamble in computer form. The standard gamble is an exercise designed to help patients measure their tolerance for health-related risks.

blind? By assessing how much you're willing to wager in order to avoid or achieve a given outcome, you can calculate how heavily specific factors are affecting your thinking or contributing to your psychological distress.

CONSIDERING YOUR PARTNER

Though you're the one who's been diagnosed with prostate cancer, the illness affects your loved ones, too. This is especially true of your significant other. Partners share the same worries. Can this illness be cured? What if it can't? What will treatment entail? How will he/I/we deal with side effects? What impact will all this have on our physical and emotional relationship? Our lifestyle? Our future?

Your partner's emotional distress could be as acute as yours, or even more so. In some ways it's easier to be squarely in the spotlight than waiting anxiously in the wings. You'll receive the care and attention. Your needs are far more likely to be noted and addressed. In stark contrast, your partner may be challenged to assume unaccustomed roles and responsibilities while subverting his or her own emotional needs.

Many men are uncomfortable expressing what they feel. If that describes you, be aware that bottled-up emotions can manifest in unfortunate ways. It's human to take out your fears and frustrations on the people you most love and trust. Unfortunately, this only magnifies their distress, while doing precious little to alleviate yours.

Millions of patients and their partners have weathered prostate cancer together and emerged with their relationships intact, or even strengthened. Other partnerships have unraveled. Based on numerous personal accounts, the key to success seems to be approaching this problem as a team, recognizing that you're in this together and that by pulling together, you'll have a far smoother, easier course.

STRATEGIES TO HELP YOU AND YOUR PARTNER TO COPE

WORK TOGETHER

Both of you should learn as much as is necessary to make rational decisions about this disease. Seek expert input together. Ask all the questions that are relevant to both of you. Do a comfortable amount of research, while avoiding information overload. Make sure you both understand the nature and possible consequences of the disease. Be sure to discuss your options as well as the pros and cons of each available approach with your partner before you settle on a treatment plan. "Once I read a few books and spent some time searching the Internet, I felt so much more on top of this thing," observed one patient's wife. "Once I calmed down a bit, he did, too."

COMMUNICATE

Tell your partner what's on your mind and encourage the same in return. Discussing sensitive issues like erectile dysfunction or incontinence can go a long way toward defusing such concerns. Explore together what can be done about sexual, urinary, or bowel side effects if they should happen to you. Keep in mind that prostate cancer treatment need not mean the end to pleasure, intimacy, or an active sex life. "I was afraid that I wouldn't know how to help him, and he was afraid that I wouldn't want to. When we finally got all that out in the open, I felt as if we'd come out from under a dark, giant cloud," one partner recalls.

Unspoken worries can loom larger than the ones you look hard in the eye. It's useful to discuss fears about survival or—from the partner's perspective—being left alone. It's positive to explore worries about what impact this disease and its aftermath could have on your relationship. If your foundation feels shaky or you think you might benefit from outside support, this is an excellent time to seek professional help.

MAKE SURE YOU'RE ON THE SAME PAGE

Don't assume that you know what your partner wants or feels. One patient decided he was content with the size of his family and opted not to bank sperm before his radical prostatectomy. After the surgery, his wife admitted she regretted losing the possibility of having another child at some future time. "I should have told him how I felt, but I didn't want to make things even more difficult for him. Now it's too late," she says.

TAKE APPROPRIATE STEPS TO EASE THE SITUATION

Try not to take on too much. Get the rest and support you need. That goes for *both* you and partner. Don't be afraid to seek or accept help from friends, relatives, neighbors, colleagues, or professionals. Don't expect your partner to deftly take on responsibilities you may need to shelve for a time. If you normally pay the bills or cook dinner, maybe there's an alternative to asking your partner to take over if it feels too difficult. Watch for signs of serious anxiety or depression, and seek help if the situation seems out of control for either of you. Even if you're coping well, counseling or support groups may prove useful. There can be comfort in shared experience and in having a safe place to air difficult feelings.

REMEMBER, THIS IS TEMPORARY

Try to keep things in perspective. The trauma of diagnosis passes. The trials of decision-making continue for only a short while. The rigors of treatment are temporary, and most side effects resolve on their own or can be overcome effectively. Chances are excellent that you will soon be able to put this disease behind you and get on with your lives.

IN SUMMARY

Dealing with prostate cancer can take a serious psychological toll on you and your partner. Getting the help you need will enable you to cope wisely and effectively with this disease.

12

■

Deciding How to Treat Localized Prostate Cancer

READ THIS CHAPTER TO LEARN:

- Which treatments are available, and what are the risks and benefits of each one?
- What factors should you consider in evaluating your treatment options?
- Is the type or quality of the treatment you get more important?

The patient, I'll call him Steve F., expected no problems when he went for his annual physical last year. Steve was 62, feeling fine, and his physical exams, including his digital rectal exam (DRE), had always been perfectly normal. When the doctor called a few days later to report that his PSA had risen from its usual low level to over 5, Steve was stunned. Still, he felt confident this had to be a false alarm. A close friend had recently been through just such an episode, and the cause had turned out to be a minor inflammation.

A few weeks later, when a biopsy found a Gleason 7 cancer on both sides of Steve's prostate, he was, in his words, "totally at sea." He and his wife spent well over an hour in the urologist's office, discussing his medical options. They talked about radiation, hormones, radical prostatectomy, watchful waiting, and new forms of therapy available through clinical trials. But Steve had a hard time absorbing any of it.

The doctor explained the situation with the help of a brightly hued plastic model of the prostate. There it was—a small, irregular orb nestled deep in the pelvis amid a daunting tangle of erectile nerves, bladder, urinary sphincters, and bowel. In measured tones, he described Steve's prognosis. There was good news and worrisome news: Right now, the cancer appeared to be contained and curable, but if left alone it would eventually escape the prostate, spread to the hips and spine, and one day, prove lethal. Suddenly, this obscure organ that Steve had barely ever given a passing thought loomed inside him like a ticking time bomb.

What I desperately wanted was the right answer—immediately! But the doctor refused to say, "This is what you should do." He told me there was no single correct response. He said I'd have to consider the possibilities and make the choice myself. So I talked to men I knew who'd had prostate cancer, did research online, read dozens of articles, and asked a doctor friend to help me interpret the medical jargon. I got tons of well-intentioned advice. But the more I found out, the more confused I felt. It took me weeks to reach the conclusion that in my case, surgery to remove the gland made the most sense. The surgeon could check my lymph nodes to tell whether the cancer had spread. If there was no spread, I had an excellent chance for a cure. And if I wasn't cured, I might have a second chance with radiation. Once I got past the initial terror, I was able to process what I'd learned and figure out the right way to go for me.

When it comes to prostate cancer, there is no magic bullet or sole acceptable response. To arrive at the action plan that's best for you, you have to balance the seriousness of your disease against the potential risks and benefits of available treatments.

For each man, the calculation is different. Prostate cancers vary enormously, as do the men who have the disease. Only you can decide what chances you're willing to take and which potential outcomes would have the greatest impact on your quality of life. Ultimately, the best measure of treatment success may be what is known as risk-adjusted quality of life. How long you live is important, but perhaps not as important as how long you live happily and well.[1]

Prostate cancer gives you the opportunity to make a deliberate, considered choice. In the overwhelming majority of cases, the disease is very slow-growing and is never a medical emergency. If you have a heart attack, medical personnel are trained to stabilize the situation quickly and then do what seems necessary to prevent or minimize damage. Some cancers grow with wildfire rapidity, and immediate intervention is essential. With prostate cancer, however, you have ample time to assess the situation, evaluate your particular needs and resources, and devise the most sensible, strategic plan of action.

When you're first diagnosed with a cancer, it's perfectly normal to be frightened and want to get rid of the tumor quickly, no matter the cost. But given the nature of this disease, you'll likely live with the consequences of your treatment decision for a long time. Taking some time to step back and think things through carefully is the best way to ensure that you will not be plagued by sorrowful regrets down the road.

You may be wondering why a doctor, the supposed expert in all this, can't simply make the decision for you. Some men view it as frustrating and immensely unfair to be burdened with such a difficult choice, especially at a time when they're feeling vulnerable, beleaguered, and scared. Unfortunately, medical science has no way to assess your very specific needs in all their striking complexity. Doctors can and should help you to understand the nuances of your medical situation, but only you can ultimately decide what trade-offs you can tolerate, what level of risk you find acceptable, and which potential sacrifices you're willing to make.

KEY FACTORS TO CONSIDER

How serious is the cancer? This is a prime consideration. A high-risk, poorly differentiated tumor calls for faster, more aggressive intervention than does a small, moderately differentiated, or low-risk cancer. Scientists in a major Swedish trial found that radical prostatectomy provided a clear advantage over watchful waiting in preventing metastatic spread, especially in men with localized tumors that were intermediate- or high-grade.[2] Studies have also determined that **brachytherapy (seed implantation), when used alone**, is less effective than surgery, external beam radiation, or a combination of seed implants and external beam radiation for intermediate or high-risk prostate cancers (Gleason score 7 through 10 in men with a PSA greater than 10).[3]

The risk posed by the cancer must be balanced against your **life expectancy**, which depends upon your age and state of health.[4] The shorter the time a patient has left to live, the less chance a tumor has to grow, spread, and cause harm. We rarely recommend a biopsy, much less treatment, for any man whose life expectancy is less than five years. Even a man who can be expected to live for a decade or more might reasonably elect to monitor, rather than treat, this disease, depending on how serious the cancer appears to be.

Calculating how this applies to you can be tricky. For one thing, no one likes to look his own mortality in the eye. Most people presume that they are going to live a long time, regardless of what the life expectancy tables suggest.

Such optimism is not necessarily unfounded. Expectations and outcomes are frequently at odds. Life expectancy tables are nothing more than statistical assessments of probability. They neither guarantee you a minimum number of years nor set a limit on your remaining lifetime. Many factors affect the estimate, including your general health, lifestyle, and family longevity, as well as a number of imponderables, including that most unscientific but undeniably key issue: luck. Still, in consultation with your doctor, you should be able to make a reasonable assessment of whether active treatment in your particular case makes sense.

A key consideration is whether you have serious health issues other than prostate cancer, medically known as **comorbidities**. Depending on their severity, chronic problems with obesity, hypertension, and diabetes or problems with your heart, kidneys, liver, or other major organs can reduce your life expectancy by 20 percent or more. To gauge what this means in your case, your doctor can measure the current state of your health against a standardized comorbidity scale, such as the Charlson Comorbidity Index, the Cumulative Illness Rating Scale, or the Index of Coexisting Disease.[5]

The importance of having active treatment would be considerably different for a 70-year-old with serious medical conditions than for a healthy man of 50. Given a normal life span, the latter might be exposed to the risk of the cancer spreading over several decades. It seems a Faustian bargain to bet that you will die of something else before this disease causes severe problems. Whether putting off treatment is a smart bet or a sucker's gamble is a crucial piece of the decision you have to make.

Based on life expectancy tables and his excellent general health, Bill R. realized that he was likely to live for another twenty years or more. "My prostate cancer was a Gleason 7 with a PSA of 5.2, and two biopsy cores positive. I decided to have surgery that could get rid of this thing for good. I certainly didn't want this disease hanging over my head for decades."

Once you've calculated the risk your disease poses, given your life expectancy, another important element to consider is: **How likely is your cancer to metastasize and eventually lead to your death without treatment?** If evidence points to a high probability that you would eventually suffer the bone pain and other symptoms of metastatic prostate cancer, treating the disease would make far more sense than watchful waiting.

If active treatment seems appropriate in your case, your next calculation should be to consider: **What is the likelihood that each available treatment would cure your cancer?** If your tumor extends beyond the prostate in a way that can be included in the radiation field, external beam therapy may offer you the best odds. On the other hand, a bulky tumor may be difficult to eliminate with radiation even if the cancer has not invaded beyond the tissues immediately surrounding the prostate, and surgery might be preferable.

All medical treatments involve a mixed bag of positive effects and side effects. Before you settle on a course of action, it's wise to consider both the potential benefits in terms of curing or controlling the cancer and the risks of long-term damage to urinary, sexual, and bowel function.

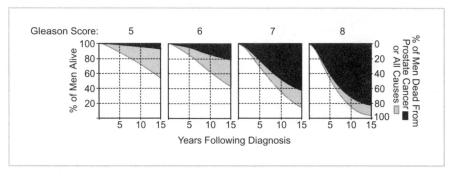

The lifetime risk of dying of prostate cancer versus some other cause, for a man age 60 to 64, the Gleason score at the time of diagnosis, for men on a watchful waiting program.*

NOTE: In about a third of cases, the seriousness of prostate cancers is underestimated on biopsy. A tumor that appears to be a low-risk Gleason 6 or less turns out to be less favorable when a pathologist examines the prostate after it has been removed to treat the disease. Remember that a biopsy only samples a tiny amount of tissue. Prostate cancer tends to be multifocal, meaning it arises in several parts of the gland at once. Areas of aggressive, poorly differentiated cancer can be missed by a biopsy. That's why I strongly recommend a repeat biopsy, oftentimes after an MRI of the prostate, for a man considering watchful waiting for what appears to be a low-risk cancer on the first biopsy.[6]

---

*Source: Modified from P. C. Albertsen et al. "Competing Risk Analysis of Men Aged 55 to 74 Years at Diagnosis Managed Conservatively for Clinically Localized Prostate Cancer." *JAMA* 280, no. 11 (1998): 975–980. © 1998 American Medical Association.

AGE (YEARS)	ALL MEN AND WOMEN	WHITE MEN	BLACK MEN
40	38.9	37.1	32.3
45	34.4	32.6	28.1
50	30.0	28.2	24.2
55	25.7	24.0	20.7
60	21.6	20.0	17.5
65	17.9	16.3	14.5
70	14.4	13.0	11.7
75	11.3	10.1	9.4
80	8.6	7.6	7.3
85	6.3	5.5	5.7

LIFE EXPECTANCY FOR MEN AGED 40 TO 85 YEARS (AVERAGE YEARS REMAINING)*

GENERAL GUIDELINES

Surgery to remove the prostate appears to confer a survival advantage in the long term (twenty, fifteen, or even as early as ten years after diagnosis), partly because recurrences can be detected very early and treated effectively with low-dose irradiation.[7] For this reason, radical prostatectomy is typically the preferred treatment choice for a young, healthy man in his 40s or 50s. Brachytherapy (seed implants) is probably the least disruptive treatment in the short term and is most appropriate for men with a small prostate that are having no trouble with urination and have a low-risk cancer. Men over 70 are generally better served by radiation, though surgery may be a reasonable option for the occasional vigorous, healthy, older man with an aggressive cancer, who wants the tumor removed and accepts the increased risk of side effects that accompanies his age. For still older men in their late 70s or 80s, most doctors would advise watchful waiting or, if the cancer is causing problems, hormone

*Source: Adapted from E. Arias, United States Life Tables, 2000. National Center for Health Statistics. National Vital Statistics Report, vol. 51, no. 3 (2002).

therapy, though some healthy older men are reasonable candidates for external beam radiation or seed implants.

These general rules of thumb leave many men in a perplexing gray area. In the final analysis, some patients base their treatment choice on decidedly nonmedical issues, such as the amount of time they might lose from work or convenient access to a good radiation facility. Understandably, some men are mired in paralyzing confusion, unable to make a choice at all.[8]

WHICH EXPERTS SHOULD YOU CONSULT?

One good way to resolve the treatment question is to seek opinions from doctors in different medical specialties. If the urologist who performed your biopsy and diagnosed your cancer recommended surgery, you may want to consult a medical oncologist or a radiation therapist, or even your primary care physician for another perspective (though keep in mind that not all doctors will have up-to-date, comprehensive knowledge of this complex disease). Most physicians are more than willing to help patients on a fact-finding mission. A doctor who is reluctant to cooperate with you as you seek further information is probably *not* someone you'd want to entrust with your care.

HOW SHOULD YOU EVALUATE EXPERT OPINIONS?

Consider the advice you get in light of its source. Despite the best intentions, doctors tend to be biased in favor of what they do. As one patient advocate aptly observed, if you visit a Cadillac dealer, don't expect him to send you across the street to buy a Lincoln. In general, radiation therapists steer patients toward external beam therapy or seed implants, and surgeons advocate radical prostatectomy. Doctors who stake their professional futures and reputations on controversial treatments, such as cryotherapy or stringent diets, would be hard-pressed to recommend anything else.

Physicians are not immune from pressures that can cloud the purity of their advice. I'd be cautious about getting a second opinion from another doctor in the same office, who might be reluctant to contradict a colleague or close friend. Keep in mind that doctors in the same community may have social relationships or rely on one another for referrals. You might want to ask your doctor to disclose any financial relationship he has that might bias what he suggests. For example, does he own an interest in the brachytherapy center where you would have seed implants or in the high-intensity ultrasound (HIFU) company he recommends?

To get the most complete and balanced input, it's best to consult with unrelated specialists and challenge them to compare the advantages and disadvantages of available treatments in *your* case. Knowing that a given therapy leads to erectile dysfunction 30 percent of the time is not nearly as useful as finding out how that statistic is likely to apply to you. Your particular risk of losing erections may be dramatically higher or lower than average depending on your age, your level of sexual function before treatment, your anatomy, and the location and seriousness of your cancer.

Be sure to ask how likely each treatment is to eradicate your tumor, and seek a comparison of long-term results. For a typically slow-growing disease like prostate cancer, what happens in the short-term can be highly misleading. Virtually no one dies from this disease in the first five years after diagnosis. If we compared the death rate at five years for men who had surgery with that of those who ate spaghetti three times a week, pasta-eating would appear to be an equally effective treatment strategy.

Insist on scientific backup for claims that sound improbably optimistic or simply too good to be true. Ask about the risks of immediate complications and long-term side effects that each option carries and what remedies are available for these problems, should they happen to you. I'd be wary of a specialist who offers you only one treatment choice and brushes off all the others. Such dogma ignores the enormous variability of this disease and the men who have it. Rarely is there only one rational way to go.

> NOTE: Be careful about information you find on the Internet, where there is no control over what is posted and where many self-proclaimed "experts" are free to tout themselves, their practices, and their "miracle cures." You can find good information about studies, medical facilities, and other resources online, but healthy skepticism is in order. It's best to start with the most reliable sites (see the Resources section at the back of this book) such as the National Cancer Institute (www. nci. nih.gov), the American Cancer Society (www.cancer.org), the National Comprehensive Cancer Network (www.nccn.org), and the major NCI-designated cancer centers, such as Memorial Sloan-Kettering Cancer Center, the University of Texas MD Anderson Cancer Center, and UCLA's Jonsson Comprehensive Cancer Center.

GETTING THE BEST ADVICE

QUESTIONS TO ASK, THINGS TO SAY, SAFEGUARDS

The answers you get can vary enormously, depending on the questions you pose. To elicit a doctor's most deeply felt conviction, try asking, "What would you do in my situation?" or "What would you recommend to your brother or son?" Also, remember that a doctor's opinion is just that: an opinion. Often, it's based on his judgment, not on proven medical facts.

LET THE DOCTOR KNOW WHAT'S ON YOUR MIND

It's important to be honest with your doctors and make them aware of central factors in your decision-making. If fear of incontinence or impotence is driving your treatment choice, say so and challenge the doctor to put your mind at ease. If you have particular concerns about anesthesia, make sure you understand what kind the doctor prefers, the reasons for that preference, and what the alternatives might be in your case.

If a doctor fails to mention an issue that concerns you, don't hesitate to bring it up yourself. Physicians tend to focus on the questions they view as most medically significant, while patients understandably worry much more about possible effects of medical treatments on relationships, lifestyle, and career. Open dialogue is the best way to clear up troubling questions and get all the information you need.

THE X FACTOR

Some element of your response to a doctor and the advice he gives may have nothing to do with credentials, approaches, or results. A certain amount of gut instinct tends to factor into the mix. You may like the way a particular specialist smiles or answers questions or how much time she spends with you. Good chemistry is certainly a plus, but significant differences in medical expertise and experience should always take precedence over whether you happen to like a doctor or even know and trust her as a friend.

This is not to suggest that you should write off your instincts. Why would you put your trust in a doctor who is too arrogant, defensive, or dismissive to answer reasonable questions? The primary focus should be on you and your disease. You should feel that she's willing to put your best interests first and not be guided by issues of her own.

SECOND OPINIONS AND EXTRA EARS

A second opinion is always a good idea. If another doctor confirms what you've already heard, that's great. If the consultations are at odds, you'll want to ask more questions or seek someone in another specialty that can help you sort things out.

It's a good idea to bring your partner along when you meet with specialists. Prostate cancer affects you both, and so will the outcome and effects of treatment. Collaborating in the information-gathering and decision-making process is important. If you don't have a significant other, ask a trusted friend or relative to back you up. Negotiating the medical maze can be frightening and stressful, and a second pair of ears will help you to keep advice and information straight. You may also want to take notes or bring a tape recorder, so you can review the conversation and confirm that your impressions of what was said are correct.

DECISION-MAKING TOOLS

Medical recommendations boil down to simple predictions. When a doctor sets your fractured arm in a cast, she's predicting that that's the best way to promote healing and avoid long-term damage to the limb. When a physician advises increased exercise or a cholesterol-lowering drug, the guess is that these changes will reduce your risk of heart disease. Such estimates are based on current scientific understanding in the field. Emerging studies lead to constant shifts in our thinking and practice.

While a doctor may appear to pluck recommendations from thin air, in fact, deciding what to do in any given case for any given patient actually involves a multi-branched and often knotty decision tree (not to mention the occasional foray onto a shaky limb). The human organism and human diseases are extraordinarily complex, and many issues must be factored into a medical calculation. How old is the patient? What are his central values and concerns? What other medical conditions does he have? How aggressive is this particular cancer? How likely is it to spread over time, if left untreated? How successful is each available treatment likely to be in arresting this disease? What are the side effects of each, how long might the problems last, and how easily can they be corrected?

USING NOMOGRAMS

More accurate predictions naturally lead to better decision-making. But increasing accuracy is no simple feat. As Yogi Berra once famously opined, "It's hard to make predictions, especially about the future."

Nomograms are mathematical tools designed to predict medical outcomes. (See Chapter 10, Understanding Your Cancer.)[9] These graphic models can gauge your odds of disease progression or cure, depending on the treatment course you choose. One man electing to undergo radical prostatectomy might lower his ten-year risk of metastatic spread by 20 percent, while another patient could have a 25 percent better shot at a cure with hormones and radiation. Prostate treatment nomograms can help you to answer crucial questions.[10] If your tumor is confined to the prostate and you choose watchful waiting, what is the risk that the cancer would spread in the next ten years? What are the chances that you have extracapsular extension (ECE) or seminal vesicle invasion (SVI)? How great a threat is there of spread to the lymph nodes? How likely would your PSA be to rise within five years after radiation therapy, indicating that the cancer was not cured? If you choose radical prostatectomy, what are the odds that you'd have a recurrence within ten years?

By combining all your relevant diagnostic features and weighting them appropriately, nomograms offer more solid predictions than we could make by looking at specific factors like your PSA, clinical stage, general health, age, family history, or tumor grade alone.[11] Nomograms also help us to avoid undue reliance on broad generalizations or such vague and often misleading categories as "risk groups." You want to know what's likely to happen to you, not what generally happens to someone who—like you—has an intermediate- or high-risk cancer. Nuances of your diagnostic profile can make a tremendous difference in your prognosis. A man with a negative DRE, a small focus of cancer, and a PSA of 4 would have a far more favorable outlook than someone with a large, palpable nodule, extensive cancer on both sides of the gland, and a PSA of 12, even though both of these patients have been assigned a "high-risk" Gleason score of 8.

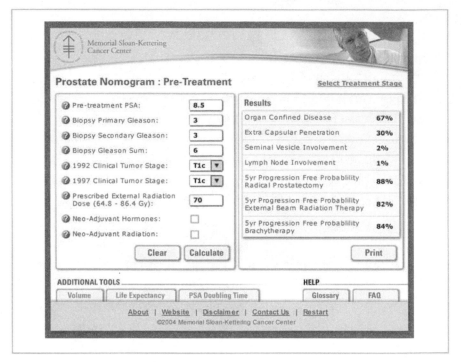

Screen shot from the Memorial Sloan-Kettering Cancer Center nomogram website showing predicted pathological stage and prognosis for each treatment alternative. Note that five-year progression-free probability percentages are approximate and vary by plus or minus 10 percent.

These nomograms can be used in paper form and can also be accessed online or downloaded to your computer. You can find them at www .MSKCC.org (search the site for "prostate nomograms").

THE BOTTOM LINE

Nomograms are not intended to make a decision for you, and they are not infallible. The findings were based on limited numbers of centers and doctors, and validated on large, but not universally representative, groups of patients. Any particular prediction has a built-in error rate, usually plus or minus 8 percent, so differences of less than 10 percent between treatments may be meaningless. Still, these tools can be useful in the process of choosing between competing alternatives. If external beam therapy offers you a 20 percent long-term survival advantage over seed implants, you might well choose the former.

PROSTATE CANCER CLINICAL TRIALS

For some diseases, such as breast cancer, doctors can base their treatment recommendations on extensive clinical trials. This is not true for prostate cancer. We have had no good long-term studies to determine whether or not treatment can be safely delayed (with active surveillance) until we see signs that the cancer is becoming more aggressive. Only one randomized trial (the Swedish study) compared active treatment with watchful waiting.[12] This groundbreaking investigation found that men lived longer after surgery and had much less risk of developing metastases than men placed on watchful waiting. But in Sweden, PSA screening for prostate cancer is uncommon. The men in this study presented with symptoms of advanced disease, such as bone pain or urinary problems, so the results might not apply to patients in the U.S. who are typically diagnosed early in the course of the disease. No studies have successfully compared surgery with any form of radiotherapy. Within the field of radiation therapy, randomized trials have shown conclusively that serious prostate cancers are much more likely to be cured with a high dose of radiation than a low dose. Studies have also shown that men with very serious cancers live longer when they are treated with a combination of radiation and hormones than with radiation alone.

Two important trials are under way. The SMART trial is just getting started, but for the PROTECT (a British screening) study, all the patients have been accrued. These studies are designed to help us learn whether active treatment with radiation therapy or surgery provides a survival advantage when compared with active surveillance (i.e. deferring treatment in an early, low-risk cancer until the tumor shows signs of progression). In the next few years, we also should have the results of the ongoing PIVOT trial, which seeks to compare radical prostatectomy with active surveillance.[13]

Whatever the results prove to be, we are unlikely to find a one-size-fits-all treatment for localized prostate cancer. Despite small differences in risks and benefits, any of the existing forms of treatment, including active surveillance, can be a reasonable alternative for most men diagnosed with prostate cancer in the United States today. A major goal of modern cancer research is to learn how to better characterize every case of prostate cancer, so we can determine the treatment course that will offer each individual the best chance of a cure with the fewest side effects.

HOW TO COMPARE THE TREATMENT OPTIONS

Watchful Waiting (Active Surveillance)

Traditional watchful waiting meant that a patient diagnosed with prostate cancer was told to go home and ignore the disease until he had symptoms of metastatic spread. This is no longer practiced. A more appropriate term for the approach we take today is active surveillance, a much underutilized but quite reasonable way to handle a low-risk cancer. If the cancer you have poses little risk now, it can be reasonable to defer treatment until we find evidence that the cancer is growing and becoming more serious. This treatment option involves no disruption in your normal activities and causes no immediate side effects. By opting for this, patients (especially older men who are in poor health) can avoid the complications of treatment for a disease that is unlikely to cause any problems in the near future and that can still be cured later, if necessary.

Is it for you? Active surveillance is appropriate for men with a life expectancy of less than five to ten years who have no symptoms from their tumor. It is also appropriate for men with a very low-risk prostate cancer, recognizing that most people die with, not of, this disease. The major risk is that the seriousness of the cancer has been underestimated. I always go the extra mile to rule out more serious cancer with a repeat biopsy or MRI before placing a man on active surveillance.

The downside is the very low risk that the tumor may spread while you're monitoring it. Vigilance cannot guarantee that we won't miss the window of opportunity for a cure. (See Chapter 13, Watchful Waiting [Active Surveillance], for a full discussion.) We have no established tests that signal when is the right time to switch to active treatment, so a certain amount of guesswork is involved. Also, living with a cancer, no matter how low a risk it seems to pose, provokes troublesome anxiety. Though older men with low-risk disease may be better served by a wait-and-see approach, anxiety often drives them to seek active treatment. Keep in mind that any treatment involves a risk of side effects. Also, once you have a cancer diagnosis, regardless of how it is treated, you will always have the worry about whether it will progress or recur.

BRACHYTHERAPY (SEEDS, SEED IMPLANTS)

Logistically, this is the simplest of local treatment options. After a single treatment-planning session, radioactive seeds are implanted into the prostate under anesthesia in an outpatient surgical facility. Recovery is rapid, and men soon return to normal activities.

Is it for you? Brachytherapy is most appropriate for a very narrow spectrum of cases. Seed implants are not recommended for someone with a large prostate (over 50 grams) or a man with **obstructive voiding symptoms** such as hesitancy, intermittent stream, dribbling, decreased urinary flow rate, and straining to urinate. All of these indicate that the urinary channel is partially blocked, and swelling from the needles used to implant the radioactive seeds could shut down the flow altogether. Acute urinary retention requires emergency catheterization and sometimes surgery is necessary to relieve the blockage.

A prior TURP (transurethral resection of the prostate) to alleviate the symptoms of benign prostate enlargement leaves you with inadequate tissue for proper seed placement and increases the risk of incontinence after brachytherapy. If your prostate lies behind a high pubic bone, proper seed placement may be far more difficult or even impossible. Pretreatment tests can determine this and other significant aspects of your anatomy and disease.

Because they offer the least powerful form of cancer therapy, permanent iodine or palladium seed implants are best for men with the most favorable, least risky tumors (a PSA level less than 10 and a Gleason score of 6 or less, stage T2a or lower). In these patients, the track record for long-term cancer control is comparable to modern external beam radiation or radical prostatectomy.

Seed implants, however, are technically challenging. The chances of controlling the cancer and avoiding side effects are directly related to the quality (uniformity, spacing, and dosage delivered) of the implant. While serious short-term side effects are minimal, seed implants can cause a variety of vexing problems in the long term. Brachytherapy results in about the same risk of erectile dysfunction (ED) and bowel problems as external beam radiation, but more urinary side effects, especially acute urinary retention and painful, frequent urination. Seed implants cause less immediate ED than surgery, though the risk of ED worsens over time with seeds as radiation damage accumulates.

Following brachytherapy, the PSA does not go to zero, and in about 1 in 7 patients there is a temporary, meaningless rise in PSA level, called a **PSA bounce**, which makes it difficult to diagnose recurrences promptly. By the time we are able to confirm that the cancer has started to grow again, the chance to cure the disease with salvage surgery—which has a high complication rate—might be lost.

> NOTE: If brachytherapy does not work, we're left with a difficult problem. Cancers that remain or recur are difficult to cure and side effects are difficult to treat.

External Beam Therapy

With radiation, the key to success is the dose. Curing all but the smallest, most favorable prostate cancers requires high-dose radiation. Delivering an adequate dose safely and without damage to surrounding tissue requires great precision. This can be achieved only with intensity-modulated radiation therapy (IMRT) or comparable highly sophisticated technology (See Chapter 15, Radiation Therapy.) Standard therapy, giving low-dose radiation with a conventional linear accelerator, is far less successful at curing the disease and increases the probability that you'll develop serious urinary, sexual, and/or bowel problems. I don't recommend that you go this route. If you opt for external beam therapy, choose a center that can deliver high-dose radiation (at least 75.6 Gray) using IMRT or a comparable approach. (See Chapter 15, Radiation Therapy.) The limiting factor with radiation is the ability to completely destroy the cancer, which is related to the size of the cancer or the number of cancer cells. Even at very high dose (81 Gray), about a quarter of patients have a biopsy positive for persistent cancer three years later.

After any form of radiation, patients may feel insecure about whether or not the cancer has been eradicated, since the prostate remains in place. The PSA goes down but rarely becomes undetectable. There is often a PSA bounce, a meaningless, transient rise in PSA, which can cause extreme anxiety or a critical delay in detecting a recurrence. (See Chapter 15, Radiation Therapy, for a full discussion.)

Is it for you? External beam radiation is a reasonable treatment for almost any prostate cancer, but it may be overkill for men with a very low-risk tumor who should consider active surveillance, since radiation does carry a risk of serious long-term side effects. For very serious cancers (T3 or greater, Gleason 8–10, PSA over 10) even high-dose radiation may not be enough, and it is often combined with androgen deprivation therapy. Hormone therapy can increase the cure rate, but it increases side effects as well.

Since this treatment involves about nine weeks of daily weekday therapy, the logistics can be difficult. If you don't live near a center that offers intensity-modulated radiation therapy, you might have to relocate for the duration or deal with a cumbersome daily commute to get the care that offers the best outcome with the lowest risk of side effects. On the other hand, if you have easy access to good modern radiation, the procedure involves little disruption to your normal schedule. Also, unlike surgery and seed implants, external beam radiation does not require anesthesia.

Though modern treatment has reduced the risks of serious side effects, any external beam treatment still carries some risk of bowel injury, urinary problems, and erectile dysfunction, all of which tend to worsen over time as the effects of radiation damage accumulate. Because the urethra cannot be totally eliminated from the radiation field, men with obstructive voiding symptoms are at some risk for acute urinary retention. (See the description of brachytherapy on page 241.)

If your prostate is larger than 60 grams, the radiation beam may affect more of the rectal wall, which lies immediately behind the prostate. Hormone therapy may sometimes be used to shrink the prostate, making it possible to give external beam radiation to men with large prostate glands.

Since the rectal wall lies perilously close to the prostate, patients with colitis or inflammatory bowel disease are usually not good candidates for radiation treatment. Prior radiation to the area for any reason probably means you've had your lifetime limit and further radiation would risk serious complications.

Recent studies confirm an increased risk of cancers of the rectum, bladder, and other structures adjacent to the prostate in men treated with external beam radiation compared with those treated with surgery. These cancers can be serious, or even lethal.

> NOTE: A temporary **high dose rate (HDR) implant** is sometimes recommended for men with aggressive, high-risk disease. This is a far more effective, aggressive therapy and should not be confused with permanent, low-dose iodine or palladium implants. (See Chapter 15, Radiation Therapy, for a full discussion.)

RADICAL PROSTATECTOMY

Radical prostatectomy involves the complete removal of the prostate and seminal vesicles, usually in conjunction with the pelvic lymph nodes. The procedure can be performed with an open, laparoscopic, or robotically assisted laparoscopic approach. Since surgery carries obvious side effects, I would caution against it for men with very low-risk cancers. Surgery is especially appropriate for large or high-grade cancers, regardless of the size of the prostate. With surgery, the PSA should drop to zero, so recurrences can be detected early. Many men not cured with surgery alone can still be cured with radiation therapy. Of course, surgery requires hospitalization and anesthesia, and patients lose some time from work, since full recovery can take 3 to 6 weeks. Though surgery may be the most difficult treatment in the short run, it offers excellent cancer control in the long term. For a young, healthy man, this is an important consideration.

While incontinence and erectile dysfunction are common right after surgery, only 1 to 2 percent of men operated on by top specialists still have serious, troublesome urinary control problems a year after the procedure (this can be as high as 6 to 8 percent for an average surgeon). The average time before regaining partial erections is four months, and a return to full function generally takes a year or two, though recovery can continue for three years or even longer. For men who do not recover erections sufficient for intercourse, even with oral medications like sildenafil (Viagra), several other therapies, including injections, suppositories, and penile implants, are available.

Is it for you? Radical prostatectomy is major surgery, whether performed by the open, laparoscopic, or robotically assisted method, and all of these approaches carry comparable risks. If you have serious medical conditions aside from prostate cancer or have had serious adverse reactions to anesthesia in the past, you may not be a good surgical candidate. Radical prostatectomy is a particularly good choice for a healthy young man with an aggressive, life-threatening cancer. (See Chapter 14, Surgery, for a full discussion.)

Many believe that robotic radical prostatectomy is a simple, easy, painless way to get rid of the cancer forever. In fact, head-to-head comparisons of open and robotic surgery have proven otherwise. Despite the magnificent technology, the 3-D visualization and the remarkable finesse of the instruments, the long- and short-term results with the robotic approach have been similar to or worse than the open procedure. Don't be fooled by clever marketing.

HOW TO MAKE THE CHOICE

You are not simply a pile of reports or a collection of diagnostic numbers, and your situation, in all its complexity, is unique. Try to ignore both the grisly horror tales and the stellar success stories you're bound to hear. Avoid being seduced by what a celebrity does or what worked, or didn't work, for a friend or relative. Don't succumb to a compelling sales pitch or strong-arm tactics. Your best choice will be based on your particular medical situation, preferences, and concerns.[14]

NOTE: The quality of treatment may be more critical than which treatment you choose. The success of all prostate cancer therapies hinges on the expertise of the person delivering them, and on the quality of the technology and facilities available to that expert. If you can gain access to equally excellent surgeons and radiation programs, you should opt for the treatment that offers you the best chance for a long-term cure with lowest risk of side effects. On the other hand, if you can get excellent brachytherapy but only mediocre surgery or external beam radiation, seed implants may well be your best option. Bad surgery may be worse than good radiation, even though good surgery might be better than good radiation for your particular tumor, or vice versa.

For cancer care in general, expertise can make an enormous difference in the outcome. More experienced hospitals and more experienced surgeons and radiation oncologists have fewer complications and better cure rates. *Always strive to put yourself in the best possible hands!*

NOTE: You want to be cared for by a busy, experienced doctor, but high volume alone does not guarantee optimal treatment. One highly disturbing study found that in some cases, doctors who did a procedure all the time continued to do it poorly.[15] The best defense is to seek a highly experienced expert with a wonderful reputation and an excellent track record.

Three years after his radical prostatectomy, Steve F. is content with his choice. "If I had it to do over again, I would do the same thing," he says. "I'm back to functioning mostly as I was before. And I can't tell you how nice it is to speak of the cancer in the past tense." Whatever treatment you choose, things might not end up as you had anticipated. Studies show that 15 to 20 percent of men regret their treatment choice five years later, whether they choose surgery or radiation therapy. To minimize the chances that you'll regret your decision, spend the time before treatment to get the best information you can.[16]

IN SUMMARY

All treatments for prostate cancer carry a risk of side effects.[17] Be sure your cancer needs treatment. Not all prostate cancers do. For many men, treatment can be safely delayed for many years. To decide what's best for you, you have to weigh the risks and benefits of all the available options against the seriousness of your disease and several other factors, including your life expectancy, lifestyle, general health, and personal values. In the final analysis, the quality of the treatment you receive may be more important than which option you choose. Be sure you place yourself in the care of a highly experienced expert with an excellent track record!

13

■

Watchful Waiting
(Active Surveillance)

READ THIS CHAPTER TO LEARN:

- Why might you monitor cancer rather than treat it?
- What is the difference between traditional watchful waiting and modern active surveillance?
- How should prostate cancer be monitored, and when is it appropriate to intervene?
- Does active surveillance make sense for you?

Among the many long-standing questions and controversies surrounding prostate cancer is whether it makes sense to treat the disease at all. Those who argue against active intervention point to the fact that countless men have cancer cells or minuscule tumors in their prostate glands that would never cause problems or symptoms if left alone. For every man who dies of prostate cancer in this country, seven to eight are diagnosed with the disease. For every man diagnosed, two or three others have some cancer cells in the gland that would never be detected unless their prostates were removed for some other reason, such as bladder cancer or benign prostate enlargement, and examined in the lab, or if they were subjected to a 12- to 80-core (saturation) biopsy because of a minor variation in their PSA. To put it another way, a 50-year-old man has a 16 percent chance of being diagnosed with prostate cancer in his remaining lifetime, but only about a 3 percent risk of dying of the disease. Forty-two percent of men in their 70s have some tiny clusters of cancer cells in their prostates, though the vast majority will never be discovered, much less cause any problems or harm.[1]

Most prostate tumors grow very slowly. On average, it takes two years for a cancer in the prostate to double in size. That's two years to grow from two cells to four, and another two years for those four cells to become eight, which gives you a good idea of why these cancers can take decades to become detectable (though some develop at a far slower rate, and advanced, metastatic prostate cancers can double in as little as a month or two). Often, the disease is diagnosed in older men who, as is commonly stated, are more likely to die *with* their prostate cancer than *of* it.

While it is difficult to predict with *absolute certainty* which cancers will remain small and harmless and which will prove dangerous, we can generally make this distinction by using available medical tests, including the digital rectal exam, PSA, Gleason grade, and the amount of cancer present in the biospy cores. Our level of certainty increases if we repeat the biopsy (another session of 12 cores) and get an endorectal MRI of the prostate.[2] Sometimes a repeat biopsy finds no cancer at all. In other cases a second biopsy reveals that the cancer is more aggressive than it seemed at first. By going the extra mile, we can reduce the risk of underestimating a serious cancer. (See page 253 for a nomogram used to determine the likelihood that a cancer is indolent.)

TRADITIONAL WATCHFUL WAITING

In the traditional sense, **watchful waiting** meant do nothing. Patients were advised to take no action and return to the doctor only if they developed symptoms of advanced disease, such as bone pain or urinary blockage.

At that point, men were treated with hormone therapy for bone pain or a TURP to alleviate urinary symptoms. Proponents of this approach claimed that most patients would die of other causes before they developed symptoms, and they would be spared the side effects of needless radical treatment. They argued that men who left their prostate cancers alone lived as long and did as well as men who had radiation or surgery.[3]

Recent studies have proven that idea wrong for all but the most favorable, lowest-risk cancers. In a landmark Swedish trial that compared radical prostatectomy with watchful waiting, patients on traditional watchful waiting were twice as likely to develop metastases as were men treated

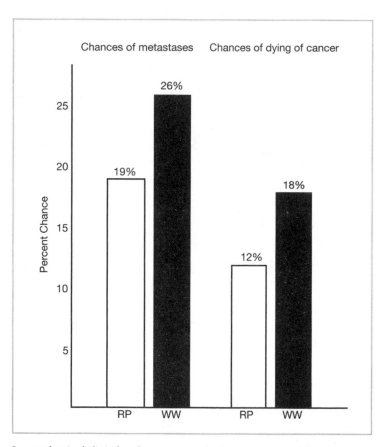

In a randomized clinical trail comparing radical prostatectomy (RP) with watchful waiting (WW) in Sweden, men who had their prostate surgically removed were much less likely to develop metastases or to die of their cancer twelve years later.

with radical prostatectomy.[4] Ironically, this finding came out of the very country where traditional do-nothing watchful waiting had been most ardently and universally embraced. In fact, the Swedish study found that men treated with surgery were less likely to die of *any* cause, prostate cancer included, within twelve years. Men treated with radical prostatectomy had fewer urinary problems, were much less likely to need hormone therapy with its many side effects, were less likely to be admitted to the hospital, less likely to have fractures caused by metastases, and overall had improved quality, as well as length, of life compared with men on traditional watchful waiting.[5]

All that aside, this study does *not* mean that all men with prostate cancer should have surgery. PSA screening is not routine in Sweden. Consequently, the men in this study had cancers that were discovered much later in their course than the typical prostate cancer we diagnose in the United States today. On average, prostate cancer detected through PSA testing is found five to eleven years earlier than the prostate cancer of the men in this study.[6] Typically, the Swedish patients' prostate tumors were found because of an abnormal digital rectal exam or because the cancer had progressed to the point of causing urinary symptoms.

DO ALL MEN WITH PROSTATE CANCER NEED TREATMENT?

With PSA testing so widespread and so many cancers detected early, it makes sense to consider whether or not your cancer really needs to be treated now. It may seem contradictory to screen for cancer and not attempt to cure it immediately, but this is often reasonable. Many prostate cancers are so slow-growing, they are unlikely to cause symptoms during the remainder of a man's natural life. If the cancer ever shows signs of becoming more aggressive, we can treat it then with a high probability of success. Remember, all the treatments we currently have for this disease carry a risk of troublesome side effects, so you do not want to have treatment unless you absolutely need it.

Watchful waiting in the traditional, do-nothing sense is unwise. But that is very different from the contemporary approach—active surveillance—where we monitor the disease closely and recommend surgery or radiation at the first sign that the cancer is progressing. This approach recognizes that prostate cancers, no matter how favorable, can change over time and require vigilance. Instead of deciding at the time of diagnosis that you will never have radiation or surgery, we keep a close eye on diagnostic indicators and switch to definitive treatment as soon as there is evidence that the risk from the tumor has increased.[7]

I've become a strong advocate of active surveillance for many patients. Every once in a while—about 1 in 100 cases—we perform a radical prostatectomy and find no cancer in the prostate at all! Far more often— 1 in 4 cases—the cancer turns out to be so tiny and insignificant when examined under the microscope that I question whether it was worth removing.

Despite this, when confronted with a problem, most Americans want a rapid solution. Our cultural value is to be proactive about problems, and active surveillance can feel like inaction. Keep in mind that that a precipitous response may only make a difficult situation worse. A sharp downturn in the investment market drives some people to panic and sell off at fire-sale prices, but taking the time to make a clearheaded

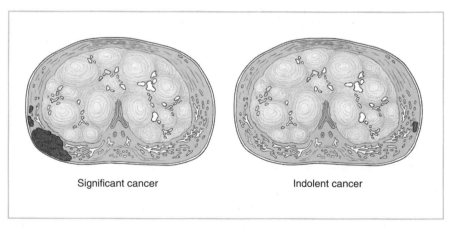

Significant cancer   Indolent cancer

Indolent cancers, which are much smaller than significant cancers, are confined within the prostate and contain no poorly differentiated Gleason pattern 4 or 5 components.

Prostate Cancer Nomogram. This computer program calculates the probability that you have an indolent (tiny, insignificant) cancer, and the extent of the cancer, and the probability that your cancer will be cured, whichever treatment you choose (surgery or radiation). The nomogram can be reached on the Internet (www.mskcc.org/applications/momgrams/prostate/PreTreatment .aspx). Simply enter your PSA, age, Gleason grade, stage, and biopsy information as instructed, then click "Calculate" to display the results.[8]

decision may be a far better way to go. This is true of prostate cancer as well. Active surveillance is not equivalent to ignoring or avoiding the problem. It requires regular checkups to track the progress of the disease and intervention with radiation or surgery as soon as the cancer shows definite signs of progression.

Be aware that doctors have many reasons to be cautious about recommending active surveillance, in addition to any skepticism they may have about the accuracy of identifying suitable candidates and detecting progression in time for effective treatment later. Economic and legal factors also play a role in medical decision-making. Medical reimbursements reward procedures such as surgery and radiation much more than they do ongoing follow-up and counseling. Also, doctors can be reluctant to actively monitor a patient, given the risk (no matter how small) that the cancer could progress and become incurable. The treating physician is rarely blamed if he carries out a therapeutic protocol conscientiously and the patient suffers a well-known side effect. But if a doctor defers active intervention and the cancer grows despite careful monitoring or the patient develops metastases, the physician may fear a lawsuit. I have always felt this was a poor excuse for recommending radical treatment, since after an honest discussion and fully informed consent, the risk of successful litigation is remote. But doctors fear medico–legal consequences of their recommendations.

Regardless of these pressures against it, active surveillance is a sound option for many men. Deciding whether you're an appropriate candidate for this approach depends on how serious and threatening your cancer is, as well as your age and life expectancy, your general health, and your level of concern about the side effects of treatment.

Before we recommend monitoring, we need a thorough evaluation of the cancer. A good candidate for active surveillance has a PSA less than 10, a Gleason 3 + 3 or less, a normal DRE, or a small palpable nodule (stage T1C or T2a). The amount of cancer found in your biopsy is also an important consideration. Someone with a small amount of cancer in one or two biopsy cores is likely to have a favorable tumor, while finding that 6 of 12 biopsy cores containing cancer suggests a large tumor. Other useful measures include your PSA density. A man with a very large gland

and a PSA over 10 could be an acceptable candidate for active surveillance as long as his PSA density is less than 0.1 (for a 120 g prostate, that
would mean a PSA less than 12. If the PSA density is 0.15 or greater, the
risk of an aggressive cancer is higher.

To help make sense of all this, we developed a nomogram that combines PSA, the stage (extent) of the tumor, the Gleason grade, the size of
prostate, and a comparison of the amount of cancer in the biopsy cores
to estimate the chance that a cancer is indolent and poses no immediate threat to life or health. (See page 253 for a nomogram, or predictive
model, used to determine the likelihood that a cancer is indolent. This
nomogram is available on the Memorial Sloan-Kettering website, www
.MSKCC.org. Search for "prostate cancer nomograms.")[9]

The indolent cancer nomogram is not perfect, but its accuracy has
been confirmed in a large European population. At best, it can predict
with 75 percent certainty that a prostate cancer can be safely monitored.
Still, anyone who scores over 50 percent on this nomogram has a highly
favorable cancer and is a potential candidate for active surveillance.

If your tumor seems favorable and you opt to monitor rather than
treat, a repeat biopsy is the next essential step. This should include taking
at least six, and preferably ten to fourteen, sample cores. If this second
biopsy shows a much more extensive tumor or any poorly differentiated (Gleason pattern 4 or 5) cancer, treatment is usually indicated. On
the other hand, if the second biopsy finds no cancer, as happens in 20
to 30 percent of cases, or the cancer is similar to that on the original
biopsy, chances are much lower that the cancer will require treatment. A
negative biopsy does not mean that the gland is cancer-free.[10] Because a
biopsy samples only about 1 percent of prostate tissue, very tiny cancers
may not be picked up. Generally, a negative repeat biopsy indicates that
the tumor is small and low-risk. Studies at Memorial Sloan-Kettering
Cancer Center have found that 85 percent of patients whose repeat
biopsy was cancer-free showed no signs of disease progression within
ten years.[11]

An MRI of the prostate can also be useful. Many doctors are not
enthusiastic about the value of MRI in diagnosing prostate cancer,
but I think this stems from a lack of expertise. While it is true that

Screen shot of indolent cancer nomogram on the Memorial Sloan-Kettering Cancer Center website.

prostate cancers smaller than 5 mm will not show up on MRI, a normal MRI finding helps us rule out the presence of an "iceberg" (a large cancer lurking that we fail to detect). Our studies have shown that when we combine MRI with other factors in a nomogram, accuracy is improved.[12]

NOTE: Rarely, despite the best state-of-the-art monitoring, a tumor will grow, spread, and become incurable. This is certainly the major risk in deferred treatment. On the other hand, the treatment of advanced prostate cancer is continually improving, and even though a cancer is not cured by radiation or surgery, it can often be controlled for the rest of a man's natural life.

WHY WOULD YOU MONITOR RATHER THAN TREAT A PROSTATE CANCER?

Side effects: Every effective treatment carries some risk of side effects, especially troublesome problems with bowel, urinary, or sexual function. Tolerance for these risks is highly individual, and some men are much more troubled by their cancer than they are by the chance that one of these problems will occur. If the potential downsides of a proposed treatment don't concern you, you may choose to have your cancer treated no matter how favorable it is or how little risk it poses.

Be wary of overly optimistic claims. Proponents of newer therapies, whether robotic surgery, cryotherapy, or HIFU (heat therapy), may suggest that their approach carries a lower chance for collateral damage. No effective treatment for prostate cancer is without risks, and there is no evidence that the risks of these new therapies are any less than with surgery or radiation. (See Chapter 14, Surgery, and Chapter 16, Focal and Other "Local" Therapies.)

Nature of the cancer: Another factor in deciding whether or not to defer treatment is the size and aggressiveness of your tumor. A man in his mid-60s who has a favorable cancer (no palpable nodule, a PSA less than 10, and a Gleason score of 6 or less in only one or two biopsy cores) may be as reasonable a candidate for deferred therapy as a healthy patient in his mid-70s to 80s whose tumor is more aggressive.

Life expectancy: Prostate cancer grows slowly, but given enough time, many cancers will enlarge, spread, and eventually, cause symptoms. Your life expectancy, determined by your age and state of health, is one important factor in estimating whether your cancer is ever likely to cause trouble. The general rule of thumb is that deferred treatment is a reasonable approach for someone whose remaining life expectancy is less than ten years, unless he has an unusually aggressive cancer with a Gleason score of 4 + 3 or above. But assessing how long you are likely to live is far from an exact science.

You can start by using the life expectancy tables available from the National Vital Statistics System or your life insurance company.[13] Most financial management software quickly calculates your life expectancy from your gender and your present age. Still, this is no more than a ballpark figure. Your health, family longevity, lifestyle, and several other factors can alter the estimate of the number of remaining years you have. Many people think that having a life expectancy of less than ten years means that there is no chance that you will live longer. The estimate actually indicates a fifty/ fifty chance that you will live that long. Some men in this group will die far sooner, and others will survive considerably longer. For active surveillance, the question is not only whether you should be treated now, but what is likely to happen over time. If we've ruled out the presence of a serious cancer, it is highly unlikely that your disease will cause any serious problems in the next ten years. Let's say your Gleason 3 + 3 cancer was present in only 1 mm of one core of a twelve-core biopsy. If that accurately represents the amount of cancer in your prostate, the tumor is likely less than 1 cubic mm. These small, early cancers double in size about every two years. In ten years, your 1 mm cancer would still be tiny—less than 50 cubic mm—harmless and imperceptible. (Keep in mind that it takes about 1 gram of cancer to raise your PSA level by 3 to 4 ng/ml.) In twenty years, the cancer would reach 2 cubic cm (or 2,000 cubic ml), enough to raise your PSA by 6 to 10 ng/ml, but still too small to metastasize or cause symptoms.

Let's run the same scenario for a cancer that starts out as 3 mm of Gleason 3 + 3. It is about 30 cubic mm now, and in ten years would still be less than 1 cubic cm. It would take fifteen years for the cancer to reach 5 cubic cm, the earliest threshold for spread to other sites, but still highly curable with modern surgery or radiation therapy.

Unfortunately, after many years with no apparent change in a tumor, patients can become complacent. Just at the point when the risk of the cancer is increasing, men can believe, erroneously, that they are out of the woods. This confusion is understandable. After treatment for prostate cancer, the risk of recurrence typically decreases over time. With active surveillance, the opposite is true. The risk from the still-present cancer *increases* as the years go on, and you would need to be especially vigilant ten to twenty years into an active surveillance program.

Age: Most doctors are comfortable recommending active surveillance or watchful waiting for men over 75 with serious medical conditions and limited life expectancy, but they are understandably reluctant to do this for a young man under 50 whose cancer might have thirty years or more to progress and become deadly. If you're between those age extremes, the decision about whether to opt for active intervention now or wait and monitor the situation closely may be much cloudier. Screening with PSA allows us to detect these cancers five to ten years earlier than was previously possible when diagnosis relied on DRE or symptoms. In many cases, we find prostate cancers twelve to eighteen years before they are likely to spread and become incurable. Men aged 60 to 75 who are diagnosed with a very low-risk cancer could opt rationally to follow the disease for a while before deciding whether to have treatment. If the tumor is small and has very favorable characteristics (**indolent**), it might take fifteen to twenty years to spread.[14] Realistically, many men in this age group would die of other causes before their prostate cancers presented any problem. In the meantime, regularly monitoring changes in the PSA, free PSA, and DRE, along with periodic repeat biopsies, would usually give us ample warning that the cancer is beginning to change and that treatment should be started. Of course, there is the remote possibility that the disease will spread no matter how vigilantly we monitor it. Many men are unable to live with that uncertainty and opt for immediate treatment instead, accepting the risk of side effects.

Sixty-six-year-old Ray F., a Massachusetts importer, chose to monitor rather than treat his favorable tumor. "My business involves a lot of travel, and it would be difficult at this point to take time off. Also, I'm hoping for advances in the field that may make treatment easier. I have a great doctor, and I'm confident waiting with him in my corner. But I must admit that living with a cancer in my body takes a psychological toll."

WHAT DOES ACTIVE SURVEILLANCE ENTAIL?

Active surveillance calls for regular, rigorous monitoring. My protocol includes a return visit to the doctor every six months for a DRE and a blood test for free and total PSA, with a repeat biopsy twelve to eighteen months after the program begins and every two to three years thereafter, as long as active treatment with surgery or radiation would be an option. While the role of imaging studies such as MRI is still being defined, I think it's wise to do one every few years.[15]

You and your doctor should be on guard and prepared to treat the cancer if there are clear signs that it is progressing. If the cancer proves to be more extensive or higher-grade on a subsequent biopsy, if it is seen to grow on ultrasound or MRI, or felt on DRE to enlarge, it's time to begin treatment. Changes in PSA are harder to interpret. The PSA normally fluctuates day to day by as much as 30 percent,[16] so we have to see a steady, persistent rise, involving at least three consecutive new peaks, to be sure that a change is significant. The rate at which PSA level increases, expressed as **PSA velocity or doubling time** (see Chapter 8, Detecting Prostate Cancer with PSA and Other Tests),[17] may give us some indication of what the tumor is doing, but this measure alone is far from completely reliable.[18]

In a large active surveillance study in which PSA doubling time less than 24 months was used to signal the need for intervention, patients were treated with surgery or radiation, and the cancer returned in more than half the cases. In my opinion, waiting until the doubling time becomes short or the velocity high is unwise. By then, the cancer has become very aggressive and treatment is no longer as likely to cure the disease.

While changes in PSA should be monitored closely and used to signal whether a biopsy needs to be done sooner than the typical two to three years, I make decisions about intervention based mostly on biopsy results, not PSA alone. Checkups will have to continue every six months, and biopsies every two to three years (even if all appears well), as long as you're healthy and would be a candidate for curative surgery or radiation. While the cancer may be stable for six or even ten years, the risk of rapid growth increases over time.

THE ADVANTAGES

The obvious advantage of deferring treatment is that you avoid the side effects of treating a cancer that currently poses little threat. For a man over 70, especially one with serious medical problems, or for a younger man with a very low-risk tumor, active surveillance is a sound approach.

Even though active surveillance makes a lot of sense for many men with favorable prostate cancers, most men are reluctant to accept it. They are unable to cope with the fear of an untreated cancer left growing in their body, so they opt for immediate treatment, even though it is often unnecessary.

NOTE: Worry about living with an untreated cancer is not a good reason to opt for immediate therapy. Men who choose radical prostatectomy or radiation still worry every six months when they return to have their PSA checked. Once you have prostate cancer, it will always be a presence in your life. The better response is learning to manage those anxieties and minimize their effects on your life. Radical treatment is not a good antidote for anxiety.

CONCERNS ABOUT ACTIVE SURVEILLANCE

While the advantages are obvious, the disadvantages of active surveillance drive some men to choose immediate therapy, no matter how favorable their cancer happens to be. The major worry—foremost in the minds of most doctors uncomfortable recommending active surveillance—is that the cancer is actually much larger and more aggressive than it appears to be on biopsy. The best way to overcome this concern is with a complete reevaluation. Repeat the PSA and free PSA six weeks after the first biopsy, have a high-quality MRI of the prostate if it is available in your area, and ask your doctor to repeat the biopsy to see if the cancer is more serious.[19] If your doctor is adamantly against active surveillance, get another opinion or have the repeat tests and biopsy done in a different office or medical center.

The most common reason men choose treatment over active surveillance (and the fear most often expressed by their spouse or partner) is the fear that the cancer will grow and spread (metastasize) before anyone realizes it, and they will miss the chance that the cancer can be cured. This is an understandable but exaggerated concern. Small, favorable cancers are typically found as a result of PSA testing six to eleven years before they would be detected by DRE or cause symptoms. If your cancer progresses over time, it would almost certainly be found during a semiannual checkup or during the biopsy we recommend every two to three years. Choosing therapy for prostate cancer requires balancing risks. The best defense is to be as certain as possible that your cancer poses very little risk at present, and to consider the real risks of treatment in light of the small risk of unexpected spread of the cancer many years in the future.

A genuine worry is the increased probability of side effects from the more aggressive treatment that may be needed to control a larger, more extensive cancer that might develop in the future. Even if the cancer can be cured five, ten, or fifteen years from now, will the surgery have to be more extensive, with a greater risk of damage to the erectile nerves, or will hormone therapy have to be used in conjunction with radiation, worsening the damage to sexual function? Offsetting this appropriate concern is the chance that simpler treatments may become available in the future, such as focal ablation of cancer, which may have fewer side effects. Again, balancing risks is the best way to arrive at the right decision for you.

Other legitimate concerns are the risks of spreading cancer to surrounding tissues with the multiple repeat biopsies required to monitor the cancer during active surveillance. This risk seems very low, but it is certainly not zero. We almost never see local seeding of a cancer after biopsy, but it would be very hard to detect.

Even with all the medical reports on the good results of active surveillance, few studies have followed patients for more than ten years. We really don't know what will happen later. How many of these small cancers will remain unchanged, and how many will grow and spread if left alone? How many men become complacent after a long period on watchful waiting and cease having their cancers monitored just at the time they may begin to pose a greater threat?

Current studies indicate that about 1 in 4 men on active surveillance end up being treated within five years and about a third do so within ten years. Much more needs to be learned about the long-term outcomes of active surveillance for early, favorable prostate cancer.[20]

WHY SOME MEN SWITCH FROM ACTIVE MONITORING TO TREATMENT

In studies of men on active surveillance, 10 to 30 percent drop out and seek treatment during the first five years, even though some of the tumors showed no sign of growth. These men simply find the anxiety of living with a cancer intolerable.[21]

One-third of the men showed signs that the cancer was changing for the worse and were referred for surgery or radiation therapy. Still, though two-thirds could have continued to monitor their disease, 1 in 6 decided to have their cancers treated. Ten years after starting active surveillance, about half to two thirds are still in the program and their cancers have shown no sign of change.

I wish I could tell you that there was a certain test result that would signal the perfect time to switch from active surveillance and treat the cancer with surgery or radiation, but we have no such test, and it remains, like so much in medicine, a matter of judgment. I find PSA testing alone unreliable, but I do use it to establish the interval between testing and biopsy. If a man's PSA appears to be rising, I will check it more frequently than if the PSA is falling or flat. In the final analysis, we get the best information from a prostate biopsy.

The Fear Factor— Refusing Necessary Treatment

Active surveillance for a small, indolent cancer can be sensible, but refusing lifesaving treatment for a dangerous cancer that poses a risk to life and health is unwise.

Despite this, I've had patients with serious tumors say that they would rather risk death from their cancer than the loss of erections or urinary control that sometimes results from surgery, or the bowel, urinary, or sexual complications that can result from radiation. Some men feel this way even though these side effects affect only a fraction of patients, are often temporary, and are generally treatable when they do occur. Fear of side effects can be paralyzing and stand in the way of a rational choice.

If concerns about side effects are driving your decision to defer treatment for a significant cancer, keep in mind that growing prostate cancer causes considerable side effects of its own. **Hormone therapy**, which eventually becomes essential to alleviate symptoms of advanced cancer, can cause a loss of erections, libido, body hair, and muscle mass, as well as osteoporosis, hot flashes, breast enlargement, and depression. As it progresses, the cancer itself can lead to erectile dysfunction and serious urinary problems, not to mention severe bone pain, a host of other systemic problems from metastases, and eventually, death.

CAN DIET AND SUPPLEMENTS STOP PROSTATE CANCER?

While active surveillance is a logical choice for the right patients, many men with potentially dangerous cancers shun proven therapies in fear of side effects and turn instead to diet, supplements, mind/body work, or alternative medicine. It's tempting to imagine that by maintaining a healthy lifestyle or following an ascetic regime, we can alter the course of this disease.

Unfortunately, though there are some factors that show promise as possibly preventing prostate cancer, such as a heart-healthy diet and an active exercise program, nothing has a demonstrated ability to change the course of this disease once it has been established.[22] We had hopes that certain supplements, such as selenium, vitamin E, lycopene, and soy, might prevent or slow the course of prostate cancer, but so far, studies have been disappointing. (See Chapter 7, Risk Factors and Prevention.)[23]

We do have a promising medical therapy that might slow the growth of some small, early prostate cancers (a process called **chemosuppression**), but I am hopeful that chemosuppression with finasteride or dutasteride will eventually prove beneficial and give men on active surveillance one way to slow the growth of their cancers and help them avoid active treatment with surgery or radiation.

DO ANY OF THE "MIRACLE" PROSTATE CANCER CURES REALLY WORK?

When it comes to prostate cancer, claims for curative miracles abound. A brief Internet search will unearth numerous extravagant, unproven, and often absurd claims that everything from diet to self-hypnosis, taking performance-boosting hormones, or even drinking one's own urine can arrest, shrink, or eradicate an established prostate cancer.

During more than three decades of reading the literature, conferring with colleagues, and practicing in the field, I have never heard of a single case in which a prostate cancer disappeared spontaneously. Though rare, instances of malignancies vanishing without treatment have been reported with certain other cancers, such as melanomas and kidney cancers, which are highly vulnerable to the body's own immune response.

Once you have been diagnosed with a clinically significant prostate cancer, only radiation therapy or surgery to remove the gland has a proven track record of curing the disease. Certainly, not every prostate cancer warrants intervention, especially low-risk cancers that have all the characteristics of being indolent. You would be much wiser to evaluate and weigh your options carefully with established experts than to put your faith in people who prey on men's fears and profit from the sale of empty promises.

THE FUTURE

Patients with a favorable, low-risk cancer face a difficult choice between active surveillance and radical therapy such as radiation or surgery. Among the most exciting developments on the horizon are techniques that will allow us to destroy a small, confined area of the gland (focal ablation therapy), while leaving the rest of the prostate intact. This may prove to be an effective way to stop a small cancer from growing into a large one without subjecting the patient to side effects of more radical treatments. (See Chapter 16, Focal and Other "Local" Therapies.)

To help men make wise decisions about immediate treatment versus active surveillance, we need more accurate ways to size up prostate cancers and separate the tigers from the pussycats. One fertile area of research is the Cancer Atlas Genome Project, a large-scale government-sponsored effort to thoroughly characterize all the genetic abnormalities in prostate cancers. We have already found genetic alterations that help us characterize the nature of prostate cancer, such as the TMPRSS-2 (pronounced *tem-press*) fusion gene, which causes parts of two genes to combine. New genomic studies can separate the highly favorable from the dangerous, aggressive canccrs by this profile on comparative genomic hybridization (CGH), which gives a fingerprint of all the genes gained or lost in a cancer compared with normal tissue. Many others are in the pipeline. Researchers are also exploring protein patterns in the blood or tissue (**proteomics**) and analyzing cancer cells circulating in the bloodstream to develop a means of predicting which cancers pose a serious threat.

Systems pathology is a new approach to analyzing tissue under the microscope that uses computerized image analysis of microscopic elements of the cancer along with precise measurement of levels of key proteins such as the androgen receptor to characterize the behavior of prostate cancer. In early studies of one such approach, a company called Aureon Laboratories has been able to classify the risk posed by some tumors more accurately than standard nomograms, though further testing is needed.

Another investigational focus is on better imaging. We don't know whether it will be MRI with spectroscopy or dynamic contrast enhanced (DCE) MRI, but the field is progressing rapidly.

Finally, some chemical cousins of PS such as free PSA, hK2, and nicked PSA, measured in a blood test, are pretty good at distinguishing the more serious from the less serious cancers. Studies are in progress to test these factors. Someday we may have a constellation of serum markers that we can track through simple blood tests. This would provide a crucial early-warning system so we'll know which men can safely continue to defer treatment and which should switch to active intervention while we can still cure the disease.

IN SUMMARY

Active surveillance is a reasonable, responsible way to deal with low-risk prostate cancer in a man of almost any age, but it requires a commitment to lifelong follow-up and periodic biopsies. In choosing this course of action, men and their doctors need to recognize that it is not foolproof, and the cancer could grow and progress before it is treated.

The promise of active surveillance is to avoid or postpone the side effects of surgery or radiation, which might be unnecessary for many men. But be cautious. Active surveillance for a serious, aggressive cancer is highly risky business. For these cancers, avoiding the side effects of treatment in the short run can lead to the need for more radical therapy, and even worse side effects, later on, with much less chance of a cancer cure.

14

■

Surgery

READ THIS CHAPTER TO LEARN:

- Does surgery to remove the prostate gland make sense for you?
- How has radical prostatectomy changed, and which type of procedure should you seek?
- How can you choose the best surgeon?
- Should you have a pelvic lymph node dissection at the time of surgery?

Given widespread screening with the PSA test, we now detect many prostate cancers very early in the course of the disease, when they pose no risk and could reasonably be monitored rather than treated right away. When we find significant cancers that do represent a serious health risk, surgery is an excellent way to be rid of the cancer for good.

In fact, when performed by a skilled, experienced urologic surgeon using modern techniques, surgical removal of the entire prostate may offer the *best* chance for a permanent cure. With surgery alone, we can even cure 40 to 75 percent of high-risk, aggressive cancers. If we follow with radiation, half of the remaining patients with high-risk cancers can be cured.

Nevertheless, radical prostatectomy is a major operation that carries the risk of side effects and complications, even in the best of hands, so electing surgery for a small, innocent (indolent) cancer may be unwise. Despite their billing as "minimally invasive," laparoscopic and robotic-assisted radical prostatectomy carry the same risks and complications as does removal of the gland by the traditional "open" method. Urinary incontinence and loss of erections, unfortunately, happen just as often with these new operating techniques.

NOTE: It pays to be cautious about new technology that may not have a proven track record. Many people find the idea of robotic surgery appealing, believing that robots are somehow infallible and more precise than procedures left in human hands. In fact, the surgical robot is nothing more than a tool. The surgeon guides the robot, and directs the operation. A robot, no matter how technologically impressive and advanced, will not make up for a lack of judgment, knowledge of anatomy, or technical skill.

Surgical treatment for prostate cancer entails complete ("radical") excision of the gland ("prostatectomy"). During a **radical prostatectomy**, we also take out the delicate tissue surrounding the prostate, including the seminal vesicles. What makes the operation so challenging is the close proximity of vital structures so important for urinary, bowel, and sexual function.

A natural question is, Why remove the whole gland for a cancer in only one part of it? Why not remove the tumor and leave the rest of the gland behind? Removing only the tumor, a common practice in breast cancer, is not an option, for several important reasons. Prostate cancer tends to be multifocal, meaning it arises in several areas at once. A pathologist examining a cancerous prostate after surgery will find an average of five to six separate malignancies, distributed in an unpredictable pattern throughout the gland. Furthermore, the prostate is located deep in the pelvis, surrounded by vital structures, including large blood vessels. An attempt to remove part of the prostate surgically would be as damaging and risky as removing the whole gland.

For breast cancer, treatment almost always involves radiation after a "lumpectomy" or excision of the cancerous nodule. Doctors rely on radiation to get rid of any remaining malignant cells elsewhere in the breast. The prostate is surrounded by delicate structures, so we usually do not give radiation unless a rising PSA signals that the cancer has recurred. Radiation to the prostate can cause damage to surrounding structures, including the erectile nerves, the urethra (which channels urine), and the bowel.

For many men, radical prostatectomy is a safe and highly effective treatment choice. If you choose surgery and all goes well, you'll be able to live out the rest of your life with no sign of prostate cancer and no life-altering side effects.

A SHORT HISTORY OF PROSTATE CANCER SURGERY

Compared with many types of surgery, radical prostatectomy is a decidedly new kid on the block. Evidence from Neolithic sites confirms that trepanning, a procedure in which a hole was bored in the skull (some say to release demons) was practiced 40,000 years ago. Amputations date to the Cro-Magnon era. Skeletal remains of a 45,000-year-old male whose arm had been amputated are on display at the Smithsonian Institution.

In striking contrast, Theodor Billroth, a renowned German surgeon, reportedly made the first attempt to remove a cancerous prostate in 1867.[1] Billroth also performed the first surgical procedures for rectal, esophageal, and laryngeal cancers; developed a new way to resect (remove) part of the stomach for gastric cancer; and devised novel methods for educating surgical residents that remain in use today. This remarkable innovator was a close friend of Johannes Brahms and an accomplished musician in his own right. Despite copious other commitments, Billroth found time to serve on occasion as a guest conductor for the Zurich Symphony Orchestra.

In the United States, removal of the prostate for cancer was not attempted until 1904, when Hugh Hampton Young, the "Father of American Urology," operated on an elderly preacher. When that patient died years later of an unrelated cause, the autopsy showed no evidence of cancer.[2]

These early surgical procedures used the **perineal** approach, in which the patient was placed in an odd, head-down position and the incision was made behind the scrotal sac. The method held blood loss to a minimum, and patients recovered quickly. Nevertheless, the surgeon's view of crucial structures was highly restricted, providing more of a meager porthole than an open window to the surgical field. Incontinence after surgery was common, and impotence was seen as inevitable.

In 1945, a British surgeon named Terence Millin pioneered a new technique involving a vertical abdominal incision to remove the prostate from its perch behind the pubic bone. Millin's procedure resulted in more blood loss, but it provided surgeons with a much better view of the operative field and far better access to critical organs. After many important refinements, **radical retropubic prostatectomy**, or **open prostatectomy**, remains the most popular and effective technique for surgical treatment of prostate cancer today.

Many men are terrified of radical prostatectomy because of horror stories that stem from the bad old days of prostate-cancer surgery. Until the early 1980s, removing the prostate was virtually synonymous with serious and sometimes catastrophic side effects. Often, the operation caused severe bleeding that, in the worst cases, could be life-threatening. The surgery left 15 to 25 percent of men incontinent, and the great majority lost their ability to have erections. Bowel injuries and urinary strictures (narrowing of the urethra by scar tissue) occurred with troubling frequency. Understandably, few patients elected to have the procedure, and most doctors were reluctant to recommend it. By the 1960s, following the development of the linear accelerator that could deliver

X-rays to a targeted organ, external beam radiation became the prostate cancer treatment of choice. Radiation remained the dominant option for nearly thirty years, even though irradiating the gland before the discovery of modern conformal therapy caused serious side effects and often failed to arrest the disease.

As in real estate, the central issue in prostate operations is location, location, location. The prostate lies deep in the abdomen, where it is difficult to access or examine. Several critical structures, including the rectum and bladder, lie perilously close to the gland. The urethra, which carries urine from the bladder and sperm from the testes through the penis, tunnels directly through the prostate. To perform a radical prostatectomy, a surgeon must sever the urethra just above the urinary sphincter and again near the bladder neck. Then, after removing the gland, the surgeon carefully connects the cut ends of the urethra to the bladder to form an **anastomosis**, which is basically what you'd need to do if you wanted to reconnect the severed ends of a rubber hose. Only three decades ago, doctors performing this highly complex, delicate surgery were seriously handicapped by incomplete and often erroneous ideas about prostate anatomy.

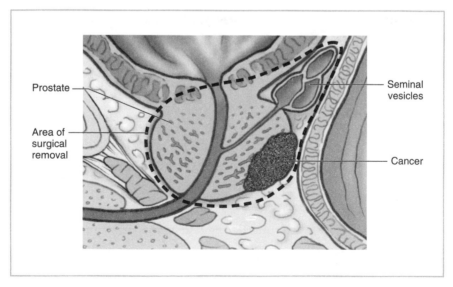

The dotted line indicates the tissue removed in a radical prostatectomy.

NOTE: Though some surgeons continue to prefer it, I see little reason to use the perineal approach today. The prostate can be removed, but given the limited visibility, the surgeon has no flexibility to excise surrounding tissues that might harbor cancer. Even advocates of this procedure support its use only for small-volume, favorable-risk cancers (a PSA level of less than 10; a Gleason score of less than 7 with a low risk of extension through the capsule; no more than two biopsy cores containing cancer). For more serious cancers, the risk of incomplete removal with positive surgical margins is just too great.

Also, while some surgeons have performed nerve-sparing perineal prostatectomy, in actual practice both nerves are almost never spared. Consequently, this procedure results in an unacceptably high rate of impotence. I consider the perineal operation reasonable only for men over 65 with no erectile function, who have a small, favorable cancer.

MODERN RADICAL PROSTATECTOMY: "ANATOMICAL" APPROACH TO PROSTATE SURGERY

When I was trained to perform radical prostatectomy in late 1970s, the anatomy of the prostate was poorly understood. We did not appreciate the major source of blood vessels in and out of the gland, the relationship between the prostate and the urinary sphincters, or the location of the nerves responsible for penile erections. In those days, the goal of the operation was to get the prostate out as quickly as possible to minimize potentially dangerous blood loss. This was true of most cancer operations. Surgeons lacked the time and knowledge to avoid damage to surrounding organs.

Since the early 1980s, there has been a renaissance in cancer surgery, including radical prostatectomy. We have progressed from a singular focus on getting the cancer out to highly controlled operations designed to remove tumors and then repair/reconstruct to minimize structural and functional damage. Accomplishing this requires clear, detailed understanding of the relevant anatomy.

We now know where prostate cancer tends to invade. We are able to identify the key surrounding structures. Using this knowledge, we have systematically devised a procedure that allows a surgeon to remove the entire prostate and all of the cancer with minimal risk to urinary, sexual, and bowel function. The goal of radical prostatectomy is complete removal of the prostate, seminal vesicles, and pelvic lymph nodes without the need for blood transfusion and without surgical complications, but with complete recovery of urinary and sexual function in all patients. This is the ideal toward which all serious surgeons strive, though no one achieves it 100 percent of the time.

NERVE SPARING

Men first strolled on the moon in 1969, but astonishing though it may seem, we did not figure out the exact anatomy of the nerves responsible for penile erections until 1981. Credit for that discovery goes to urologists Patrick Walsh of Johns Hopkins Hospital and Pieter Donker of the University of Leiden in the Netherlands. For many years, Donker had been studying the anatomy of the nerves to the urinary bladder and sphincter in stillborn babies, which have relatively large nerves compared with adults. During a conference in the Netherlands, Walsh visited Donker's laboratory, where he identified the cavernous (erectile) nerves in a stillborn baby boy, and traced the path of these nerves as they ran along the outside of the prostate, not through the gland, as experts in urology had believed.

Walsh realized that it was therefore possible to preserve erectile nerves during radical prostatectomy and leave prostate cancer patients with their sexual function intact.[3] In 1982 he performed the first nerve-sparing radical prostatectomy. Today, most surgeons routinely strive to preserve erectile nerves when removing the prostate. Doing so allows most men who were previously potent to regain erections after surgery and reduces the incidence of urinary incontinence, which also appears to depend to some degree on preserving these nerves.

Unfortunately, complete sparing of erectile nerves is not always possible. These nerves are tiny and delicate, like the tentacles of a jellyfish. As the surgeon teases them away from the gland before removing the prostate, they often suffer damage that can cause the nerves to stop functioning, though they may heal and recover in time. The farther away the surgeon can stay from the nerves and the less they are manipulated, the sooner erectile function will recover. If a cancer grows through the capsule of the gland near the nerves, wider dissection becomes necessary (partial nerve sparing) with more consequent damage. Occasionally, the cancer is so large and extensive, invading an erectile nerve, that we have to remove an entire nerve (nerve resection) to get around the tumor. Ten years ago, we removed one nerve during the operation in 1 of 5 men. Given improvements in surgical techniques today, we rarely remove a

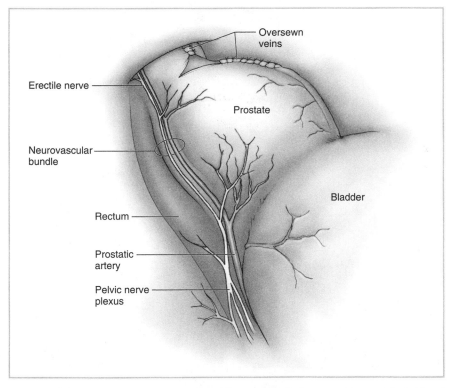

View of the surgical field from the perspective of the surgeon. The feet are at the top of the field, and the head at the bottom. The neurovascular bundle (NVB), containing the cavernous (erectile) nerves, runs alongside the rectum and passes along the prostate and the urinary sphincter, into the penis.

nerve (1 to 2 in a hundred), and then only for extensive, locally advanced T3 cancers.

NERVE GRAFTS

If, in your particular situation, one or both erectile nerve bundles have to be completely removed in order to remove the cancer, a **nerve graft** can improve chances of recovering sexual function. A section of nerve can be taken from the side of the foot (sural nerve) or from inside the pelvis (genitofemoral nerve) to replace an erectile nerve that needs to be removed.[4] Synthetic nerve grafts are also being investigated that may make it unnecessary to take a patient's own nerve to replace one removed during surgery.

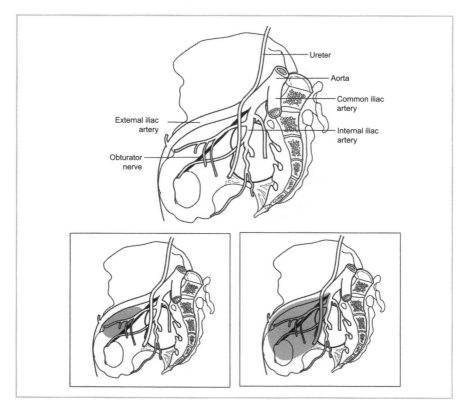

(A) Side view of the pelvis showing the major blood vessels and nerves. (B) Shaded area shows the lymph nodes removed in a limited pelvic lymph node dissection (PLND) compared with (C) the full pelvic node dissection, which I recommend.

Today, many medical centers offer nerve grafts for radical prostatectomy patients whose erectile nerves cannot be spared, and the results have been encouraging.[5] Without grafts, men who lose both nerves during surgery almost never recover erectile function. With increased experience using grafts, about 40 percent of patients with bilateral nerve grafts recover, often with the help of erection-inducing drugs such as sildenafil (Viagra). Removing one nerve substantially reduces the chances of recovering potency, depending on a person's age. In my experience with 60-year-old men, only about 40 to 50 percent regain erectile function when one nerve is removed, compared with 80 to 90 percent who do so when both nerves are spared.[6] When one nerve is resected and then replaced by a graft, about 70 percent recover. This is not as good as when both nerves are spared, but better than the outcome without grafts.[7] Operating on seven out of eight cylinders is far better than trying to run on only four or—in a truly futile enterprise—none at all. If erectile function is important to you, you may want to consider finding a surgeon who can do a nerve graft if it proves necessary to remove one or both of your erectile nerves in order to cure the cancer.

NOTE: We now use fewer and fewer nerve grafts because we have learned how to remove more tissue to cure the cancer without destroying the erectile nerves. Five years ago, 20 percent of men undergoing radical prostatectomy had an erectile nerve removed. This is down to 1 to 2 percent today.

Even a large tumor that has grown into the nerves can sometimes be cured as long as it is completely removed. Even if the cancer eventually recurs, there's a benefit to removing the primary tumor, which would otherwise be left to grow and cause symptoms. Incurable prostate cancer does *not* mean you're going to die soon or spend all of your remaining years debilitated by the disease. Most men live symptom-free for many years, and there's no reason they shouldn't be offered the chance for good erectile function and a satisfying sex life during that time.

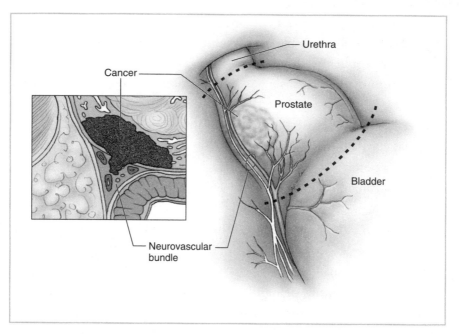

When a large cancer grows into a neurovascular bundle, the nerve must be removed along with the prostate to cure the cancer. Dotted lines show what is removed during the operation.

Some doctors are skeptical about nerve grafting, arguing that a cancer large enough to invade the erectile nerves is not curable and surgery should not be done. I disagree. In a recent randomized trial, doctors reported no better recovery of erections when one nerve was excised and replaced by a graft than if no graft was used. But this study involved many different surgeons with a range of skill and experience, and the results likely reflect poor technique rather than real lack of benefit.[8]

NOTE: These results have yet to be proven in a randomized trial.

The Downside of Nerve Grafts

Nerve grafting does involve a bit more operating time, and it can add the cost of a plastic or neurosurgeon, though in some cases the urologist performs the graft himself. If the sural nerve is taken from the foot, some patients experience inflammation or a wound infection at the donor site.

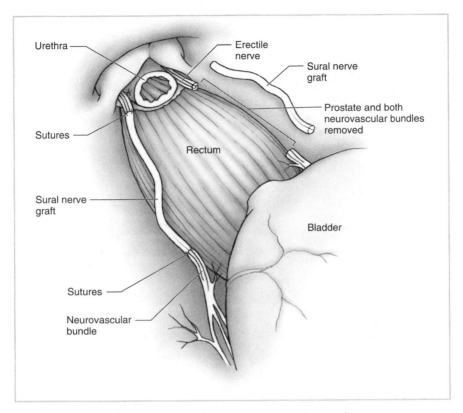

Bilateral nerve grafts to replace the erectile nerves.[*]

In 1 to 2 percent of cases, men develop pain in the area from which the nerve has been taken. If this persists, it may be necessary to operate again to reposition the cut end of the nerve. Borrowing your sural nerve will leave a small area of numbness on the top of your foot, but this does not interfere with walking or running, and shrinks over time. If we use the genitofemoral nerve for a graft, there may be a small area of numbness on your scrotum and inner thigh. Most patients don't notice this except at the time of an examination, and again, the numb area gradually gets smaller in size. Obviously, synthetic nerve grafts have the advantage of being readily available and avoiding any problems at the donor site.

[*]Modified from Edward D. Kim et al., "Interposition of Sural Nerve Restores Function of Cavernous Nerves Resected During Radical Prostatectomy," *Journal of Urology* 161, no. 1 (1999): 188–192. Reprinted with permission from Lippincott Williams & Wilkins.

NOTE: While nerve grafts mark an important step forward in reducing sexual problems after radical prostatectomy, nerve sparing—when possible—is always the better choice. Doctors should not use the possibility of a graft to justify removing nerves unnecessarily. In most cases both nerves can be safely preserved.[9]

RESULTS TODAY

The technique we currently use for modern radical prostatectomy is quite different from the nerve-sparing procedure of the early 1980s. After analyzing the long-term results of thousands of cases, we have learned how to excise the cancer completely in almost all cases, while preserving both neurovascular bundles in over 90 percent of patients. By recognizing the wide variation in prostate cancers and appreciating subtle variations in the size and shape of individual prostate glands, expert surgeons have learned to tailor the operation to each patient's anatomy and tumor.[10] We have also discovered how to minimize trauma to the **external urinary sphincter**, reducing the risk of serious, long-term urinary incontinence to 1 percent. Serious blood loss is rare today, hospital stays are as short as one to three days, and the urinary catheter is typically removed in seven to ten days. Most patients regain continence in a few days or weeks, and sexual function typically begins to return in a few weeks or months, though full recovery can take as long as two years.

The ideal outcome of radical prostatectomy is cancer cure along with recovery of normal urinary and erectile function. This is a goal that no technique (open, laparoscopic, or robotically assisted surgery) and no surgeon achieve in every case. James Eastham, the head of Urology at MSKCC, developed the concept of the "trifecta," i.e. how often, using a particular surgical technique, the operation is successful by all three measures.[11] When we first examined our results seven years ago and included all patients (average age 60), 60 percent achieved success in all three areas. For men younger than 60 with normal sexual function before surgery whose nerves were spared, 80 percent had a completely successful operation.[12] All surgeons should be dedicated to improving these results by refining their surgical techniques and meticulously measuring their outcomes.

Nevertheless, radical prostatectomy remains one of the most challenging procedures in oncology, and national results reflect the struggle that most surgeons have with this operation. Among all surgeons nationwide, positive surgical margins are reported in 25 percent of patients, serious incontinence in 8 percent, and 55 percent of men fail to recover erections.[13] The difference in outcomes between top experts and surgeons who rarely perform this operation can be enormous.[14]

LAPAROSCOPIC SURGERY— FREEHAND AND ROBOTICALLY ASSISTED

The first laparoscopic radical prostatectomy was performed in the United States in 1992, but the procedure was developed and refined in France, most particularly by Bertrand Guillonneau, a superb surgeon now at Memorial Sloan-Kettering Cancer Center. In a marvel of high-tech instrumentation, a magnifying, lighted, robotically controlled scope inserted through the navel transmits a magnified image of the surgical field to a monitor in the operating room. Despite the lack of a large "window" through the skin, the laparoscopic surgeon has an excellent view of internal structures at twelve- to fifteen-fold magnification

The abdomen is inflated with gas to make room for insertion of the surgical tools. Laparoscopic instruments are then threaded through four or five other tiny incisions, each only ¼ to ½ inch long as compared with the typical 3½-inch incision made just above the pubic bone for open prostatectomy. Because the scars are tiny, laparoscopic procedures have been dubbed "Band-Aid" surgeries. Laparoscopic prostatectomy is also referred to as "minimally invasive," though, in fact, removing the prostate requires deep invasion of the abdomen no matter what technique is used.[15]

In the United States today, most laparoscopic surgery is performed

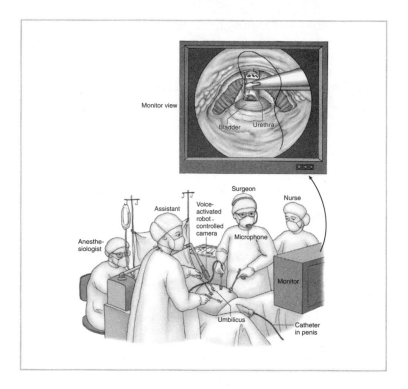

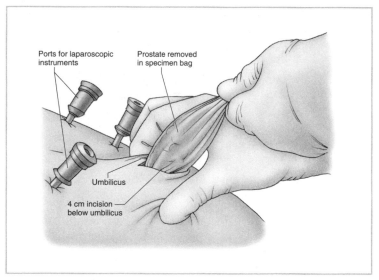

(top) Scene in the operating room during laparoscopic radical prostatectomy. Monitor view shows the urethra being sewn to the bladder after the prostate is removed. (bottom) In laparoscopic radical prostatectomy, the prostate is removed through a small incision below the belly button.

with the assistance of the **da Vinci surgical robot**, which uses computer technology to translate and stabilize the doctor's hand and finger motions, allowing control of the instruments inside the patient by remote. Theoretically, the surgeon and patient need not even be in the same room during the procedure.[16]

The surgical robot offers the advantage of magnified three-dimensional visualization. It is also much easier for surgeons to learn than freehand laparoscopy, which is technically challenging. Still, despite the growing popularity of robotically assisted prostatectomy, long-term outcomes remain to be seen As yet, we have no evidence that the tremendous expense of the robot ($1.5 to 2 million to purchase the robot plus $200,000 per year in maintenance costs) translates into improved patient care.[17]

LAPAROSCOPIC PROSTATECTOMY AND THE LEARNING CURVE

The development of laparoscopic surgery marked a major breakthrough in the treatment of certain diseases. For gallbladder disease, open surgery involved a major incision and a difficult, painful recovery. Doing this operation laparoscopically meant far less pain, a lower risk of postoperative pneumonia, and a shorter, easier convalescence. The large open scar was replaced by a tiny one with far better cosmetic results.

A number of laparoscopic procedures soon swept the surgical field. They promised less blood loss, less pain, and shorter hospital stays. In urology, kidney removal (nephrectomy) was the first procedure done using a laparoscope, and it offered a major improvement over the open operation. Everyone assumed the same would be true for radical prostatectomy for prostate cancer, but this procedure turned out to be more complicated and more difficult than kidney surgery. To remove the prostate, the surgeon must take care to avoid the rectum, the erectile nerves, and the urinary sphincter, and must reconnect the urinary tract once the gland has been excised. Early on, patients had more complications with laparoscopic surgery, and the operation took a very long time. A decade passed before laparoscopic radical prostatectomy gained wide acceptance.

During that time, surgeons changed and refined the open procedure, using smaller incisions and learning to control blood loss during the operation. Patients recovered more quickly and hospital stays were reduced. By the time robotic prostatectomy came along, the open procedure was very different than it had been ten years earlier. Open surgeons were spurred by the challenge of showing that the laparoscopic approach was not necessarily better.

Patients continue to be drawn to the laparoscopic procedure, believing that it is kinder and gentler, but the success of radical prostatectomy by any approach depends on the skill and experience of the surgeon. Thanks to the pioneering work of Dr. Bertrand Guillonneau, now director of the Minimally Invasive Surgery in Urology at Memorial Sloan-Kettering Cancer Center, we know that it is possible to achieve similar results with a laparoscopic procedure to those reported by the best open surgeons. Dr. Guillonneau has performed over 2,000 laparoscopic radical prostatectomies. Today, the results are comparable to those after open radical prostatectomy in the hands of the best experts, although recovery of urinary control is somewhat slower.[18]

But only the most skilled, experienced surgeons can achieve these results. The learning curve for radical prostatectomy is long.[19] Even with the help of a surgical robot, it takes hundreds of cases to perform the procedure well and achieve optimal cancer cure with low rates of complications and long-term side effects.[19]

Large-scale nationwide comparisons of the results of open and laparoscopic and robotic surgery confirm the shorter hospital stays (2 versus 3 days) and fewer blood transfusions with the "minimally invasive" approaches. But there were no differences in cancer cure rates or in major complication rates. Strictures (scar tissue narrowing the urethra) were more common with the open approach, but recovery of urinary control and sexual function were no better and in some cases worse after laparoscopic and robotic radical prostatectomy.[20] Today we know there is a very long learning curve for open radical prostatectomy. It takes 250 to 500 cases before the average surgeon stops improving and patients have an optimal chance of cure. Even then, there are remarkable differences between surgeons, with some experienced doctors never achieving very good results and others routinely doing so.[21] The learning curve for laparoscopic prostatectomy is even longer.[22]

COMPARING THE TECHNOLOGY

Minimally invasive surgery—done through a scope—appeals to patients because it allows surgery to be performed through small incisions, which are associated with less pain and blood loss and a faster recovery. All of these proved to be true advantages of laparoscopic tubal ligation, gallbladder, and kidney surgery. Manufacturers of the da Vinci surgical robot touted the additional advantages of 3-D vision, huge magnification, and highly flexible instruments.

But complex laparoscopic surgery is hard, requiring many years of experience. It is a bit like trying to touch a keyhole with a ten-foot pole. Freehand laparoscopic surgery allows the surgeon to feel some sense of touch (haptic feedback), but robotic surgery does not. The surgeon cannot tell how firmly he is pressing against the tissue or feel any cancerous nodule or hardening in the prostate. These limitations mattered little in the early applications, but they are highly significant in radical prostatectomy.

In this procedure, blood loss is not from the incision but from the many small vessels surrounding the prostate and seminal vesicles. Pressure from the carbon dioxide used to inflate the abdominal cavity during laparoscopic and robotic surgery keeps blood loss down. Delayed bleeding, once the pressure is relieved, has turned out to be a bigger problem than anticipated.

The loss of touch is also a problem when operating for prostate cancer. Most cancers cannot be seen within the prostate or even when they extend out microscopically into the neurovascular bundles. These cancerous nodules can be felt, guiding the surgeon to excise all malignant tissue with the open procedure. The magnified view with laparoscopic and robotic surgery is impressive, but not equivalent to direct visualization. A digital video image of a face provides less detail and clarity than sitting next to someone and looking at his face directly. Open surgeons often use magnifying loupes and a headlamp to achieve superb, detailed visualization of the intricate anatomy during radical prostatectomy.

Finally, removing the pelvic lymph nodes is a challenge with robotic surgery because the instruments are designed to operate straight ahead or below the camera, not from side to side, where the lymph nodes lie. For this reason, few robotic surgeons perform a lymph node dissection. When they do, it is often limited to the easily accessible areas, not where the malignant nodes usually lie. Vincent Laudone and his colleagues at MSKCC are committed to developing a way to perform a full lymph node dissection laparoscopically, a procedure essential for men with an intermediate or high-risk cancer.

> NOTE: The lack of supporting data has not deterred hospitals and companies marketing the surgical robot from claiming that the device offers advances in cancer control, urinary continence, and potency.

CHOOSING WHICH KIND OF SURGERY TO HAVE

Surgery is more an art than an exact science. The technique a surgeon uses matters far less than his ability and track record. You'd be wise to opt for the best surgeon rather than a particular technique (open, laparoscopic, or robotic).

Open surgery is preferable for a man with a large, high-grade cancer (stage T2b or higher, a Gleason score of 3 + 4 or greater) overlying the neurovascular bundle. The crucial decision in such cases is not whether to preserve the nerves entirely or to remove them, but whether it is feasible to dissect widely enough around the cancer without removing some or all of the nearby nerve. With magnifying loupes and a headlamp, the open surgeon can manipulate the prostate, expose the nerves, feel any cancerous nodules, and decide exactly how widely to dissect to completely remove the cancer while maintaining normal urinary function and preserving the nerves to promote the recovery of sexual function to the maximal possible extent.

For any man, I would recommend laparoscopic radical prostatectomy, whether freehand or robotically assisted, *only* if it can be performed by a highly skilled surgeon who has a great deal of experience with this procedure and is capable of achieving the same low rate of positive surgical margins, incontinence, and erectile dysfunction as the best open surgeon. While many surgeons today are performing robotically assisted laparoscopic radical prostatectomy, very few surgeons have measured their results and can demonstrate that they have mastered the approach.

If your cancer is intermediate or high-risk, removing the lymph nodes is important. Sometimes, we can cure cancers that have spread to the lymph nodes by surgery alone. Laparoscopic surgeons have developed techniques to remove lymph nodes, as have open surgeons. The inability to perform a thorough lymph node dissection is a major problem with the robotically assisted approach.

IS SURGERY RIGHT FOR YOU?

The first, and most important, decision involves whether a prostate cancer needs to be treated now or if treatment can be safely deferred. (See Chapter 13, Watchful Waiting [Active Surveillance].) I estimate that a third to a half of all cancers diagnosed today do not need to be treated immediately.

Radical prostatectomy may be the right treatment choice if your cancer shows signs of being large and palpable (stage T2b or higher) or aggressive (Gleason grade 7 or higher), or if your PSA is high or rising rapidly but you have no sign of distant spread. If you have a Gleason 6 and a PSA under 10, surgery is appropriate only if the cancer is in multiple biopsy cores and fills most of a core. We also consider a patient's age and general health. A young man, under 60, with multiple cores of Gleason 6 cancer, should probably be treated. But a man at any age found to have only one or two cores with a tiny amount (3 mm or less) of cancer in any one core can reasonably opt for active surveillance. (See Chapter 10, Understanding Your Cancer.)

For significant cancers, surgery offers an excellent chance of a cure. If the tumor is aggressive (with a Gleason score of 7 or more in the biopsy), over 80 percent of men are cured with surgery alone as long as the cancer is still confined to the prostate. If your test results raise the possibility of local spread of the cancer, radical prostatectomy may still be a good treatment option, but the surgeon will have to modify the operation to make sure all of the cancer is removed. In long-term results from my own patients and from other surgeons at Memorial Sloan-Kettering Cancer Center, 6 of 10 men whose cancer extends through the prostate into the surrounding tissue (extracapsular extension) and 1 of 3 with seminal vesicle invasion remain free of cancer recurrence ten years after surgery, if they've had the proper operation. Even 15 to 20 percent of cancers that have spread to the lymph nodes can be cured by removal of the prostate and lymph nodes.

The common suggestion that surgery is only effective for men with cancer that is confined to the prostate underestimates the real power of radical prostatectomy to stop this disease. In fact, more than 50 percent of men with a cancer that has spread locally can be cured with radical prostatectomy alone. On the other hand, in 10 percent of radical prostatectomy patients whose cancer appears to be confined, the PSA eventually rises again. The important question is not whether a man's cancer is confined to the gland but whether the tumor is *contained* in the prostate area and can be removed completely. (See illustration on page 272.)

Few men treated surgically die of their cancer. In a series of over 11,000 patients treated with radical prostatectomy, whose average age at the time of surgery was 61, the risk of death from *any* cause fifteen years later, at the average age of 76, was 33 percent. This is exactly what one would expect in any group of men, including those who never had prostate cancer. Only 12 percent of our surgery patients eventually died of prostate cancer. Even men with seminal vesicle invasion or lymph node metastases—the most aggressive tumors—had only a 23 to 29 percent risk of dying of their cancer in the next fifteen years.[23] The risk of death from cancer within fifteen years for men with low-risk cancer was only 2 percent. For intermediate risk (Gleason 7 or PSA 10 to 20) the risk of death within fifteen years was 10 percent, and for high-risk cancers (Gleason 8 to 10 or PSA greater than 20 ng/ml) the risk was 19 percent.

Radical prostatectomy is effective even for cancers that extend through the capsule of the prostate or have limited seminal vesicle invasion seen on MRI. Surgery alone, however, will not cure an extensive T3 or T4 cancer with obvious seminal vesicle invasion. Hormone therapy followed by radiation or participation in a clinical trial of new chemotherapeutic agents (see Chapter 21, Treating Advanced Prostate Cancer) may be better treatment choices.

Except in the rare case of a localized but very aggressive tumor that might spread soon and cause serious symptoms, I would not recommend radical prostatectomy for a man whose life expectancy is less than seven to ten years. Even aggressive prostate cancers tend to grow slowly enough that radiation and hormone therapy can control the disease for years. Some of the side effects of surgery are age-related. The rate of incontinence increases in men over age 70,[24] and the risk of erectile dysfunction is higher after age 60.[25] For surgery to make sense, you need to be young and healthy enough to come through the operation well and benefit from the long-term survival advantage that removing the gland may provide.

Serious medical conditions, such as active heart or lung disease, uncontrolled high blood pressure or diabetes, or a prior history of thrombophlebitis (blood clot in the legs) or pulmonary embolism (blood clot in the lungs), put you at increased risk for major surgical complications. So does the presence of urinary incontinence, which strongly predicts more serious incontinence after surgery. Diabetes, high blood pressure, smoking, and heart disease increase the incidence of postoperative erectile dysfunction. You may not be a good surgical candidate if you've had a serious adverse reaction to anesthesia during a previous operation.

PELVIC LYMPH NODES

Prostate cancers today are usually found at an early stage, when spread to the pelvic lymph nodes is uncommon, thought to occur in only 1 to 3 percent of men. Consequently, a complete pelvic lymph node dissection (removal of the nodes), which used to be a routine part of radical prostatectomy, has been abandoned by many surgeons and is often recommended only for patients with the most serious, aggressive cancers.

I believe this is a mistake. The pelvic lymph node dissection (PLND) widely performed in the United States is extremely limited and fails to remove the nodes at highest risk of containing prostate cancer cells. When a full PLND is performed, the chance of finding a positive node is 6 to 8 percent. By removing these nodes, the cancer can sometimes be cured with surgery alone. A complete PLND for prostate cancer should include all the lymph nodes in the area into which prostatic lymph fluid typically drains. The average number of nodes removed by most surgeons is 6 to 8. A full node dissection removes 12 to 20 nodes on average.

DISADVANTAGES OF SURGERY

Radical prostatectomy by any technique—open, freehand laparoscopic, or robotically assisted—is major surgery and requires a hospital stay of one to three days. Full recovery of your normal energy level can take as long as six to eight weeks, though most men can return to work and most normal activities after two to three weeks (except heavy physical labor, which should be avoided for up to six weeks).

Blood loss during this operation has been greatly reduced by modern surgical techniques.[26] Only about 2 percent of men need a blood transfusion with laparoscopic approaches compared with about 5 to 10 percent with open prostatectomy. Some patients still lose enough blood to require transfusion. This does not mean your doctor has done a bad job. In fact, doing the *best* procedure can involve more blood loss than one aimed at minimizing the need for transfusion at all costs. Clamping or cauterizing every tiny bleeder near the neurovascular bundles can increase the risk of damage to these exquisitely sensitive erectile nerves. If your surgeon believes that you may need blood during or after surgery, the blood supply in this country is so safe, it's no longer considered advantageous to bank your own. In fact, the overall risk of banking your own versus receiving blood from the blood bank are identical. There is no good evidence that blood stimulators such as erythropoietin (EPO) or epoetin alfa (Procrit) reduce the need for transfusions, except in men who are chronically anemic, and they pose some risk.

SURGICAL COMPLICATIONS

Any surgery carries a small risk of lethal complications, which can result from either the procedure itself or the anesthesia. Radical prostatectomy is no exception, though thankfully, the instance of surgically related deaths is low.[27] According to a Medicare database from the 1990s, the mortality rate for prostate cancer patients ages 65 to 79 was about 1 in 200.[28] Widespread statistics are hard to find for younger men, but reported outcomes from several Centers of Excellence worldwide suggest that for men below age 65, the risk of death from radical prostatectomy is about 1 in 1,000. The death rate for all surgical procedures in this country is about 1 in 3,000. The risk is greatest for older men and those with serious medical conditions (**comorbidities**) aside from prostate cancer. Severe complications within the first thirty days after surgery, called the **perioperative period**, are uncommon. The ones we watch for are bleeding, infection, blood clots (thrombophlebitis or pulmonary embolism), and arrhythmias (abnormal heart rhythms). Pneumonia is a concern after general anesthesia and a major reason that patients are encouraged to breathe deeply and to get up and walk as soon as possible after surgery. These complications occur in 4 or 5 percent of men with modern surgical and anesthetic techniques.

Other potential problems that may occur soon after this operation include wound infections (which affect 1 to 2 percent of patients), urinary tract infections (3 to 4 percent), and excessive bleeding (2 to 3 percent). Some men also experience urethral stricture (narrowing of the tube by scar tissue) at the site of the anastomosis (where the urethra is rejoined). Repairing a stricture may require dilation in the office or incision through a cystoscope under anesthesia.

> NOTE: On average, strictures occur in 15 percent of men, but the incidence ranges from 0 to 75 percent, depending on the skill of the surgeon.[29] This is another important reason to find an experienced—and busy (see, however, the caveat to this on page 246)—specialist to perform your radical prostatectomy.

SIDE EFFECTS OF RADICAL PROSTATECTOMY

INFERTILITY

When you have an orgasm after your prostate is removed, no seminal fluid will be released. The orgasm will be "dry," with no ejaculation. Consequently, you will no longer be able to father children through sexual intercourse. If this is an issue for you, make arrangements to bank sperm before your operation. The more you bank, the better, but you should not contribute more than once every three days or the sperm will be too dilute. Give yourself ample time to bank six to twelve deposits before surgery.

Sperm are still produced after radical prostatectomy, but, as happens after vasectomy, they are no longer released. Instead, they migrate as far as the **epididymis** (the ducts that drain the testicles), where they slowly deteriorate and are reabsorbed with no negative effects.

INCONTINENCE

Many men facing prostate cancer surgery worry about losing urinary control. Fortunately, severe, permanent incontinence is largely a thing of the past.[30] Most men are dry within a few days or weeks after the catheter is removed. (See Chapter 17, Urinary Side Effects.)

It's a good idea to bring a few absorbent pads when your catheter is removed. About half of our patients stop wearing pads after two or three days. By six weeks after surgery, 6 out of 10 patients no longer need pads for leakage. By one year, 9 out of 10 men never need them, and the other 1 out of 10 wear a pad a day at work or while engaged in intense physical activity. Only about one man in a hundred has troublesome urinary leakage a year or more after the operation serious enough to warrant medical intervention. And there are ways to correct problems that do arise. With modern treatment, men are not doomed to live with severe incontinence after radical prostatectomy.

Many doctors advocate **Kegel (pelvic floor) exercises** once the catheter is removed. Several randomized clinical trials showed better continence with regular use of these exercises,[31] but I suggest waiting to see if you quickly regain control on your own, which most men do, before starting them. You don't need to do Kegel exercises if you have no urinary leakage.

The probability of incontinence after radical prostatectomy varies. Men over 70 are at increased risk, as are those who had any stress incontinence prior to surgery. Incontinence rates are higher in patients with large cancers, whose neurovascular bundles have to be removed. Intact erectile nerves appear to play some role in urinary control. The single greatest predictor of urinary continence, however, is the skill of the surgeon performing the operation.

SEXUAL DYSFUNCTION

Along with the fear of incontinence, prostate cancer patients worry most about a loss of erections. Today, in the hands of the best surgeons, the majority of patients who were potent before surgery eventually recover erections sufficient for intercourse. As with incontinence, the outcome hinges heavily on the skill of the surgeon, not the surgical technique, so make sure you're in the best possible hands. Recovery of erectile function also depends on your age, the quality of your erections before the operation, and the preservation of erectile nerves during the operation. (See Chapter 18, Sexual Side Effects, for a full discussion.)[32]

Erections typically take longer to recover than urinary control. The average man experiences his first workable erection about four months after surgery, and erections can take two to three years to recover fully. If both nerves are spared, about 85 percent of our patients at MSKCC recover erections sufficient for intercourse, and about 55 percent say they are functioning as they were before surgery by two years after a radical prostatectomy.

After radical prostatectomy, about 10 percent of men complain of a noticeable shortening of their penis or of **Peyronie's disease**, the development of fibrous tissue that causes a curve in the erect penis. The reason for these changes is unknown, but they occur less often when both nerves are spared and when erections return early after surgery.

EJACULATION AND ORGASM AFTER SURGERY

Erection, **ejaculation**, and **orgasm** are independent—though interrelated—sexual functions. Infertility (the inability to conceive children) is not synonymous with erectile dysfunction, and a loss or lessening of erections does not mean you can no longer have sexual pleasure. Even

> NOTE: If left untreated, prostate cancer can cause erectile dysfunction and much worse, not only by growing directly into the nerves that lie close to the prostate but also by requiring further treatment—radiation or hormone therapy—that can cause loss of erections and (in the case of hormones) decreased libido as well.

men who can't have erections continue to have normal sensation in the penis and can experience orgasms, though they no longer ejaculate. (See Chapter 18, Sexual Side Effects.)

THE BOTTOM LINE

The discomfort and negative effects of radical prostatectomy are typically temporary. Disruption in your normal activities usually lasts a week or two, your energy level may be reduced for a month or two, incontinence usually resolves in a few weeks or months, and erections begin to return within the first year. Recovery is largely a matter of time, and the chances that your cancer will be cured are excellent!

CHOOSING A SURGEON

Radical prostatectomy is a delicate, complex, and technically challenging surgical procedure that should *only* be undertaken by an experienced, board-certified urologist. Ideally, you'll want to be in the hands of a surgeon who specializes in the procedure, has done it many times, still performs it routinely, works in a top-notch facility with the latest medical technology and techniques, and has a proven track record of successful results.

While the risk of fatal complications from radical prostatectomy is uniformly low, regardless of the surgeon's skill level, expertise can have a huge impact on major postoperative complications, including blood clots, pneumonia, and cardiac arrhythmias. A highly skilled surgeon knows how to reduce the risk of urethral strictures, incontinence, erectile dysfunction, and positive surgical margins.[33] The **surgical margin** is the outer surface of the tissue—that is, the very edge—of what a surgeon removes. A **positive surgical margin** means the pathologist found cancer cells right at that cut border. This can happen for two reasons: either you had a very large cancer which was sending out microscopic roots beyond the prostate that the surgeon couldn't see, or the surgeon has not taken out enough tissue to excise all the cancer. Positive margins greatly reduce the probability that the tumor has been cured and increase the risk that you'll need further treatment, such as radiation therapy, down the road.[34]

Getting to the right doctor can require homework, legwork, and persistence. Thankfully, prostate cancer is almost always slow-growing and poses no imminent threat. Once you decide to have surgery, you have ample time to evaluate surgeons carefully and make a thoughtful, considered choice. Waiting a few months to have the operation will not make a significant difference in your chance for a cure.

To start the process, you might ask your primary doctor and any specialists you see to recommend top surgeons in the field. To get the most heartfelt response, try asking whom they would go to if they had prostate cancer, or whom they would trust to operate on someone in their family.

Many men seek recommendations from family, friends, or acquaintances. It's comforting to know someone or, better yet, several people who have had a good experience with the doctor you plan to use. If you lack such contacts, you can ask the surgeon(s) you're considering for referrals to patients who might be willing to talk with you about their radical prostatectomies.

Several magazines and books publish annual lists of "best doctors" by location and specialty.[35] Generally, these selections are based on the opinion of other physicians in the field (akin to a Zagat guide for doctors). These listings can be useful, though they may be biased somewhat by issues such as familiarity or popularity, which have nothing to do with professional skill. I would not rule out a surgeon solely because he is absent from such a list, but it can be reassuring to confirm that the doctor you're considering is highly regarded by his peers.

Finding out which surgeons have a negative record can be much trickier. State medical boards keep records of complaints against physicians, but this information is generally not available to consumers. You can find out about serious disciplinary action that's been taken against a doctor by contacting the state medical board, but such records may not alert you to major infractions that occurred years ago or in another jurisdiction the doctor may have left under a cloud. Rules governing disclosure of such matters vary from state to state, and as yet there is no national registry of medical complaints or misconduct by doctors.

Because of the intricacy and complexity of radical prostatectomy, you might want to seek a physician who has a regional, national, or even international reputation as an expert in the field. Staying close to home and dealing with doctors and hospitals you know might offer a measure of comfort and ease, but getting the best available procedure with the fewest side effects will have a far greater long-term impact on your quality, and possibly quantity, of life. I'd urge you to consider carefully what price you're willing to pay to avoid some temporary inconvenience.

Be sure to interview surgeons you're considering, and check their credentials. Though it doesn't guarantee expertise, it's fair to assume that a doctor who has trained at a Center of Excellence for prostate cancer has been exposed to good surgical technique. **Board-certified** means the surgeon has achieved a level of professional training in his chosen specialty, but being a board-certified urologist does not necessarily mean that a doctor has the training and experience required to remove a prostate well. Some urologists specialize in kidney stones or benign prostatic enlargement and rarely perform prostate cancer surgery. Others have a more general practice and highly limited experience with radical prostatectomy, though given the opportunity they may be willing, or even eager, to do the procedure.

Ask how many radical prostatectomies the doctor has done and how often he does them. I'd avoid someone who performs this operation less than once a month, which is not often enough to develop or maintain a high level of skill. Twenty to fifty radical prostatectomies a year should be the minimum acceptable number, and busier, more experienced surgeons are likely to have better results.[36] Gaining competence in the modern, anatomical, nerve-sparing approach requires considerable experience and regular practice. Ideally, you should seek someone who specializes in radical prostatectomy and performs the procedure several times a week.

Few surgeons track their own results. Collecting information about the rates of positive surgical margins, incontinence, and erectile dysfunction is laborious and expensive. Outside of major medical centers, few doctors can afford the resources to collect this data. So when they are asked about side effects and surgical successes, most doctors quote statistics from textbooks or medical journals. The best physicians, whose professional reputations depend on a candid analysis of their own outcomes, carefully monitor how their patients fare and report those outcomes in respected professional journals. If you are eager to find a recognized expert, you might ask whether the doctor you're considering can steer you to papers he has published on his radical prostatectomy results.

In considering surgical outcomes, be sure you're comparing apples to apples. Some doctors define incontinence as having to wear any pads on a regular basis, while others deem a patient continent unless urinary leakage has a serious impact on quality of life.

Some surgeons are rigorous about patient follow-up, using standardized interviews and questionnaires, while others report success rates based on very limited data. It's important to know where the quoted numbers come from and how they are likely to apply to you. Is your risk of side effects greater or less than this doctor's average patient? Hearing that a surgeon's patients have an 80 percent potency rate doesn't mean much if you're destined to be in the unfortunate minority. If your cancer is large and one nerve must be removed, your chances of recovering erections can drop to less than 30 percent, depending on your age. If both nerves need to be excised, return of erectile function is virtually zero. Given that a nerve graft or grafts could increase your odds considerably, you might want to consider a doctor who does grafting when nerves must be excised.

NOTE: While it's generally true that busier surgeons have better outcomes, this is not universally the case. Some surgeons continue to do the same procedure badly, even though they do it all the time.

NOTE: Even the best reported results are not an absolute guarantee of surgical skill. Some surgeons limit their caseloads to only the most favorable patients, artificially inflating their record of good outcomes. Adequate due diligence and several credible recommendations are your best route to a good surgeon.

OPEN PERINEAL VERSUS RETROPUBIC

Ask whether the surgeon uses the more widely accepted retropubic approach or performs radical prostatectomy through the perineum, which lies between the scrotum and the rectum. Perineal prostatectomy makes it far more difficult to spare erectile nerves, to customize the procedure to suit the individual cancer, or to do a pelvic lymph node dissection (PLND). It is a more limited cancer operation than the retropubic procedure. Less tissue is removed, and the chances of a positive surgical margin are higher. Doing a lymph node dissection would require a separate incision and a second procedure.

When the risk of positive lymph nodes is more than minimal (1 percent), 13 to 15 percent of men have spread to the lymph nodes. (Visit www.MSKCC.org and search for "prostate nomograms.") If the risk of spread on the nomograms is less than 2 percent, we find positive nodes in 7 of 1,000 men and a PLND can be avoided.

OPEN VERSUS ROBOTICALLY ASSISTED SURGERY

If the doctor's approach is robotic, ask how long he's been practicing this technique and how many cases he has done. I'd be skeptical of someone who has less than several hundred of these operations under his belt. The learning curve for this very challenging procedure is long and slow. You don't want to be a guinea pig.

If you're considering a robotic or laparoscopic prostatectomy, be sure to get details about the surgeon's approach and his results. How often does he perform a pelvic lymph node dissection (PLND), and how many lymph nodes, on average, does he remove? Most robotic surgeons do not do a PLND, because it is difficult and time-consuming to perform with the robotic instruments.[37] They justify this by the apparent low incidence of positive nodes, but we can cure prostate cancer in 15 to 20 percent of men with positive lymph nodes by removing these nodes during surgery. With the open procedure, a thorough PLND is easy to perform, adds only about 45 minutes to the operation, and should certainly be done in anyone other than men with favorable, low-risk prostate cancers.

Ask how long the operation typically takes. What is the surgeon's rate of positive surgical margins, bowel injuries, serious bleeding, and internal urinary leakage? How often do his patients need to return to the hospital or have further surgery to deal with complications? How quickly do they regain erections and urinary continence? You'll want to find a surgeon who can offer outcomes at least as good as you could expect with an open procedure, which has a longer, stronger track record.

Be leery of the surgeon who shows you a table of results comparing his unpublished claims against other surgeons' results that have been published in medical journals. It takes years to accumulate data on large numbers of patients to get an accurate picture of outcomes, and published medical reports are subject to the scrutiny of other doctors, while an individual doctor's own unpublished results can not really be verified.

I'd be skeptical of anyone who dodges questions about his results. Doctors are ethically bound to keep careful records about new procedures like robotic radical prostatectomy. If the program is too new to have statistics about recovery of erections, which can take years, the doctor should be able to tell you about his rates of urinary continence and positive surgical margins, which are available soon after each man's operation. Finally, you might ask if he would choose his robotic procedure over open surgery for himself or his close family.

Do age, obesity, the size of the prostate gland, or serious other health (comorbid) conditions affect whether you're better off with one approach than another? We used to believe that laparoscopic prostatectomy was less risky than open surgery for older, sicker patients, but studies have found no real difference in the complication rates between these procedures based on age, serious medical problems, body weight, or the size of the prostate.[38] The same things that make open surgery difficult are true for the robotically assisted or freehand laparoscopic procedure. In general, with larger, more serious cancers, we favor the open procedure, but the right operation can be done with any of the techniques.

Open prostatectomy can be done under spinal, epidural, or general anesthesia. Laparoscopic surgery requires general anesthesia because the abdomen is filled with carbon dioxide, the patient is tipped down, and breathing is difficult, so patients have to be placed on a ventilator.

Be aware that surgeons and hospitals can be highly susceptible to marketplace issues. When a new approach like robotic radical prostatectomy comes along, there's pressure to offer the procedure in response to patient demand. To get a new program up and running, and because of the high cost of equipment, doctors and hospitals may place an overly optimistic spin on results.[39]

NOTE: In three years of comparing the results of open and laparoscopic surgery in the hands of top experts at Memorial Sloan-Kettering Cancer Center, we found that the rates of positive surgical margins and recovery of erectile function were similar for both procedures. Recovery of urinary continence was a bit slower for laparoscopic surgery and fewer men reported complete continence without the need for any pads. With strict attention to detail, these results may improve as surgical margin rates did.[40]

NOTE: In the final analysis, the quality of the surgical procedure is the most critical issue, and this depends on the quality of the surgeon. Shop for the *surgeon,* not the approach. In the best hands, freehand laparoscopic, robotically assisted and open surgery can offer excellent results.

NERVE SPARING

You'll want to know whether you're a good candidate for nerve-sparing surgery and how often the surgeon you're considering actually spares the erectile nerves. If your cancer is advanced, extending to a nerve, does he offer nerve grafts when these nerves must be removed to cure the cancer? Even if sexual potency is not an issue for you, nerve-sparing surgery can help you recover urinary continence.

Some surgeons always remove the nerves on the side of a positive biopsy, especially if the Gleason score is 7 or more. Others never remove the nerves and recommend radiation therapy later if the surgical margins turn out to be positive. I would avoid anyone who espouses either of these all-or-nothing approaches. What you want is a surgeon whose guiding principle is to remove the cancer completely with the least damage to the erectile nerves. Today it's rarely necessary to excise the nerve completely in order to get around a cancer.

PREPARING FOR SURGERY

It's generally wise, though not mandatory, to wait about six weeks after your biopsy for the prostate area to heal before having surgery. While you may be understandably anxious to get rid of the cancer quickly and put the operation behind you, the delay will not endanger your life or reduce your chance for a cure.

It's important to stay as active as possible before radical prostatectomy. Being in good shape facilitates recovery, so exercise is valuable. If you've been involved in a regular fitness program, keep it up. If not, get the go-ahead from your doctor, and then try to get more physical activity in the weeks before surgery.

Maintaining a healthy weight is always desirable, but I don't recommend crash diets to slim down or beef up before the operation. Dietary imbalances can have a negative effect on healing, so you don't want to be depleted of essential nutrients. Strive to maintain a normal, well-balanced diet, but don't make drastic changes. If you're overweight, you can aim for a moderate reduction in your overall caloric intake and increase your exercise with the goal of losing about a pound a week.

Be sure to tell your surgeon and anesthesiologist about any medications you're taking. This includes over-the-counter drugs, nutritional supplements, and herbal, homeopathic, and so-called "natural" remedies. A recent study found that some seemingly innocent substances, including vitamin E and saw palmetto, may interfere with commonly used anesthetics and increase the risk of operative bleeding.[41]

You'll be told to stop taking vitamin E and anything containing aspirin ten days before the operation. Blood platelets take ten days to turn over, and if you use these substances, every platelet in your body becomes less sticky and takes longer to coagulate. This increases your risk for serious bleeding during and after surgery. Forty-eight hours before the operation, stop taking nonsteroidal anti–inflammatory agents (NSAIDs), such as ibuprofen (Advil, Motrin) or naproxen (Aleve).

Make sure your surgeon knows about any previous surgery or major injury you've had to the penis, prostate, or pelvic area—including a hernia operation, appendectomy, bladder, colon, or rectal surgery, or a penile prosthesis. Scarring and fibrosis from such operations or injuries, even if they happened long ago, could make a radical prostatectomy more difficult. This may not be a contraindication to surgery, but you don't want your doctor to be surprised.

The same holds true for minor procedures. Tell your doctor if you've ever had a Foley catheter placed in your penis, or if you had surgery for hypospadias (small penile opening) as a little boy. Also, indicate if you've had gonorrhea or other sexually transmitted diseases. Any of these could increase the chance that you have a urethral stricture. If the surgeon is aware of this, he can arrange to view the area with a cystoscope and dilate or treat any stricture that exists (which can hinder the return of urinary continence after surgery).

Radiation effects last a lifetime, so be sure your surgeon knows about radiation treatments you have had to the pelvic area for any reason, no matter how long ago. Irradiated tissue could substantially increase the difficulty of the procedure and slow the healing process.

Banking your own blood before an operation (autologous donation) was frequently recommended in the past, but in the last five years, blood loss from the operation has decreased and blood from the bank has proven just as safe as banking your own. If your surgeon recommends it anyway, then follow his advice. You may not be able to bank your own blood if you have active hepatitis or other infectious conditions, or if you are anemic or have a cardiovascular problem that could be worsened by anemia. Blood banked by patients for their own use is discarded if transfusion proves unnecessary. If you're unable to give blood, you may want to ask friends or relatives to donate for you. If you don't need blood that's been banked in your name (directed donation), it will be used for somebody else. There is always a chronic shortage and critical need.

The day before radical prostatectomy, most patients are put on a clear liquid diet. You will probably be told to take a self-administered Fleet enema at home on the night before surgery. It's not necessary to go through rigorous bowel preparation involving strong laxatives and multiple enemas, because bowel injuries are so rare nowadays. They occur in less than 1 percent of patients, and when they do, they can be closed uneventfully and treated with antibiotics to prevent infection.

For the two weeks before surgery, keep alcohol intake to no more than one to two glasses of wine (or the equivalent) per day. Heavy alcohol ingestion makes you relatively resistant to the effects of some anesthetic agents and pain medications. It's essential to stop smoking two weeks before the operation. Smoking is associated with a substantially increased risk of pneumonia, partial lung collapse, and prolonged coughing, which can be painful postoperatively.

Typically, preoperative testing will include a blood hemoglobin test (to anticipate your need for a blood transfusion) and a urinalysis (to make sure you don't have an active urinary tract infection). Other blood levels will be checked if you're taking medications for conditions such as high blood pressure or diabetes. The specific tests you get will depend on your age, general health, and the kind of anesthesia your doctor uses. If you're scheduled to have spinal or epidural anesthesia, pre-op tests will include coagulation studies and a careful history of any bleeding problems. If you're over 50, you'll probably have a chest X-ray and electrocardiogram. The exam will also include a careful medical history, and you will be asked to sign an informed consent giving permission for the surgery. These forms tend to detail every conceivable dire possibility, no matter how improbable or rare, so they can be frightening. (If you read the package insert that comes with any over-the-counter drug, including aspirin, you'd find similarly hair-raising worst-case scenarios.)

Try to get a good night's sleep before your operation so you don't feel sleep-deprived. On the night after surgery, a nurse will awaken you every two to four hours to check vital signs and make sure you're doing well.

Note: Clinical trials to understand the causes and cures of prostate cancer depend on the good will of patients with the disease. Your doctor may ask for permission to save your tissues for use in future research. I would encourage you to cooperate. This usually involves no change in normal testing or treatment, but could make a tremendous difference to future generations and help us to understand this disease.

THE OPERATION

Typically, you'll be admitted to the hospital on the day of your surgery. You should not eat or drink anything within six hours of your operation. Anything in your stomach can cause vomiting and aspiration when you are given anesthesia. If you're taking medications for high blood pressure, diabetes, heart disease, or other serious medical problems, be sure to ask your doctor or anesthesiologist whether you should continue them on the morning of your operation. Some medicines should be stopped (e.g., drugs to treat diabetes can drastically lower your blood sugar if you are not eating), while others, such as medicines for a heart arrhythmia, should be continued.

Make sure to see your surgeon briefly before the operation. It's comforting to know that the doctor you've chosen is actually there. Also, it's important to make sure that you are properly identified and scheduled for the right procedure. Serious mistakes happen rarely, but extra vigilance can help to ensure that they won't happen to you.

Be aware that a good anesthesiologist is as important as the surgeon in ensuring a safe, smooth operation. You should have your surgeon's reassurance about the anesthesiologist who is going to take care of you. If you meet an anesthesiologist as part of your pre-op checkup, it's not likely to be the same person who will be with you during surgery. Most anesthesiologists work in groups and rotate in the operating room, but you can seek your surgeon's recommendation and request a particular doctor. Ask if your surgeon would be comfortable using this particular anesthesiologist personally or for close family. Most patients put a great deal more stock in choosing the person who will perform the operation than the one in charge of anesthesia, but, in fact, the anesthesiologist, not the surgeon, has the responsibility for vital functions that could be a matter of life and death.

Radical prostatectomy can take anywhere from one and a half hours to as long as five, depending on the surgeon's technique, your anatomy, and the nature of your cancer. A pelvic lymph node dissection adds time to the procedure, but it can also provide valuable information for planning future treatments if they prove necessary in your case. Patients tend to presume that a longer procedure is undesirable, but that is not necessarily the case. Modern radical prostatectomy is more like brain surgery than traditional urology: the erectile nerves must be handled with exquisite delicacy, and that requires cautious deliberation, not speed. The procedure should take as long as necessary to ensure optimal results.

NOTE: Anesthesia for open radical prostatectomy can be general, spinal, epidural, or a combination. All are safe and effective. I'd advise that you go along with the protocol regularly used by your surgical team. They'll be most adept at what they do routinely. For laparoscopic and robotic surgery, general anesthesia is essential to control the pain caused by the gas used to distend the abdomen to allow introduction of the surgical tools. Also, the head-down position required to perform these techniques requires a breathing tube, so regional or local anesthesia would not be adequate.

DURING OPEN SURGERY

I begin by making a 3½-inch vertical incision in the abdomen, starting just above the pubic bone to a point about two thirds of the way to the belly button. A surgical retractor holds the tissues apart, allowing a good view of the bladder and the pelvic lymph nodes. At this point, I remove the nodes in the prostate drainage area to check for spread of the cancer if diagnostic signs point to that possibility. There are thousands of lymph nodes in the body, so you won't miss these few, and removing these nodes rarely causes swelling or other side effects.

The next step is to isolate the prostate from surrounding tissues, taking care to dissect widely enough to excise all the cancer and leave no malignant cells at the edge (surgical margin) of what is removed. On the top of the prostate, covering the urethra, is a group of blood vessels that must be controlled, tied off and divided to expose the urethra. This is the first delicate step of the operation, where the surgeon's judgment is extremely important. The surgery must be tailored to each patient's unique anatomy and the nature of the cancer. In 1 of every 4 patients today, the largest area of cancer lies just under these blood vessels. Cutting too close can risk positive surgical margin, cutting too far away can impair recovery of urinary continence.

Once these blood vessels are divided, I can see the urethra and the neurovascular bundles and determine where I must dissect to get safely around the cancer, while preserving the erectile nerves to the maximum possible extent. First, I tease the nerves away from the prostate near the apex or tip of the gland, divide the urethra, and then tease the nerves away from the prostate all the way to the base or top. Next, I remove the prostate and the entire seminal vesicles, and reconnect the bladder to the cut end of the urethra.

NOTE: **Shortcut Prostatectomy.** Some surgeons believe that it's adequate to remove the prostate, leaving the seminal vesicles and the pelvic lymph nodes in place. They focus on speed and convenience, rather than maximal cancer control. I would be wary of this simplistic approach, which may be easier for the surgeon but will too often leave cancer behind, saddling the patient with the need for radiation or hormone therapy and the side effects of these treatments later on. If your cancer is so minimal that the surgeon would contemplate shortcut surgery, you should seriously consider watchful waiting instead of surgery.

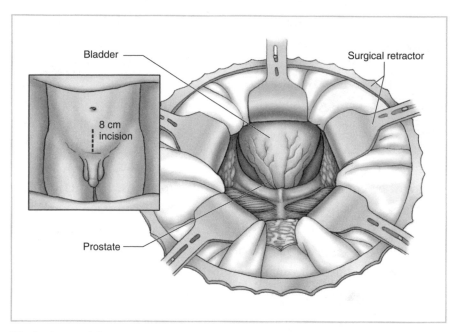

The incision used for open radical prostatectomy and the exposure of the bladder and prostate as seen by the surgeon. A surgical retractor holds the incision open.

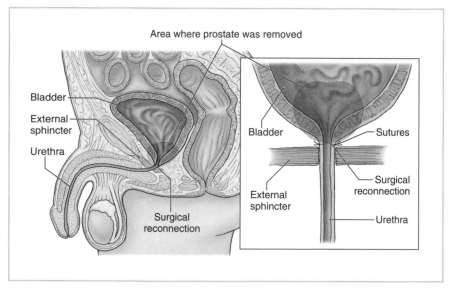

After a radical prostatectomy, the bladder is brought down and reconnected to the urethra just above the external urinary sphincter.

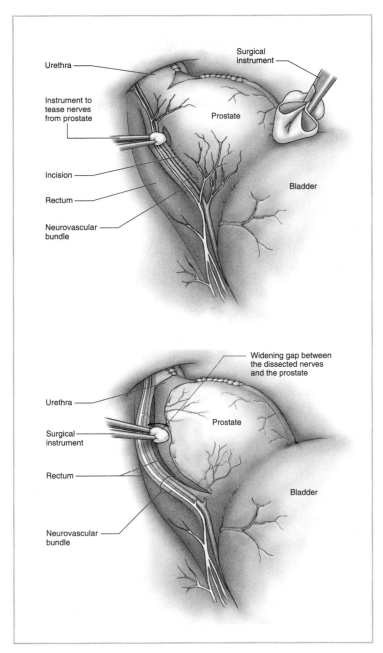

View of the surgical field from the perspective of the surgeon. The feet are at the top of the field, and the head at the bottom. The surgical technique for dissecting the neurovascular bundles (NVB) away from the prostate is the most delicate phase of the operation, where the surgeon must dissect widely enough to completely remove the prostate and the cancer without damaging the erectile nerves in the neurovascular bundle.

Done properly, the removal of the seminal vesicles does not increase the risk of incontinence or erectile dysfunction. Since 5 to 10 percent of patients have seminal vesicle invasion and more have extension of cancer cells around the seminal vesicles, these sacks should always be removed. Some surgeons mistakenly believe they need to preserve the bladder neck to retain urinary control. But in fact, continence does not depend on sparing the bladder neck. It's far more crucial to divide the bladder neck well away from the prostate to avoid leaving cancer cells (or normal prostate tissue that could later grow or develop cancer) behind.

If I'm concerned that one or both neurovascular bundles have been damaged, I use a neurostimulator called the CaverMap to be sure they are functional and intact. If they aren't, or if I've had to remove one or both nerves to control the cancer, I do a nerve graft.

I then make sure the new end-to-end connection (anastomosis) between the urethra and bladder is watertight. Next, I insert the urethral catheter. A balloon the size of a large marble in the bladder holds the catheter in place until the urethra heals around it. Finally, I close the wound with internal absorbable sutures that do not need to be removed.

DURING LAPAROSCOPIC SURGERY

The surgeon begins by placing a needle just below the belly button to fill the abdominal cavity with carbon dioxide. The gas is used to distend the abdomen, so the surgeon can see and work around the internal organs.[42]

The patient is in a head-down position, so the intestines move into the upper abdomen, away from pelvic organs. Next, the surgeon inserts ports (tubes), through which the operation is performed. The largest is a 3- to 4-cm incision made just below the belly button. Three to five additional puncture sites are made on the left and right side to allow surgical instruments to be inserted.

A camera placed through the largest port site below the belly button projects onto multiple screens in the operating room, which the surgeon and assistants use to view the procedure as they work. First, the surgeon divides the lining of the abdominal cavity over the tips of the seminal vesicles beneath the bladder. The seminal vesicles are freed from the surrounding tissue, and the surgeon then dissects between the bladder and the pubic bone, dropping the bladder out of the way as he works on the front of the gland. Next, the prostate is divided from the bladder, and the seminal vesicles, previously freed, are grasped. Working from the top of the prostate (base) toward the bottom (**apex**), the surgeon gains control of the large blood vessels, dividing them from the prostate to expose the neurovascular bundles. These bundles are teased away from the prostate all the way to the apex at the tip. Finally, the surgeon divides the blood vessels in front of the prostate, divides the urethra, and sets the prostate to the side to be removed later. The final step is to reconnect the bladder neck to the urethra and insert a catheter into the bladder. The prostate is then placed in a plastic bag and pulled out through the 3- to 4-cm incision. (See illustration on page 282.)

Robotic prostatectomy is a variation on the laparoscopic procedure. The difference is that the surgeon sits at a console and controls movement of the laparoscopic instruments through the robot.

AFTER SURGERY: COMMON PROBLEMS, REMOVING THE CATHETER, RECOVERING

Whether the surgery was open, laparoscopic, or robotic, you'll remain in the recovery room for a few hours after the operation, where you'll be monitored closely to make sure that you recover fully from the anesthesia and that your blood pressure is stable, your breathing and heart rate are regular, and you show no sign of bleeding. Hospital policy varies, but close family can usually visit with you briefly while you're in recovery.

You should expect to awaken from the operation without severe pain. Most hospitals today have a pain management service, which sets the standards for postoperative pain control. The goal is to avoid severe pain while still keeping you alert. Overmedication can lower your blood pressure, reduce your respiratory rate, increase the risk of postsurgical complications, and make it harder for you to get up and around (which is important for healing). This does *not* mean you have to suffer a lot of discomfort. Patients do better and return to normal activities sooner when postsurgical pain is well controlled.

Pain tolerance and perception vary widely. Some men experience little or no pain after radical prostatectomy, while others require more pain relief. Today, **patient–controlled analgesia (PCA)** is common. By pressing a button, you can administer exactly the amount of pain medicine you need. Studies have shown that patients actually require less medication with these systems, and there is no risk of accidental overdose. Many surgeons prefer to prescribe powerful anti-inflammatory drugs such as ketorolac (Toradol), which also acts as an effective, non-narcotic pain reliever.

From recovery, you'll be sent to your room. Most men are awake and alert the evening of the operation. A family member or close friend can stay with you if you like and if the facility allows. Having somebody around to help you do simple things, like reach for the water, can be reassuring at first, and I encourage this. Rarely would your medical condition warrant a full-time, private-duty nurse.

As soon as possible after the procedure, hospital personnel will get you to sit up on the side of the bed and, shortly afterward, in a chair. Depending on the time of your operation, this could happen later the same day or the following morning. This may seem difficult at first, but it's important. Pain medication will help reduce any serious discomfort. Be sure to tell your doctor if you're not getting sufficient relief.

The day after surgery, most men no longer need any strong injectable narcotic pain medication. Powerful oral analgesics like acetaminophen with hydrocodone (Vicodin or Percocet) are usually sufficient for the next few days.

Your intravenous line will stay in for a day or two, until you're able to take liquids and solid foods. You'll have one or two small plastic drains in the side(s) of your abdomen until the wound drainage decreases, to avoid the accumulation of fluid that could become infected. You may also have compression boots or elastic stockings on your legs to encourage blood circulation and reduce the risk of clots, though the best prevention is leg exercise and walking. I leave the urethral catheter in for eight to ten days, until the new connection between the bladder and urethra is well healed.

You may have a few strips of sterile tape across the incision, and a gauze dressing for the first day or two to catch any seepage. If your doctor uses metal clips or conventional stitches instead of absorbable sutures, you'll need to have them removed about a week after surgery.

The morning after the operation, you should be up and about, able to walk the halls with little support or assistance. Physical activity will lower the risk of blood clots and pneumonia and help you to recover intestinal function. To prevent blood clots, it's important to keep the circulation moving in your legs. Avoid standing still for more than a few minutes, and keep your feet elevated when you sit. The more you move around, the sooner you'll be able to eat, pass gas, and have a bowel movement— all part of normal recovery.

You can start most regular oral medications the evening of or the morning after surgery, but some drugs are best avoided at first. Your blood pressure will likely be lowered by bed rest in the hospital, so blood pressure medication should not be necessary for the first couple of days. If you take aspirin regularly to prevent heart disease, you can start this again by the second or third day after surgery.

Once your lines are out (except the catheter), there's no danger in showering. Soap, water, and exposure to air will help the wound to heal. A tub bath, which could allow water to seep in and increase the risk of infection, is *not* recommended until after the catheter is removed.

Generally, it takes four to five days after surgery to have a bowel movement and a week to ten days to regain your normal regularity. I recommend a stool softener such as Colace for six weeks after the operation. If you're constipated, don't hesitate to take a mild laxative such as Dulcolax or milk of magnesia at bedtime until your bowel movements are regular. Because a prostatectomy is performed in close proximity to the rectal wall, you shouldn't take an enema for three weeks after surgery, but suppositories are safe. In any event, avoid straining at stool, which exerts pressure on the wound and could increase your risk of a pulmonary embolism.

Early activity soon after the operation is not dangerous. Given modern wound-closure techniques, you needn't worry about pulling out your sutures or tearing the incision. I discovered one of my patients, a marathon runner, running up and down twelve flights of stairs in the hospital two days after surgery without doing himself any harm (though I didn't and wouldn't recommend this). Moderate exertion and regular activity, like climbing stairs or walking a few miles, are not risky after the surgery and are likely to be beneficial. The only things you'll need to avoid are extreme abdominal straining and dangerous physical activities, like playing tackle football or mountain climbing, for at least three to six weeks after the operation. You should not drive until the catheter is out, you are off all strong analgesics such as Percodan, Percocet, and Vicodin, and you have no pain that would limit your ability to move your legs or react quickly. If you need to fly soon after surgery, remember to drink a lot of fluids, avoid dehydrating substances such as caffeine and alcohol, walk around frequently during the flight, and keep your legs elevated when you sit. Short of these restrictions, regular activity is good for you once all your tubes have been removed.

Walking is good exercise while the catheter is in place. During the day, you'll attach the catheter to a small leg bag, which won't be noticeable under loose-fitting trousers.

The catheter requires some care and attention. Twice a day, clean the tip of the penis with soap and water. Half-strength hydrogen peroxide diluted with water can remove any crusting or blood. Placing a lubricant like bacitracin or K-Y Jelly around the penile opening (**meatus**) will keep the skin lubricated and reduce irritation.

It's not unusual or dangerous to have some blood pass around the catheter or in the urine. Small blood clots in the catheter bag are perfectly normal and nothing to worry about. If you see clots, or if your urine looks dark or cloudy, increase your fluid intake until the urine returns to normal.

Some patients experience bladder spasms, typically caused by irritation from the balloon in the bladder, which holds the catheter in place. But a spasm could also mean that the catheter is twisted or blocked. To keep the tubing straight, it's useful to anchor the tube loosely to your leg with a Velcro strap or a piece of tape. Bladder spasms that persist can be treated with anticholinergic medications, such as long-acting tolterodine (Detrol LA) or oxybutynin (Ditropan), after a blockage has been ruled out.

At night, be sure to switch to a large drainage bag. The volume of

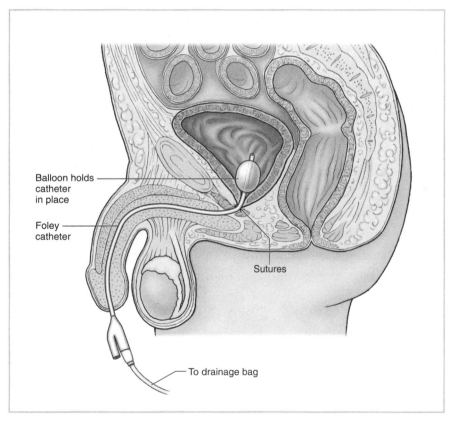

A urethral catheter through the urethra is held in place by a balloon in the bladder. The catheter allows the urine to drain into a drainage bag until the reconnection heals.

urine will be too much for a small leg bag to accommodate, and the urine will back up, causing a distended bladder, painful urinary retention, and a greater risk of urinary tract infection.

COMMON PROBLEMS AFTER SURGERY

IN THE TESTICLES

Some men have pain or aching in their testicles after the operation. This can last for four to six weeks or, in rare cases, a few months. Often, testicular pain will respond well to anti-inflammatory medicines such as ibuprofen (Motrin) or to scrotal support with a loose jockstrap. Some men also find soaking in a hot tub bath helpful, which is fine once the catheter is removed. Most often, this discomfort goes away on its own. Rarely, it's a bona fide infection, requiring antibiotics. Signs of infection include increasing swelling and pain, exquisite tenderness, and fever.

IN THE PENIS AND SCROTUM

Swelling and discoloration of the skin over the penis and scrotum are common after radical prostatectomy. While alarming, this is usually caused by a harmless accumulation of wound fluid that makes its way by gravity to the lowest point—the genitalia. Mild swelling can be relieved by elevating the area with a rolled washcloth under the scrotum while sitting or lying in bed and by the use of a loose scrotal support or jockey shorts when standing. Severe scrotal or penile swelling is fairly uncommon and usually results from excess intravenous fluids you were given during and right after the operation to increase blood volume and reduce the need for blood transfusions.

WEIGHT GAIN

While most patients weigh a few pounds more the day after surgery, some gain ten, fifteen, or even twenty pounds of fluid weight. This excess salt water, administered intravenously to keep you hydrated during the operation, can show up as swelling in your genitals, feet, and ankles. Since gravity carries fluid to the lowest point, the swelling often increases on the second or third day as you spend more time up and about. I ask my patients to weigh themselves every day while they're in the hospital. If I detect troublesome swelling and a man's weight is up ten pounds or more compared with his preoperative level, I'll recommend a daily diuretic such as furosemide (Lasix), which promotes the excretion of water. If you need a diuretic for more than 2 or 3 days, you may need to replace potassium, which is essential for heart rhythm and is washed out by most diuretics. Because of the fluid weight gain and abdominal soreness from the incision, be sure to bring boxer shorts and sweatpants or other loose-fitting pants without a belt or zipper to wear home from the hospital.

REMOVING THE CATHETER

Many men dread having the catheter removed, imagining a painful trauma. In fact, it's a simple maneuver, usually done in the nurse's office, and most men are so tired of the catheter that having it out is a tremendous relief. I ask patients to start a short course of antibiotics the day before to reduce the risk of a urinary tract infection. An effective way to take out the catheter and immediately test whether a patient can urinate is called a fill-pull-flow test. The nurse fills the bladder with water through the catheter until you feel the need to urinate, the balloon holding the catheter in place is deflated, and the catheter slides out while you are standing. Then you void into a container, so the nurse can measure how much you have eliminated.

Bring a pad along to wear home. Most men experience some leakage at first. Small absorptive pads such as Depend Guards for Men are available at most drugstores.

RECOVERING

ACTIVITY

It's important to keep active after you go home from the hospital. For the first two to three weeks, get up every hour or so to walk and keep the circulation flowing in your legs. Being active will help you heal and regain a normal energy level sooner.

That said, you are likely to feel some fatigue, which will worsen late in the day. Get the extra rest you need, and take a nap in the afternoon, if necessary.

DIET

You can eat a normal diet, but try to get extra iron from foods such as beef and spinach for the first few weeks to make up for any blood loss during surgery. Iron supplements can make you constipated, so I rarely recommend them unless a man has a measured iron deficiency.

THE PATHOLOGY REPORT: WAS THE CANCER CURED?

THE SURGICAL PATHOLOGY REPORT

A pathologist will examine the tissue removed during surgery, and you should have the report within a week or two. One of the advantages of removing the gland is that we can get more detailed and accurate information about the nature of your cancer. One third of the time the Gleason grade in the surgical specimen turns out to be higher than it appeared to be on biopsy. In 5 percent of cases, the grade is lower. In some instances, a tiny focus of more serious cancer is found.

The key thing to learn from the pathology report is your final Gleason score. After surgery, the Gleason score will be reported as a single number between 6 and 10. This represents the Gleason patterns of the two most common tumor cells present, not necessarily the worst ones. It's important to know whether the pathologist found any poorly differentiated tissue (Gleason pattern 4 or 5) in the gland. If such aggressive elements were found, you should ask about their size and extent.

From the pathology report, you can also learn whether your cancer was confined to the prostate. If you had extracapsular extension, was

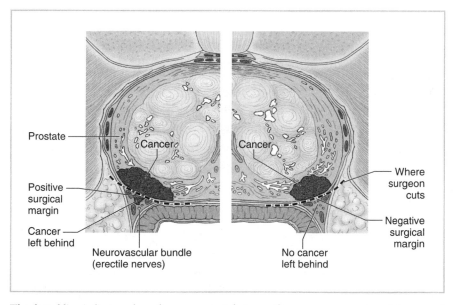

The dotted line indicates where the surgeon cuts between the cancerous prostate and the normal tissue. In the panel on the left, the margin is too close to the prostate, so cancer cells may have been left behind (positive surgical margin).

it focal (small) or established (more than two microscopic high-power fields)? Was there seminal vesicle invasion? If so, did this grow directly from the prostate tumor—as happens in 80 percent of cases—or did you have a microscopic amount of cancer in the seminal vesicles that grew separately and has a more favorable prognosis? Did the cancer spread to the lymph nodes? If so, how many were involved? How many were removed? Did the cancer grow through the capsule of the lymph nodes (extranodal), or was it contained? Was there a positive surgical margin, and if so, how many, and where were they located? A positive margin means that some cancer may have been left behind, and you may need further treatment to cure the disease.

All of these factors will determine whether you need further treatment and, if so, what kind. By plugging the specifics into our postoperative nomogram (decision-making tool), you can estimate your prognosis. (Nomograms are available online at www.MSKCC.org. Search for "prostate nomograms.")

PSA TESTING AFTER SURGERY

Six to eight weeks after surgery, you should have your PSA level checked. If the cancer has been completely removed, the PSA will be *undetectable*. Since it is impossible to measure zero PSA, the laboratory will report your PSA level as "less than" some very low level. This is less than 0.05 in our laboratory at Memorial Sloan-Kettering Cancer Center, though other labs count less than 0.1 as undetectable. Some labs use ultrasensitive PSA assays that measure as little as 0.001 ng/ml, but at such low levels, some men will have false positive results that can be anxiety-provoking and may not indicate the presence of cancer. Such low levels should be interpreted cautiously unless the test is repeated and the PSA is definitely rising on two or three subsequent occasions. A detectable and rising PSA after the operation is a sign that cancer is still present or that normal prostate tissue has been left behind, and further treatment may be indicated (see Adjuvant Therapy on page 321).

If the PSA is undetectable, you should have your level measured every six months for the first five years, and then annually for the rest of your life, as long as you are healthy and further treatment would be indicated if the PSA rises. I see patients every six months for a checkup during the first year and annually after that. Further tests, such as bone scans, are not necessary unless your PSA rises. (See Chapter 20, Rising PSA After Surgery, Radiation, or Other Therapy.)

ADJUVANT THERAPY: WILL YOU NEED ANY OTHER TREATMENT?

Adjuvant therapy is defined as additional treatment required because you are at high risk for cancer recurrence, though no clear evidence exists that some tumor remains. Deciding whether you should have such treatment depends on a careful analysis of the potential benefits weighed against the risk of side effects from the treatment.

The most common form of adjuvant therapy after surgery is external beam radiation. Hormone therapy is rarely recommended as an adjuvant, as long as the PSA is undetectable, despite some studies that suggest that men with lymph node metastases may live longer with immediate hormone therapy after surgery. Those studies were done before the era when PSA testing was widely available. Since some men with spread to the lymph nodes will never develop a rising PSA after surgery, we recommend waiting to use hormone therapy until the PSA is measurable and rising rapidly. (See Chapter 20, Rising PSA After Surgery, Radiation, or Other Therapy.)

Bicalutamide (Casodex), a drug that inhibits the action of male hormones, has been shown to delay progression of the disease, and studies are under way to determine whether that will translate into a prolonged survival advantage. I would be cautious for now, since this drug actually shortened survival in a study of watchful waiting patients. We do not routinely use bicalutamide after surgery, regardless of the risk of recurrence.

Chemotherapy, which is commonly used after surgery for breast cancer, is not a standard part of therapy for prostate cancer after radical prostatectomy. However, studies are under way to examine the role of chemotherapy in combination with hormone therapy before radical prostatectomy in patients with very high-risk cancers. This is called neoadjuvant therapy. If you have a very high-risk cancer (Gleason score 8 to 10, and clinical stage T3, and a PSA well over 10) you may want to ask your doctor if you are eligible for such a clinical trial. Generally, this would apply to men whose probability of recurrence is greater than 40 percent on the preoperative nomogram. (For more on the preoperative nomogram, visit www.MSKCC.org and search for "prostate nomograms.")

Adjuvant External Beam Radiation

For men with positive surgical margins, extracapsular extension, or seminal vesicle invasion, routine adjuvant radiation therapy reduces the risk of recurrent cancer after radical prostatectomy. And the chances of dying from prostate cancer.[43]

Why, then, don't we recommend adjuvant radiation for all men found to have extracapsular extension, seminal vesicle invasion, or positive margins after surgery? Both of the randomized, controlled trials that proved the benefit of routine postoperative adjuvant radiation were conducted before the era of routine use of PSA, so the patients who did not receive radiation had no treatment for a rising PSA until relatively late in the course of their disease. Unless radiation is given before the PSA level reaches 2 ng/ml, it is unlikely to help. Early radiation, given to men with a rising PSA after surgery, is highly likely to reduce the PSA to undetectable levels if started before the PSA reaches 0.5 ng/ml, regardless of the Gleason grade or local extent of the cancer or the rate of rise of PSA. PSA is such a sensitive indicator of recurrent cancer that most doctors still recommend waiting to give radiation, even in men with high-risk cancers, until the PSA begins to rise. (See Chapter 20, Rising PSA After Surgery, Radiation, or Other Therapy.)

If you have positive surgical margins, adjuvant radiation therapy may still make sense even if your PSA is undetectable. In an important analysis of the European study of adjuvant radiation therapy, men with positive margins benefited, but those who had negative surgical margins with extracapsular extension or seminal vesicle invasion did not.[45]

I turn to the postoperative nomogram to determine the risk of recurrence without adjuvant radiation. If the surgical margins are positive and the risk of recurrence is greater than 30 to 40 percent, early radiation makes sense rather than waiting for the PSA to rise. (For more on nomograms, visit www.MSKCC.org and search for "prostate nomograms.")

Adjuvant radiation normally begins three to six months after the operation, when the incision has healed and you've regained urinary control. If return of urinary continence takes longer, therapy can be delayed until nine months to a year after surgery. Because the treatment is meant to eradicate microscopic clusters of cancer cells rather than a large tumor, a low radiation dose of 70 Gy (see Chapter 15, Radiation Therapy, and page 327 for a full discussion) is delivered to the prostate area, and only in some cases to the area of the pelvic lymph nodes. It is not usually necessary to give hormone therapy along with radiation in this situation unless there is a large amount of cancer left behind.

THE FUTURE

While current results with robotic surgery are no different from results with laparoscopic or open surgery, in the future, if the technology improves, the surgical robot could offer exciting new ways to improve this operation that would be more difficult with the open technique. One possibility is the "glowing margins" project, in which the cancer could be illuminated with a special chemical. The edge of the tumor would then glow when excited by a laser. This approach could make it easier to remove the cancer and the prostate completely, improving cure rates and avoiding positive surgical margins. Today, the surgical robot offers no tactile feedback, and the instruments are rigid, making it difficult for the surgeon to tailor the operation to a patient's specific anatomy or to do a pelvic lymph node dissection. If future versions offered surgeons tactile feedback and greater flexibility, the operation might eventually lead to better results than open surgery. An improved future version of the robot might also allow an imaging study of the cancer to be superimposed on the surgeon's field of view, so he knows exactly where the tumor resides within the gland.

At the time of surgery for breast cancer, it is possible to identify the first ("sentinel") lymph node into which breast fluid drains and examine that node for signs of cancer spread. We have never found these sentinel nodes in prostate cancer. Hopefully, in the future, we'll be able to inject a radioactive tracer before radical prostatectomy and then use a PET-CT fusion study or a probe with a Geiger counter to track which pelvic lymph nodes take up the radioactivity. Removal of pelvic lymph nodes containing cancerous cells can increase our ability to arrest the spread of prostate cancer and cure the disease with a less extensive operation.

Being able to see the cancer better before surgery would help us plan a more effective operation. Imaging studies are constantly being improved. We use endorectal MRI enhanced by spectroscopy, but there is great interest in other MR techniques that can better identify the size, location, and extent of the cancer.

IN SUMMARY

For a healthy man who likely has many more years to live, radical prostatectomy, which offers the best proven long-term results, can be an excellent treatment choice for localized prostate cancer that needs to be treated. Though this is the most disruptive approach in the short run, with modern nerve-sparing surgery most men soon regain normal urinary control and recover normal sexual function over time. The quality of the surgery is critical, far more important in the long run than the type of procedure you have. Be sure to put yourself in the hands of an experienced specialist with an excellent track record.

15

■

Radiation Therapy

READ THIS CHAPTER TO LEARN:

• How does radiation work, and what does radiation therapy for
  prostate cancer entail?
• What are the types of radiation, their advantages and disadvantages, and which might be best for you?
• What should you look for in a radiation therapy program?

Simply put, radiation kills cells. Exposure to enough radioactivity damages the cell's genetic blueprint: DNA. Lacking these critical instruc-
tions, irradiated cells die off when they try to divide. As a result, rapidly
dividing cells are eradicated sooner than those which multiply slowly.

Radiation can also control cancer by cutting off the blood supply a
tumor requires to survive and grow. The cells lining blood vessels are
extremely vulnerable to high-energy X-rays. Even with relatively low-
dose therapy, a tumor's blood supply can be destroyed, leading to the
cancer's demise.

Recent experiments at Memorial Sloan-Kettering Cancer Center
indicate that radiation can induce programmed cell death (**apoptosis**),

effectively causing cells to commit suicide.[1] Normal cells regularly die off, and new ones arise to take their place. Lacking this innate control, untreated cancer cells multiply and spread in a mounting swath of destruction. By robbing the tumor cells of their immortality, radiation heads off this dangerous overgrowth.

Radiation effects are fractional, meaning the tumor is killed by degrees. With each day's dose, a small proportion of the cancer is destroyed, and then a portion of what remains is killed, and so on. If we get the number low enough, the body can naturally eliminate the remaining malignant cells on its own. Treatment failures in radiation do not usually represent growth of a new cancer. More often, the original tumor has been dealt a stunning blow but not knocked out. Over time, the remaining cancer cells regroup and multiply until they are large enough to cause a rising PSA, which signals that the cancer has returned.

If you douse a lawn with powerful herbicides, you'll kill both the weeds and the grass. Radiation oncologists face a similar conundrum. They need to administer enough destructive rays to eradicate the cancer without inflicting unacceptable damage on normal surrounding tissues. When the therapeutic target is the prostate, which lies perilously close to the bladder, urethra, erectile nerves, and the bowel, the challenge is especially daunting.

To make matters worse, tissues in the body have widely varied radiation tolerance. The intense therapy required to kill prostate cancers would destroy the adjacent rectal wall if a large enough area of the rectum was hit by a high dose of radiation, where the normal cells divide far more rapidly and are, consequently, exquisitely susceptible to radiation effects.

Modern radiotherapy can be administered via **external beam therapy (EBT)** or **seed implants (brachytherapy),** and sometimes the two are combined. Since radiation works best and is safest for a small tumor in a small prostate, hormones are sometimes recommended to shrink a large cancer or a large gland before treatment.

The amount of radiation energy received by the target organ is expressed in **Gray (Gy)**, named for Louis Gray, an English radiologist and physician. The **rad**, an earlier way of describing dose level, was shorthand for radiation absorbed dose (100 rads equal 1 Gy). Treating prostate

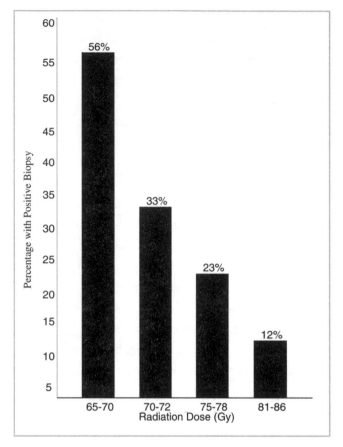

The higher the radiation dose, the lower the chance that the cancer will recur, as indicated by a biopsy of the prostate three years after radiation therapy.

cancer requires a minimum of 70 Gy, sometimes expressed as 7,000 **centi-gray (cGy)**. The cancer cure rate increases with the strength of the dose.[2]

Some patients ask why all the radiation can't be given at once. In fact, early on, some radiation therapists advocated saturation, with one large exposure of the tumor to a radioactive source, over **fractionation** (many smaller doses). They found that delivering the treatment over time markedly improved results and reduced side effects. This is comparable to the difference between brief regular exposures to northern sunlight and many hours spent baking under a blazing tropical sun. Minimal sun exposure in the first case provides some important, cumulative benefits, such as helping the body to synthesize vitamin D. In more intense, concentrated doses, the sun's rays can cause serious burns and permanent cell damage.

Nevertheless, researchers are now investigating the possibility that, given highly precise modern techniques, saturating the tumor with fewer radiation doses or even one large dose (**hypofractionation**) may prove particularly lethal to cancer. With **image-guided radiation therapy (IGRT)**, the physician can constantly look at the tumor being irradiated. This works very well in treating metastatic cancer in the brain, bones, and lung. It has also been used in clinical trials for pancreatic cancer, but it has not yet been used for prostate cancer.

A BRIEF HISTORY OF RADIATION THERAPY

In 1895, William Roentgen, a German physicist, discovered a strange greenish light that could pass through soft tissues in the body but not through most metals or bones. He dubbed his discovery the X-ray, with *X* meant to indicate that the source of this astonishing phenomenon was unknown.

News of Roentgen's breakthrough spread quickly and fueled the imaginations of scientists around the world. In little over a year, the mysterious rays earned a place in medical treatment and diagnosis. For the first time, doctors had a way to visualize some of the body's internal structures without having to operate. In recognition of this landmark achievement, Roentgen was awarded the first Nobel Prize in physics in 1901.

Inspired by the X-ray and the accidental finding of uranium rays soon afterward, Marie Curie, then a young graduate student in Paris, resolved to study a variety of chemical compounds and to find ways to unleash their radiation. The research she did with her husband, Pierre, led to the discovery of radium and its potential use in the destruction of cancer cells. Mme Curie went on to become France's first female university professor and the first person to be named a Nobel laureate twice.

Unfortunately, the Curies' pioneering research brought them more than accolades. As a result of their frequent, unprotected exposure to radioactive materials, the couple suffered chronic, debilitating health problems, including skin lesions, weakness, and intractable pain. The Curies not only helped introduce the world to the potential positive power of radioactivity, they were also among the first to demonstrate its alarming side effects.

Studies in the early twentieth century confirmed that radiation could kill rapidly dividing organisms, such as bacteria, and could slow the growth of rapidly dividing cancer cells. Investigators inserted radioactive pellets into tumors in test tubes or animals. As they had hoped, the treatment caused cancers to shrink.

The first radiation therapy for prostate cancer in humans was performed at Johns Hopkins University by Dr. Hugh Hampton Young.[3] Young, who also pioneered surgery for prostate cancer, implanted very high-intensity radium or radon pellets in patients with prostate and bladder cancers. These primitive attempts at brachytherapy did yield some temporary remissions, but they came at a considerable cost of radiation injuries to patients and medical personnel. Until work was done on the atom bomb during World War II, the dangers of handling radioactive materials were not fully appreciated, and shielding techniques were woefully inadequate.

Early on, seed placement was freehand and imprecise. Doctors would operate to implant six to eight radioactive pellets in a cancerous prostate. Typically, certain areas of the gland received inadequate radiation to kill the tumor (**cold spots**), while other sites received too large a dose (**hot spots**), causing an unacceptable incidence of serious side effects, especially damage to the rectum and bladder.[4]

The first external beam therapy, developed in the 1940s, involved taking radioactive cobalt, putting it in a machine fitted with lead shields, and then opening a shield like a camera shutter to expose the target to destructive gamma rays. Cobalt radiation worked well for highly sensitive cancers such as testicular seminomas that could be killed off with a very small amount of radiation, but it proved too diffuse and hard to control to give in the much higher doses needed to wipe out prostate cancers. Severe side effects, including bladder damage and dramatic injury to the rectum, overwhelmed the limited benefits of the treatment. Because of constraints on the dose that could be given safely, most tumors soon recurred.

The development of the linear accelerator in the late 1950s allowed radiation oncologists to deliver external radiation with greater safety and precision than was possible with cobalt. Dr. Malcolm Bagshaw at Stanford University championed the new approach, treating thousands of patients. Bagshaw proved that radiation could cure some prostate cancers, though, by modern standards, cancer control remained woefully inadequate and side effects unacceptably high.[5]

As a result, the 1970s saw a renewed interest in seed implants. Radiation effects from an implanted seed fall off quickly as you move away from the source of the energy rays. Brachytherapy appeared promising as a way to concentrate high doses in the prostate while minimizing damage to surrounding tissues. Theoretically, it seemed possible to administer 120 to 180 Gy of radiation using iodine-125 seeds, or a combination of radioactive gold seeds and external beam therapy, instead of the standard 65 to 70 Gy being given at the time by external beam therapy.

People were seduced by those higher numbers, but despite highly optimistic expectations, seed implants did a dismal job of curing cancers.[6] In fact, studies showed that cancer control with brachytherapy was hardly better than that for patients on watchful waiting, who received no treatment at all.

Further study turned up two wild cards. One was cold spots. With brachytherapy, some areas of the cancer were simply missed or received too low a radiation dose to kill the malignant cells. Also, the high expected overall dose failed to materialize. When 140 Gy was delivered over six months with iodine seeds, the biological effect on cancer cells proved to be no greater than giving 70 Gy of external beam treatment over seven weeks. Seed implants acted like a time-release capsule that delivered the medication slowly but didn't increase its overall strength or effectiveness.

RADIATION TODAY

Given the best modern equipment in the hands of the best practitioners, it's now possible to give powerful, effective radiation therapy with a slim risk of serious side effects. For many men with prostate cancer, radiation is an excellent treatment choice, but, as with surgery, it's important to understand the particulars and make sure you're in the best possible hands. All radiation is definitely *not* created equal.[7]

For each strategy, different centers offer a wide range of technology and expertise.

EXTERNAL BEAM RADIATION THERAPY

CONVENTIONAL THERAPY

In this approach, a linear accelerator (a machine that produces high-energy radiation) administers the minimum acceptable dose of 70 Gy over about seven weeks of daily weekday therapy sessions. Treatment targets the prostate, seminal vesicles, and sometimes the pelvic lymph nodes. Depending upon the precision with which the radiation physicist calibrates these complex machines, the actual dose a patient receives can vary, affecting cure rates and the risk of complications.[8]

Conventional radiation therapy irradiates a box-shaped area around the plum-shaped prostate. Parts of surrounding organs—the rectum, bladder, and urethra—are in the radiation field. Some of these tissues, especially the rectal wall, are extremely vulnerable to radiation damage. As a result, one third of men suffer immediate side effects such as rectal bleeding, diarrhea, bowel urgency, and urinary urgency and frequency.

The prostate is a notoriously difficult organ to target accurately within the radiation beam. Varying amounts of gas or stool in the rectum, the amount of urine in the bladder, even the act of breathing can alter the position of the prostate during treatment, diverting radiation from the intended target. Some areas of the gland can receive too small a dose to kill the tumor (cold spots), and the local recurrence rate, especially for moderate- or high-risk cancers, is high.

Conventional radiation packs an insufficient wallop for any but the most favorable cancers. We now know that 70 Gy is too small a dose for almost any prostate cancer.

3-D CONFORMAL RADIATION THERAPY (3D-CRT)

The development of **three-dimensional conformal radiation therapy (3D-CRT)** in the late 1980s took a giant step toward solving these problems. A computer program, aided by a CT scan or MRI, accurately measures the gland in three dimensions and computes precisely, in three dimensions, how the intended dose of radiation should be delivered. Radiation to surrounding organs and damage to normal tissues are markedly reduced. Using 3-D conformal radiation therapy, the risk of serious side effects at 70 Gy went down to less than 1 percent, allowing some radiation oncologists to safely increase the dose to a more effective 75 or 76 Gy.[9]

As the dosage level increases, so does the probability that the cancer will be completely wiped out. In a study by Memorial Sloan-Kettering radiation oncologists, nearly half of men given a low 68 Gy dose had a cancer in their biopsy two to three years after treatment. At the minimum acceptable dose for prostate cancer (70 Gy), 33 percent of men had a positive biopsy after therapy, 23 percent at 75.6 Gy, and 12 percent tested positive for cancer after treatment at 81 Gy.

The software required for 3-D conformal radiation is widely available, affordable, and compatible with any modern linear accelerator. No one in a developed country should be treated with radiation for prostate cancer without 3-D conformal technology.

NOTE: Better local cancer control translates into better cure rates. Increasing the dose to 75 Gy left 81 percent of men cancer-free in the long term, as opposed to a 59 percent success rate at 70 Gy. Similar gains were seen for men with intermediate- and high-risk cancers. Simply put, bigger guns pack more firepower and can bring down bigger game. A little .22 might be fine for hunting rabbits, but you'd need a high-powered .30-06 caliber rifle if you were out for big bear.

INTENSITY-MODULATED RADIATION THERAPY (IMRT)

Intensity-modulated radiation therapy (IMRT) fine-tunes 3-D conformal technology even further. By using sophisticated computerized algorithms, this technique delivers the treatment dose at varying intensities throughout the targeted field. Cancer cells in the prostate and surrounding area (within 1 centimeter of the edge of the gland) can be zapped with more damaging rays, while delicate adjacent tissues are spared. The extraordinary precision of IMRT allows radiation therapists to further increase the treatment dose to 81 or 86 Gy, while holding serious side effects to a minimum. Pioneering this technology, the radiation oncology team at Memorial Sloan-Kettering Cancer Center—Zvi Fuks, Steven Leibel, and Michael Zelefsky—were able to reduce serious intestinal complications from 17 percent to 2 percent while substantially increasing cure rates. These high doses are so effective that most men can avoid adjuvant hormone therapy, with all of its side effects, which are often used to enhance cure with conventional doses of radiation (see page 322).[10]

In addition to software, IMRT requires the addition of sophisticated hardware, involving slim tungsten plates that open and close to control the radiation intensity. The technology is relatively expensive but is now available in the U.S. at most radiotherapy centers. In my view, no man should accept radiation for prostate cancer unless it is delivered with IMRT.

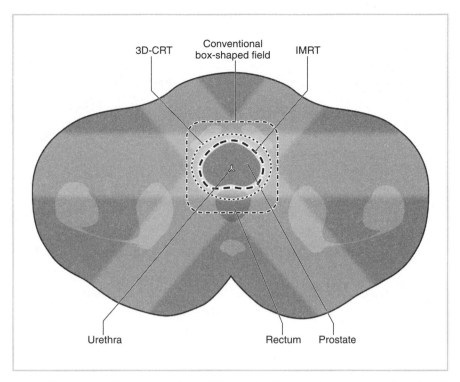

More of the surrounding tissue receives a full dose of radiation with conventional (box-shaped) radiation therapy than with 3-D conformal radiation therapy (3D-CRT). In intensity modulated radiation therapy (IMRT), even less tissue is exposed to the full dose.

CYBERKNIFE RADIATION

CyberKnife is a commercially produced, proprietary (private) technology, meaning it is a particular company's brand of IMRT. It is not, as the name implies, a surgical procedure, and no knife is involved. The company that developed and is aggressively marketing this device uses it to administer hypofractionated radiation dosages, meaning the therapy is delivered in a few weeks instead of the standard eight or nine weeks. Knowledgeable radiotherapists prefer standard IMRT to the CyberKnife variation for prostate cancer therapy.

PROTON BEAM RADIATION

Proton beam radiation was developed shortly after World War II as an out-growth of research into particle accelerators and first used experimentally in cancer therapy in the mid-1950s. The approach was popularized in a small number of centers where it was touted as a means to treat aggressive tumors in deep internal organs, including the prostate and brain, more effectively and safely than conventional external beam radiation.

Proton beams can be delivered to the precise contours of the target, where they abruptly deposit their energy, avoiding spillover into adjacent tissues. Because damage to surrounding organs is minimized, proponents also claim that high, extraordinarily effective treatment doses can be administered. The safety and efficacy of proton beam therapy has been demonstrated for many childhood cancers and for brain tumors, but its value for other adult tumors is highly controversial. Extravagant claims have been made that the therapy can boast a 100 percent success rate without complications or side effects, but there are no credible studies and no long-term data to support this.[11] Experts question whether proton beam therapy offers any advantage over modern high-dose IMRT for treating prostate cancer.

The technology is extraordinarily cumbersome and expensive, and not widely available. If you happen to live near one of the twenty or so centers worldwide that has a proton beam unit, it can provide good state-of-the-art therapy, but I would not travel to get proton beam therapy if IMRT is available.

NEUTRON BEAM RADIATION

Neutrons were discovered in 1932, and research into their potential therapeutic benefits began in 1938. As with protons, gigantic, prohibitively expensive equipment is required to accelerate these particles to the velocities necessary to release their powerful energy.

To treat cancers, high-energy neutron beams are thrown into the target organ, delivering a powerful, damaging blow. The therapy is designed for high-risk, aggressive tumors that would likely prove incurable with other forms of radiation.[12]

On the downside, any contact of the beam with normal tissues causes extreme injury, so neutron treatment carries a high risk of serious side effects. Like proton beam treatment, the equipment is available in few centers. In the limited experience published with neutron beam therapy, there are no convincing advantages over modern IMRT.

IS EXTERNAL BEAM RADIATION RIGHT FOR YOU?

External radiation can be an excellent choice for men over 70 and for younger men with health problems that make them poor candidates for surgery. Because the prostate is permanently removed with radical prostatectomy, avoiding local recurrences decades later, most experts agree that surgery is the better choice for men in their 40s and early 50s. Between those ages, the decision about whether to opt for surgery or radiation may hinge on your general health, sexual and urinary function, the nature of your cancer, personal preference, and lifestyle issues. (See Chapter 12, Deciding How to Treat Localized Prostate Cancer.)

Radiation may be contraindicated if you've had a prior TURP, or if you have a prostate gland larger than 80 grams or a urethral stricture. Radiation is not recommended for anyone with inflammatory bowel disease or those with prior rectal surgery that have had reconstruction using the small intestine. Any previous radiation to the pelvic area may make a full course of radiation challenging to deliver without excessive complications. Be sure your doctor knows about any such treatments you've had for whatever reason, no matter how long ago. The damaging effects of radiation last a lifetime, and irradiating an area again can be dangerous.

The Advantages of External Beam Therapy

If your cancer poses a health risk and requires treatment, radiation is a reasonable choice. In this country as many men are treated with radiation therapy as with surgery. The main attractions are avoiding surgery, with the need for a hospital stay and anesthesia, and the short-term risk of erectile dysfunction and urinary incontinence. In most cases radiation involves only minimal disruption to normal activities. For men who are not good surgical candidates because of health or age, radiation offers an excellent chance to control the cancer.

Because of the low risk of immediate side effects, external radiation has generally been preferred over surgery to treat the primary tumor in the prostate in men who have metastatic spread of the cancer to lymph nodes or other sites. If they have local symptoms of prostate cancer, radiation is usually combined with hormone therapy. (See Chapter 21, Treating Advanced Prostate Cancer).

The Disadvantages of External Beam Therapy

After surgery, you get a pathology report containing detailed information about the nature of the cancer and the risk of recurrence. This can be important in determining whether further (adjuvant) treatment may be necessary to cure or control the cancer. With radiation, no tissue is removed, so we gain no knowledge about the tumor or whether additional therapy might be indicated.

If surgery is effective, the PSA soon falls to zero. A rising PSA after surgery is an early warning of a recurrence that can offer men another chance to cure the cancer with further therapy. Typically, additional treatment, when needed, begins about a year after surgery. With radiation, the PSA should fall, but it does not reach zero. While PSA typically declines over time as radiation kills cells, it is difficult to know for sure whether the cancer has been eradicated or whether it will recur. Since the gland remains in place, a rise in the PSA after radiation could result from normal prostate tissue. It takes much longer—typically 5 years—to confirm that the cancer has recurred and offer additional treatment.

It might seem logical to use biopsies to determine whether the cancer has been eliminated by radiation. But the effects of radiotherapy on prostate cancer cells are slow. It may take 2½ to 3 years for a lethally irradiated cancer to disappear. A biopsy done earlier is very difficult to interpret. Are the cancer cells the pathologist sees alive and poised to regrow, or are they in the act of dying off?

In surgery, we remove the cancer and the prostate. With radiation, the gland remains in place and a new cancer can develop in the prostate at a later time. If there is a recurrence, further radiation might not be possible. Irradiated organs are given the maximum allowable lifetime dose and changed permanently. Radiation effects are cumulative, and exposing a treated area to more damaging rays is risky, although clinical trials are actively examining its feasibility.

NOTE: While a second course of radiation has rarely been used, clinical trials are under way to study the safety and efficacy of using brachytherapy to administer a second dose to some patients if the cancer recurs. These trials are in the earliest stages. And while preliminary results suggest that it might be possible to give further radiation safely, we have no idea whether it will prove effective.

In the event that radiation fails to control the cancer, there is no proven, safe, effective technique that provides a second chance to cure the disease. Any further treatment to try to the prostate is hazardous. Cryotherapy, HIFU, and a variety of other technologies have shown limited benefit and a substantial risk of erectile dysfunction, urinary incontinence, and damage to the rectum. (See Chapter 16, Focal and Other "Local" Therapies.) In my opinion, the only real chance of cure after radiation failure is salvage radical prostatectomy, a difficult procedure that should only be attempted by highly skilled, experienced surgeons. Even in the best of hands, the incidence of complications and side effects is considerably higher in salvage surgery than for radical prostatectomy on a gland that has not been irradiated. (See Chapter 20, Rising PSA After Surgery, Radiation, or Other Therapy, for more details.)

In some cases, the logistics of external beam therapy can be troublesome. IMRT requires daily treatment five days a week for nine to ten weeks. Once you start a course of radiation, you are committed to completing it. You cannot take time off in the middle or defer your remaining treatments if something comes up.

Radiation therapy using IMRT is not available everywhere. Treatment at a lower dose would increase your risk of side effects and limit your chance for a cure. If you do not live near a center that offers good modern technology, a long commute or even a temporary move might prove necessary.

While the immediate side effects are less than surgery, long-term side effects can develop over time as radiation damage accumulates. This includes serious bowel problems in 2 to 3 percent of men, troublesome urinary symptoms in 4 to 5 percent, and loss of erections in 50 percent over five years. (See Side Effects of External Beam Radiation, page 344.)

Radiation can destroy cancers, but it can also damage the DNA of healthy cells and induce cancers (as we know from the malignancies that arose in people exposed to radiation in Hiroshima and Chernobyl). Men treated with radiation may be at increased risk of developing serious invasive cancers of the rectum, bladder, or other organs. Rarely, unusually aggressive cancers such as carcinosarcomas grow in the irradiated prostate. Some have speculated that these secondary cancers may pose a greater risk of death to men with low-risk prostate cancers than does the original tumor. This is another good reason for men with small, early prostate cancer to consider active surveillance rather than immediate treatment.

HOW TO CHOOSE
A RADIATION PROGRAM

The likelihood that you'll be cured and your risk of serious side effects will hinge heavily on where you get radiation. Be sure to have your treatment with highly trained doctors who use approved modern equipment. This is especially critical with the very high-dose radiation required to destroy prostate cancer.

Effective external beam treatment depends on scrupulous treatment planning, followed by precise, consistent administration of the daily prescribed dose. You'll be best off at a center that uses modern IMRT. Meticulous maintenance of the machines is essential. If you are scheduled to receive 2 Gy (equivalent to 200 centigray or cGy) per day, you don't want to get 2.1 Gy one day and 1.9 the next, and you certainly don't want to receive less than the optimal dose overall. The hospital's radiation team should include a computer planner and a radiation physicist who calibrates the machines frequently to ensure that they're emitting the proper amount of energy.[13]

Radiation disasters happen very rarely, but you don't want them happening to you. Just as you wouldn't expect to see an airline's maintenance record before boarding a plane, you aren't likely to be privy to the center's equipment history or its incidence of serious burns or fistulas (open holes). Your best defense is a busy, state-of-the-art facility with an excellent reputation.

THE TREATMENT

One to several weeks before you start treatments, you'll be scheduled for studies to map the size, shape, and location of your prostate. The best centers use a CT scan or MRI to picture your prostate in three dimensions in relation to surrounding tissues. More conventional studies using plain X-ray films and contrast dies to outline the bladder do not offer nearly as precise information about prostate anatomy. In modern centers, a high-tech simulator is used to chart exactly where and how the therapy will be delivered in the three-dimensional field.

A mold of your torso will be made to ensure that you're placed in exactly the same position every day and held in that posture as the radiation is delivered from varying angles. To further ensure consistency, a few tiny dots will be tattooed on your abdomen and back as landmarks.

A long-standing concern about radiation for prostate cancer is that the gland moves from day to day, or even hour to hour, depending on the fullness of the bladder, the amount of stool or gas in the rectum, and even as a patient breathes. This makes it very difficult to ensure that the dose is delivered the same way each time and that the entire gland is being irradiated uniformly during every treatment session. In response, radiation oncologists enlarged the field to avoid undertreatment. But a wider radiation field meant greater side effects. Using IMRT, the targeted area can be narrowed, but the dose could be inadequate on days when the

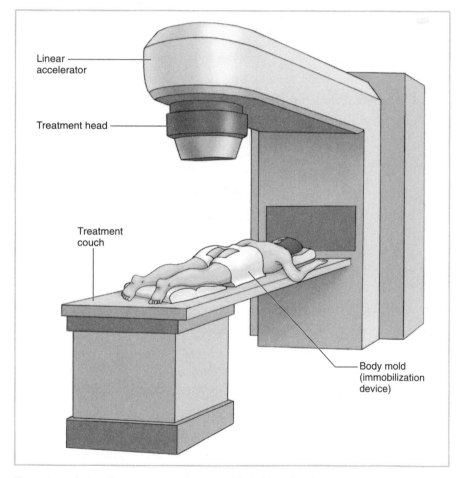

To receive radiation therapy, a patient lies on a table, held in place by a plastic immobilization device, while the radiation is beamed from a linear accelerator.

gland has moved. To avoid this, many radiation therapists place small, nonradioactive metal pellets in the prostate (**fiducial markers**). These pellets can be seen with simple X-rays when the patient is placed on the table, allowing precise location of the prostate. We refer to this procedure as **image-guided radiation therapy (IGRT)**. Some commercial vendors use the term "TomoTherapy" to describe IGRT that uses CT scanning in lieu of plain X-rays to locate the prostate before each treatment session

You'll be scheduled to receive radiation every weekday for about two months. Treatments last only a few minutes, and the entire process, including check-in and trading your street clothes for a hospital gown, should not take more than about a half hour. You will not feel any pain when the radiation is being given. Aside from this and some basic suggestions that your radiation oncologist will make regarding skin care, no changes in your normal routine should be necessary. You will not be radioactive during the course of treatment, and close contact, including sexual intercourse, is not a problem.

PSA and External Radiation

Because the prostate remains in place after radiation, the PSA drops, but not to zero. It's hard to know what level is low enough to indicate that the cancer has been destroyed, but the lower the PSA at its lowest point (PSA nadir) the greater the chance that the cancer has been cured. A nadir less than 0.5 ng/ml is optimal.

The definition of "biochemical recurrence" after radiation is a PSA level that rises 2 ng/ml above its nadir (assuming no hormone therapy was used).[14] This **nadir + 2** definition predicts the chances of eventual metastases better than the previous ASTRO definition (3 consecutive rises in the PSA). But it delays the recognition that the radiation has failed to destroy the cancer within the prostate.

If the PSA starts to rise, a biopsy may be necessary to determine whether cancer cells are present. (See Chapter 20, Rising PSA After Surgery, Radiation, or Other Therapy.) If we find a tumor, it's tough to treat.

If we do not, it's difficult to tell whether the biopsy missed cancer cells within the prostate, whether the cancer cells had already spread elsewhere, or whether the PSA is rising from benign growth of the remaining normal prostate tissue. In some men, the PSA level rises after a time and then falls again without treatment. This **PSA bounce** is difficult to interpret and can cause considerable anxiety.[15] While we wait the necessary interval to determine whether a rising PSA represents a meaningless artifact or a real recurrence, we may miss the window of opportunity for a cure. Interpreting PSA levels becomes especially confusing in a man treated with hormones in addition to radiation. Hormone therapy drives the PSA down to a very low level. When hormones are stopped, the PSA typically rises again until the full effects of radiation kick in and lower it again. For two and a half to three years after radiation, it's virtually impossible to tell for sure whether the cancer has been controlled.

Side Effects of External Beam Radiation

During the course of external beam radiation, about 15 percent of men complain of decreased energy, altered appetite, weight loss, and fatigue, but the vast majority have no such problems. Skin irritation or burns should never occur with modern radiation techniques. Ten percent of men will have some troublesome (grade II) gastrointestinal problems, such as the urge to defecate with no stool in the rectum (**tenesmus**), dietary intolerance, or rectal bleeding during or soon after treatment. In addition, 40 to 50 percent experience urgency, frequency, and other urinary symptoms. Medication can provide symptomatic relief. Most of these problems clear up about two months after treatment.

Over the long term, the biggest concern with radiation therapy is bowel injury, which may range in severity depending on the type of radiation, the precision of the technique, and the intensity of the dose. **Radiation proctitis** (inflammation of the rectum) can cause diarrhea, tenesmus, bleeding, or ulceration of the rectal wall over the prostate. These problems develop gradually, as treatment effects accumulate. The incidence of bowel injuries, especially serious ones, has been greatly reduced to 17 percent by modern 3D-CRT, and the incidence with IMRT is only 2 to 3 percent.[16]

Radiation proctitis, though rare, tends to be chronic and difficult to treat. Steroid foam or rectal suppositories may offer some relief, as can dietary changes and medications that soften bowel movements. With modern therapy, a bowel injury severe enough to require a colostomy should almost never occur. (See Chapter 19, Bowel Side Effects, for a further discussion.)

Six to seven percent of patients treated with conventional therapy develop radiation cystitis, an inflammation of the bladder that can cause urinary frequency, burning, and blood in the urine. Very rarely the bleeding is severe enough to require transfusions. IMRT greatly reduces the risk of serious urinary side effects by reducing exposure of the bladder to radiation.

Over the first five years after radiation therapy, 40 to 50 percent of patients experience erectile dysfunction. The risk is higher for older men, those who receive hormone therapy along with radiation, and for those whose erections were somewhat impaired before treatment. Seventy-five percent of patients with postradiation erectile loss find medications such as sildenafil (Viagra) helpful.[17]

Over time, radiation causes a reduction in prostate secretions and reduced ejaculatory volume. Sperm production and the passage of sperm to the prostate are also curtailed by scarring and fibrosis. Even though you may continue to ejaculate, it would be rare to be able to father a child after radiation (though this *does not* mean that it's perfectly safe to cease using birth control). If fertility is an issue, you may want to bank sperm before treatment.

BRACHYTHERAPY

The term **brachytherapy**, also known as interstitial therapy or seed implants, derives from the Greek for "short treatment," meaning the dose is delivered at close range. A radiation source—the seed or pellet—is placed directly into the target area, as opposed to external beam therapy, where the dose is delivered from outside the body. The idea is to hit the cancer cells with the bulk of the damaging rays while reducing the effects to surrounding structures. Radiation effects fall off with startling rapidity. When you move a ¼ inch from the source, there's a sixteenfold reduction in radiation energy.

Almost all brachytherapy today involves the permanent implantation of radioactive iodine or palladium seeds. Each seed is contained in a tiny titanium capsule, shaped like a piece of pencil lead. Five of the implants laid end to end would measure about 1 inch. Each seed emits very low radiation energy, and the therapeutic effect depends on the interaction of multiple seeds positioned in a three-dimensional grid. The required radiation dose depends on the type of seed. With iodine, the minimum radiation dose delivered to the periphery of the prostate must be at least 145 Gy; with palladium it's 125 Gy. This measure, called the **minimal peripheral dose (MPD)**, ensures an adequate dose throughout the gland. Because the energy is time-released over many months, 145 Gy of brachytherapy with iodine seeds is the equivalent of 70 Gy delivered externally, though this could approach 75 or even 81 Gy when therapy is administered expertly. The typical implant involves 50 to 150 tiny seeds, with the highest concentration in the peripheral zone of the prostate, where most cancers arise.

NOTE: Occasionally, **high-dose-rate (HDR)** brachytherapy, using a temporary, very powerful radiation source, is used to treat very large, advanced, or recurring tumors. For this intense treatment, patients are kept in the hospital for 24 to 36 hours, during which time high-energy radiation is delivered through a number of slim tubes inserted into the prostate. The procedure—sometimes called the "Andy Grove method" because the Intel cofounder elected to have his prostate cancer treated by HDR in conjunction with external beam therapy—is repeated several times for a few minutes each time. The advantages are delivery of very high doses over a short period of time and, when combined with external beam therapy, a shorter course of treatment.

Is Brachytherapy for You?

Brachytherapy is *not* for everyone. With the exception of the temporary high-dose iridium implant mentioned above, most experts agree that seed implants are only appropriate for men whose cancers are low-risk, with all favorable features (a low clinical stage of T1 or T2a, a low Gleason score between 2 and 6 with no aggressive Gleason pattern 4 or 5 components, and with a PSA under 10) and with cancer in less than half of the biopsy cores. Patients with *any* high-risk features should opt for surgery, external radiation, or a combination of brachytherapy plus external beam, all of which offer a greater chance of long-term cancer control.

NOTE: It is sometimes said that brachytherapy is a good form of treatment for prostate cancer that doesn't need treatment. If you really fit the criteria for brachytherapy, you have a low-risk cancer, and it might be wise to consider whether you need treatment at all. You should discuss with your doctor whether your tumor is of such low risk that it would be reasonable to monitor the situation carefully and postpone treatment until there is evidence that the cancer is becoming more threatening. Like all currently available treatments for this disease, brachytherapy does carry a risk of side effects.

Your prostate anatomy is a major consideration. The larger the gland, the harder it is to saturate with seeds. The ultrasound report from your biopsy will include a measure of your prostate size that is far more accurate than the estimate we can make from a digital rectal exam. A small prostate weighing less than 40 grams is ideal. Anything over 60 grams, even in the most skilled hands, may be too large to treat safely with seeds alone, increasing the risk of acute urinary retention after the implant and adding to the risk that the prostate will not be saturated with enough seeds to effect a cure. To treat a large prostate with seeds, hormone therapy would be required to shrink the gland before treatment, and that can cause troublesome side effects of its own. (See Hormones and Radiation on page 359.)

If you're considering brachytherapy, you will need an ultrasound, CT scan, or MRI of the prostate to establish the precise size and configuration of your gland. In some men, the prostate has large median or lateral lobes that extend into the bladder. In other cases, the prostate sits high under the arch of the pubic bone, making it hard to access. Either of these situations would add to the risks and technical difficulty of an implant. External therapy or surgery may be the better choice.

Whether or not your prostate is enlarged, if you are having difficulty urinating, you would be at high risk of developing acute urinary retention after seed implants, which occurs in 4 to 10 percent of brachytherapy patients nationwide and in 2 percent at Memorial Sloan-Kettering. Bleeding from the multiple needles used to insert the seeds and swelling from the radiation could block the flow of urine completely. Many patients are treated with alpha blockers, such as tamsulosin (Flomax) or alfuzosin (Uroxatral), to relax the prostate and ease voiding.

If you do have difficulty urinating, **urodynamic testing** before the procedure can gauge whether you have urinary obstruction. The test involves passing a catheter into the bladder through the penis, so it's mildly invasive. Also, the test is not available in every community. Another reasonable measure of obstructive symptoms is the speed of your urinary stream (flow rate). A flow-rate test, in which a patient urinates into a special funnel, can be done in the doctor's office. Another good indicator of urinary blockage is the amount of urine that remains in your bladder after you urinate (post-void residual urine). Ultrasound—a noninvasive, widely available, inexpensive imaging technique—can measure this. Finally, a score over seven on a simple questionnaire like the International Prostate Symptom Score (IPSS; see pages 00–00) indicates that you may have urinary obstruction, and the higher the score, the greater the risk of acute urinary retention after seed implants. (See Chapter 5, BPH [Benign Prostatic Hyperplasia]).

Seed implantation is generally not advised for men who have had a previous TURP (commonly dubbed a "Roto-Rooter" procedure) to relieve symptoms of benign prostate enlargement. The operation leaves a shell of the gland rather than a solid sphere. The remaining real estate is typically insufficient to allow effective seed placement.

Brachytherapy is not recommended for men with inflammatory bowel disease, previous radiotherapy to the area, or evidence of extra-capsular extension of the cancer.

THE TREATMENT

Before the implant, you'll have routine preoperative testing, including blood and urine tests. Depending on your age and health, your doctor may order a chest X-ray and an electrocardiogram. Because the radiation dose depends on the interaction of multiple seeds, precise placement of each one is critical. Before brachytherapy, the radiation oncologist will make a detailed, three-dimensional map of your prostate using a CT scan or MRI. These tests will determine the volume of the gland, which areas of the prostate and how much surrounding tissue should be targeted (target volume), the dose of radiation you'll receive, how many seeds you'll need, and exactly where each one should be placed.

In many centers, these tests are performed one to three weeks before the seeds are implanted. In the operating room, it can be a challenge to match the precise conditions of the planning session. Proper implants require an active collaboration between the radiation therapist who implants the seeds and either a urologist or a radiologist who is expert in using ultrasound. In expert centers more sophisticated dynamic treatment planning is performed during the implant in real time, allowing the radiation oncologist to make subtle adjustments to ensure an optimal result.[18]

DURING THE IMPLANT

Seed implants can be done under general or regional (epidural or spinal) anesthetic. As a rule, it's wise to go along with the method your doctor prefers and knows best.

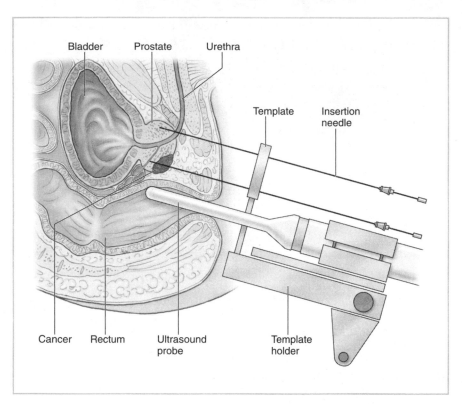

The setup in the operating room to use ultrasound guidance to place brachytherapy seeds into the prostate.

You'll be on your back with your feet raised in stirrups. A metal template is placed on the perineum (between the scrotum and the rectum), and sixteen to twenty hollow needles are inserted through holes in the template at prescribed intervals. Guided by ultrasound through a rectal probe, the radioactive seeds are then loaded through the needles and dropped in place.

After the implant is completed, an imaging study is done in the operating room or within the next few days to calculate the actual dose of radiation you've received. If the dosage is inadequate, some radiation oncologists will implant more seeds, but this increases the risk of side effects. Experienced practitioners would rarely have to do this.

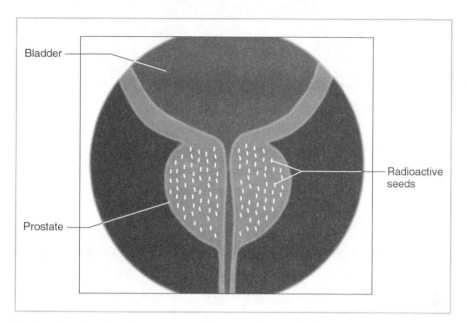

Bladder

Radioactive
seeds

Prostate

The location of seeds in the prostate on a fluoroscopic image after brachytherapy implantation.

Typically, patients go home the day of the implant and return to work and normal activities soon afterward. Before your discharge, you'll be given information about the radiation safety precautions you'll need to take. You may be asked to urinate through a strainer for several days in case any seeds are discharged. If you do pass a seed, use a spoon or tweezers to place it in a small closed container and deliver it to the doctor at your earliest convenience.

A seed can also pass in the ejaculate. For this reason, and because you may experience some pain on orgasm shortly after the implant, doctors sometimes advise that you have five or so ejaculations in private before resuming sexual relations. Some doctors suggest using a condom during intercourse for anywhere from two weeks to a year after brachytherapy. If you are instructed to do this, it's reasonable to question why and whether it's really necessary.

PSA After Brachytherapy

With successful eradication of the cancer, the PSA should drop to an almost undetectable level (preferably less than 0.5) and remain there indefinitely. Sometimes, because the prostate is still in place or the tumor has not been fully destroyed, your PSA may not sink to that ideal low. And it may take as long as three years for PSA to reach its lowest level, which is called the PSA **nadir**. The higher the nadir, the greater the risk that the cancer will eventually recur.

A major source of confusion and anxiety is the PSA bounce, a meaningless rise in the PSA level, which falls again without treatment. Seen in up to 15 percent of patients at about a year and a half to two years after brachytherapy, the bounce phenomenon makes it very difficult to identify a cancer recurrence, and a delay in further treatment may result.[19]

In radiation, treatment is not officially deemed a failure until the PSA level rises 2 ng/ml above its nadir (nadir + 2).[20] Unfortunately, this definition delays the recognition of local regrowth of cancer within the prostate. A better measure of local recurrence would be 3 rises or peaks, whether or not they are consecutive and whether or not the level rises by 2 ng/ml. If you see three new peaks in your PSA, I'd recommend having a serious discussion with your radiation oncologist and urologist about whether you need a biopsy of the prostate to find out if the cancer is present and growing. Using the current definition of recurrence after radiation, we rarely recognize a failure with brachytherapy or external beam radiation until three to four years after treatment, when the window of opportunity for a cure has passed in most patients.

The Advantages of Seed Implants

The major attraction of brachytherapy is convenience. You can have the seeds implanted and be home the same day or the next. After the procedure, you will not need a catheter. Typically, you'll have no pain beyond some soreness in the perineal area that can be managed with a simple over-the-counter analgesic such as acetaminophen (Tylenol).

The treatment has few immediate complications and minimal short-term impact on quality of life.

THE DISADVANTAGES OF SEED IMPLANTS

Though side effects are far from inevitable, problems with urinary, bowel, and sexual function develop slowly over months or even years as radiation damage accumulates. While serious side effects are uncommon, especially in the hands of top experts, almost all patients develop urinary frequency and some develop urgency, burning, and urge incontinence that can often be alleviated with the use of alpha-blocking drugs.

While the radiation from seeds generally is not harmful to others, you will be told to avoid close contact with small children, young animals, and pregnant women for a few months after the implant, until the radiation dissipates. Being in the same room is not a problem. To expose someone else to radiation from your seeds, you would need to hold the person on your lap or sit right beside them for a prolonged period. Some doctors suggest placing a pillow between yourself and your partner if you like to sleep in the "spoon" position, though others feel that the pelvic bones provide enough natural protection.

Given heightened security in airports and at border crossings, you may want to carry a card that identifies you as an implant patient. Despite the low level of radiation brachytherapy implants emit, you might set off a Geiger counter or other detection device.

Until the radiation is no longer active, it's wise to avoid elective medical procedures, such as a colonoscopy, and elective surgical procedures, such as a hip replacement or dental work, that might put the doctor or dentist at risk of radiation exposure. If you require such procedures, medical personnel should take appropriate precautions.

Treatment results are highly variable and operator-dependent. It takes a very experienced, very meticulous radiation oncologist to do a good job of implanting the seeds. Since side effects and cancer recurrences can take many years to develop or detect, getting reliable information about a particular doctor's track record can be tricky.

Some seeds can migrate out of the prostate, invading adjacent tissues or even distant organs, such as the lungs. Because the energy of individual seeds is very low, stray seeds don't pose a significant health risk.

If treatment fails to control the tumor, it is risky to receive further radiation. Radiation damage has lifelong effects and is cumulative. Doctors have reported giving external radiation after seeds fail or implanting seeds after an external radiation or brachytherapy failure. I'd warn against these approaches, outside of a clinical trial in a highly specialized center. Additional radiation carries a serious risk of damage to the bowel and urinary tract, unless you are enrolled in a formal clinical trial to carefully study the side effects. We have no good evidence that a second radiation dose can control a recurrent cancer in the long run.

Salvage surgery can be done after seed implants, but the procedure is more difficult and riskier than radical prostatectomy on a gland that has not been irradiated. Only a highly experienced surgeon should attempt salvage radical prostatectomy. (See Salvage Radical Prostatectomy in Chapter 20, Rising PSA After Surgery, Radiation, or Other Therapy.)

The Side Effects of Brachytherapy

Immediate side effects are similar to those for a prostate biopsy. There may be some blood in the urine for a few days and some blood in the ejaculate for as long as six to eight weeks. The needles used to implant the seeds can cause mild pain or soreness in the perineum, which usually responds to over-the-counter pain medications such as acetaminophen or an anti-inflammatory drug such as ibuprofen.

The seeds emit their radiation gradually. **Half-life** refers to the number of days required for the radiation source to lose 50 percent of its original strength. Palladium has a shorter half-life (thirty-five days), so it delivers radiation more quickly than iodine, for which the half-life is sixty days. It takes about four to six months for seeds to give off virtually their entire dose of radiation, but it can take years for the damaging effects to accumulate.

It was hoped that modern brachytherapy would yield the same low rates of side effects as early seed implants, but as the dose was increased in an attempt to improve cure rates, complications increased as well. Even in men who have no previous urinary problems, swelling from the implant can cause frequent urination, burning, urgency, or the need to strain to urinate. The symptoms often respond to alpha-blocking drugs such as alfuzosin (Uroxatral), tamsulosin (Flomax), silodosin (Rapaflo) or doxazosin (Cardura), and most men receive one of these drugs before and after implantation to relax the prostate and bladder neck.

In about 5 to 13 percent of cases (less in the hands of a top expert), irritation and swelling from the implants trigger acute urinary retention, especially in men who have obstructive voiding symptoms before brachytherapy. This sudden inability to urinate could require long-term use of a catheter, the insertion of a suprapubic tube (above the pubic bone at the base of the abdomen), or a transurethral resection of the prostate (TURP) which could cause incontinence.

A month to three months after seed placement, when radiation effects start to accumulate, 25 to 45 percent of patients experience symptoms of radiation urethritis (painful urination, frequency, urgency, and urge incontinence) or radiation prostatism (a prostate inflammation that causes burning at the tip of the penis), and perineal or lower abdominal pain. Incontinence persists in 4 to 6 percent of patients one to two years after treatment, and 18 percent have moderate or severe distress from overall urinary symptoms at one year.[21] These problems are more frequent in men with a large prostate and are difficult to treat. Anticholinergic drugs and alpha blockers may provide some relief. When partners of patients were surveyed, as many were bothered by the patient's incontinence after brachytherapy as after prostatectomy (5 percent in both cases) and even more (7 percent) were bothered by their partner's other urinary symptoms.

Like external beam radiation, brachytherapy causes troublesome bowel problems, including bleeding, pain, frequent bowel movements, and fecal incontinence, in 3 to 10 percent of patients. The likelihood of bowel problems relates mostly to the amount of the rectal wall that is exposed to high radiation doses, which is why precise technique in administering the radiation is so crucial.

As radiation shrinks the prostate, the amount of fluid produced by the gland diminishes, reducing the volume of ejaculate. Some patients experience painful ejaculations, and virtually all men lose the ability to father children (though this does not mean it's safe to give up birth control unless you've been tested to be sure no viable sperm are present). If fertility is a concern, you may want to bank sperm before the implant.

Over time, there is a gradual loss of erections because of damage to small blood vessels and the erectile nerves. Few good long-term studies have looked at potency after brachytherapy, but those that did observed a troublesome loss of erections in 30 to 40 percent of patients. Nevertheless, in a survey of partners, less than 13 percent reported distress related to the patient's ED two years after brachytherapy, compared with 44 percent after radical prostatectomy and 22 percent after external beam radiation.[22] Some doctors still cite antiquated data from the era of low-dose seeds, when only 10 percent of previously potent men lost erections after brachytherapy, but those numbers do not apply to the higher radiation doses delivered by seeds today. The nerves are so close to the edge of the prostate, and cancer so often grows right at the edge of the gland, that it is impossible to dose the entire prostate adequately without exposing the nerves to the same high dose of radiation. (See Chapter 2, Normal Male Function.)

THE BOTTOM LINE

Brachytherapy is a reasonable option for men with prostates smaller than 60 grams and a favorable cancer that is confined to the prostate, especially when convenience is a central issue. Even with modern improved techniques, I hesitate to recommend brachytherapy for any patients with a PSA over 10, a Gleason score of 7 or greater, a palpable or visible cancer larger than a centimeter or so, or for patients with more than half of their biopsy cores positive for cancer. However, in an ongoing nationwide study, the Radiation Therapy Oncology Group is comparing brachytherapy alone with brachytherapy combined with external beam radiation for men with more serious cancers, so in time, we will know whether high-dose seed implants will work for intermediate-risk cancers.

NOTE: At Memorial Sloan-Kettering Cancer Center, Dr. Michael Zelefsky has pioneered a more accurate approach to brachytherapy that uses a sophisticated real-time computer program in the operating room for dose distribution.[23] The program guides seed placement, ensuring an optimal radiation dose to the entire prostate while minimizing damage to the urethra and rectum. By increasing accuracy, this approach has reduced urinary and bowel side effects substantially while obtaining cancer control rates comparable to those offered by high-dose external beam therapy. But these results are early. Long-term effects on erectile, urinary, and bowel function remain to be seen.

COMBINATION EXTERNAL BEAM RADIATION AND BRACHYTHERAPY

With conventional therapy (70 Gy radiation delivered externally by a standard linear accelerator), 15 to 20 percent of men experience serious bowel or urinary complications. In an attempt to improve the cure rate for men with serious cancers while reducing the side effects, some radiation therapists have combined temporary or permanent seed implants with external beam radiation therapy. The first such program was developed by Drs. Phil Hutchins and Eugene Carlton at Baylor College of Medicine in 1965. Following their lead, many major centers started using the combination treatment in the late 1970s and early 1980s.

Current advocates of this belt-and-suspenders approach claim that it can deliver higher radiation doses, and, indeed, cure rates with combination therapy for large, risky cancers have been good.[24] The advantage of combined therapy is that it delivers a more homogeneous dose to a broader area than seeds alone and eliminates cold spots. This treatment can be offered to people with higher-grade, larger, more extensive cancers. By keeping the external beam dose lower, radiation oncologists using this approach hope to avoid some of the bowel, urinary, and sexual side effects of high-dose external beam radiation used alone.

Unfortunately, combination therapy carries a higher risk of serious complications compared with seeds or IMRT alone. While randomized clinical trails are under way to determine the risks and benefits of combination therapy, experience in institutions around the world generally show troublesome long-term bowel or urinary side effects in 15 percent of patients. Erectile dysfunction is common, especially if hormone therapy is added to the program, and long-term radiation proctitis (irritation of the bowel), sometimes followed by rectal ulcers, occurs in 2 to 4 percent of men. Mild ulcers may respond to anti-inflammatory drugs or steroids, but surgery may be necessary in the rare severe case.

The problem is prostate anatomy. The gland lies perilously close to the erectile nerves and the rectal wall. At a sufficiently high dose to kill cancers, the combination approach exposes these delicate structures to excessive and highly damaging radiation.

Radiation therapy involves complex decision-making by the oncologist and subtle variations in technique. A certain percentage of error, in which normal structures are exposed to damaging X-rays, is inevitable. When both seed implants and external beam therapy are administered, the error rate and resultant side effects may be multiplied. While many radiation oncologists are enthusiastic, there is not enough evidence that cancers are cured more effectively with combined approaches. Generally, combination therapy is a riskier substitute for modern, high-dose, intensity-modulated conformal radiotherapy. Its main advantage is logistical. It shortens the time required to deliver the external radiation dose from ten weeks to four or five.

HORMONES AND RADIATION

Radiation works best against a small, manageable adversary. It's easier to wipe out two hundred mosquitoes than two thousand, and the same holds true for cancer cells. Killing off a few insects with a shot of insect repellent has less effect on the environment than saturation crop dusting from a plane. By the same token, a small, highly targeted radiation dose risks less damage to normal surrounding tissues.

Frustrated with the poor cure rates with conventional (70 Gy) external radiation, oncologists designed studies to test whether shrinking the cancer with hormones before radiation would improve the results. Indeed it did, especially for cancers with any aggressive features. In fact, studies clearly showed better survival rates for large (T2b or greater) or high-grade (Gleason 8 or higher) cancers when hormones were combined with conventional doses of radiation. In most studies, hormones were started several months before radiation and continued until the last day of treatment. For particularly aggressive cancers, the best effects were achieved when hormones were continued for two to three years or permanently.[25] In these studies, hormone treatment involves shutting down the production of male hormones with drugs called **LHRH agonists**, administering **antiandrogens** to prevent the cells from absorbing these hormones, or prescribing a combination of the two, known as a **total** or **complete androgen blockade**.

We still don't know whether hormones work by shrinking the primary tumor and increasing the probability that the radiation will kill every cell or by eliminating tiny, undetectable areas of spread, called micrometastases. The latter seems unlikely, since hormones add nothing to cure rates with surgery. We do know that the beneficial effect of adding hormones to radiation can not be achieved by giving patients hormones alone. In a large randomized trial in Sweden, men with locally advanced prostate cancer treated with hormone therapy alone had shorter survival and more complications from their cancer than men treated with external radiation and hormones.[26]

Several studies have shown that hormones plus radiation improve cancer control, but the reason is unclear.[27] By shrinking the cancer, hormones may increase the likelihood that a given dose of radiation will completely eradicate the cancer. If so, the same result could be achieved with modern high-dose IMRT. Expert radiation oncologists estimate that combining hormones with radiation is comparable to adding 5 Gy to the dose and may not be necessary for most patients in centers where doses of 81 or 86 Gy can be given safely. If this is the only benefit, it is hard to understand why giving hormones permanently, or for two to three years, cures more patients than when hormones are given for a few months before radiation.

Another reason patients may be asked to take three to six months of hormone therapy before radiation is to shrink a large prostate and reduce the size of the field that must be irradiated. Minimizing the area that must be hit with destructive X-rays lowers the risk of damage to the rectal wall.

Unfortunately, hormone therapy carries risks of its own. Cutting off the androgen supply can cause troublesome side effects, including hot flashes, loss of libido and erections, loss of muscle mass, changes in the distribution of body hair, breast swelling, and depression. When radiation is combined with hormone therapy, the incidence of permanent erectile dysfunction is greater, though how much greater has not been well studied.

Most men regain normal testosterone production following a short course of three months to a year on hormone therapy, but some don't. Older men, those who take hormone therapy for several years, and those who started out with low testosterone levels may not regain hormone levels sufficient to restore erectile function or relieve the other side effects.

THE FUTURE

Dose painting. We now know that most cancers that recur after radiation grow back in the area in which they started, rather than arising in a new part of the gland.[28] Dose painting shows promise as a way to refine radiation treatments, allowing radiation oncologists to target highly specific areas of the gland containing cancer, while selectively protecting vulnerable adjacent structures, including the erectile nerves, urethra, and rectal wall.

Higher radiation doses. The chance of curing a cancer is directly related to the doses of radiation administered. With modern IMRT, doses of up to 86 Gy have been delivered safely. Such high doses can be achieved with commercially available equipment, excellent medical physics, and careful treatment planning, and can eliminate the need for hormone therapy in many patients.

Single-Dose Therapy. Dr. Zvi Fuks at Memorial Sloan-Kettering Cancer Center and other radiation oncologists have been investigating the feasibility of giving radiation in fewer fractions (hypofractionation) over five days, two days, or even a single day, as opposed to ten weeks. There is strong evidence from laboratory research and preliminary clinical trials that 22 to 24 Gy, given in a single day, can permanently eradicate cancer at least as well as a longer course. We now use this method routinely to treat prostate and other cancers that have metastasized to the brain, bones, and lung. Plans are under way for a new clinical trial to study single-dose radiation followed by radical prostatectomy in patients with high-risk cancers.

Sensitizing and protective agents. A number of substances currently under investigation are designed to increase the effect of radiation on target tissues and reduce the damage to normal adjacent tissues.

IN SUMMARY

Depending on a man's age and the nature of his disease, good modern radiation can be a highly effective treatment for localized prostate cancer. The dose and precise method of delivery are crucial to maximize your chance for a cure and minimize the risk of side effects. When adjacent organs are exposed to excess radiation, urinary, sexual, and bowel function can be damaged over time. The serious full consequences of radiation injury to normal tissue can take a decade or more to appreciate. Late recurrences of cancer after radiation are also a concern, since the gland is left in place. Nevertheless, radiation is a safe and highly effective way to treat most prostate cancers. If you opt for radiation therapy, be sure to choose an expert radiation oncologist and an excellent, state-of-the-art facility.

16

■

Focal and Other "Local" Therapies

READ THIS CHAPTER TO LEARN:

- What other ways are there to treat cancer within the prostate (local treatment)?
- What are the effects of cryotherapy and HIFU?
- What are "investigational" treatments, and which are approved by the FDA?
- What is focal therapy?

After a prostate cancer diagnosis, the first question is whether your cancer needs to be treated at all. If you have a tiny, low-risk tumor, the most reasonable option may be careful monitoring in an active surveillance program.

If your prostate cancer is serious enough to warrant active treatment now, both surgery and radiation offer an established track record of safety and good long-term cancer control. Radiation has the fewest side effects in the short run, and surgery provides the best results in terms of controlling the cancer. For any other local therapy (treatment directed at the prostate) to make sense, it would have to be as safe yet more effective than radiation, or as effective yet safer than surgery.

Researchers are constantly seeking better ways to search out and destroy prostate cancers. Because the gland is so devilishly difficult to access and the risk of damage to nearby vital structures accompanies all currently accepted treatments, the quest to discover a kinder, gentler, but still effective therapy continues.

Some treatments, such as destroying the tumor with heat (**thermal therapy**) or light (**photodynamic therapy**), or injecting altered genes into the prostate (**gene therapy**), are under intense study as experimental treatments, meaning they are not yet approved by the FDA for routine use in the U.S. They are being explored in clinical trials, which means their safety and effectiveness have yet to be proven.[1]

Winning FDA approval does not put an end to scientific scrutiny. Until a new treatment has been thoroughly tested, proven safe and effective, and practiced for enough time to yield convincing, durable results, it is not considered a standard of care. Several alternative treatments are currently available for localized prostate cancer. **Cryotherapy** (freezing the prostate) has been used off and on for over thirty years and is now approved by the FDA, but long-term results remain uncertain.

In considering any of these approaches, keep in mind that they lack an established track record. While some might eventually earn a place in standard practice, at this point we don't know how safe they are or how successful they will ultimately be in arresting cancers and preventing recurrences. Prostate cancer is typically slow to progress, and it can take many years, or even decades, to demonstrate whether a particular type of treatment stops the spread of cancer and prolongs survival. Also, just because a treatment seems "less invasive" or otherwise easier than standard surgery or radiation therapy does not ensure that it will cause fewer side effects in the long run or yield better cure rates down the road.

A major problem with HIFU and cryotherapy is that doctors sometimes try to treat cancers that are too big or too serious for these approaches. None of these treatments are particularly effective for anything but favorable, low-risk cancers with a PSA below 10, a Gleason grade below 7, and stage T1 or T2a. Men typically shy away from surgery in fear of side effects, but remember, a promise of low side effects may mean the treatment is limited and unlikely to cure a life-threatening tumor.

Establishing a new program or center to administer an investigational approach involves considerable expense, time, and energy. Doctors who embrace a novel treatment may stake their financial and professional future on its success. It's wise to be mindful of this as you evaluate these methods and weigh reported outcomes. Physicians studying experimental treatments in clinical trials are ethically bound to disclose whether they or their institution have a financial stake in the outcome of the study. You are well within your rights to ask if a doctor you are considering has such an interest in the treatment he recommends.

> NOTE: While treatments for cancer may have different side effects, the best bet is to cure the cancer with the first attempt. If the first treatment does not work, the second try is likely to be more complicated and less effective. In balancing risks and benefits, the best bet is to have the treatment that has the best chance of getting rid of the cancer the first time.

FREEZING THE GLAND (CRYOTHERAPY)

Freezing is a well-established way to destroy cancer cells. For the prostate, modern cryotherapy is done under anesthesia and requires a short hospital stay and a tube through the abdomen to drain the bladder for a few weeks.

Guided by ultrasound, probes are placed in the prostate through the **perineum** (behind the scrotum). Argon gas is delivered through the probes to freeze the gland and surrounding tissues, creating an ice ball. As it forms, the ice ball can be observed by ultrasound, so the surgeon has some control over the extent of tissue damage. Cancer, along with the blood vessels that feed it, are damaged by freezing below -40 degrees centigrade and further damaged by subsequent thawing. Typically, the treatment involves two cycles of freezing and thawing, though in some cases, additional cycles may be required.

Proponents tout cryotherapy as a minimally invasive treatment that causes little disruption to normal activities and can be repeated if the cancer recurs. Given modern ultrasound guidance, cryotherapy now has a lower rate of serious complications such as a rectourethral fistula (hole between the rectum and urethra), which occurs in 0 to 3 percent of patients, or serious incontinence, 0 to 13 percent. Immediate mild to moderate complication rates are much higher. Forty-seven to 100 percent of men have erectile dysfunction after treatment. In men with normal sexual function before cryotherapy, only 10 to 15 percent will recover full erections, and one third will recover some function over three to four years. One to 19 percent experience urinary incontinence.[2] Cryoablation can also result in scrotal swelling, penile pain or numbness, pelvic pain, and urinary obstruction. Results are highly operator-dependent, varying with the skill and experience of the doctor performing the procedure. Unlike external beam therapy, the damaging effects of treatment do not build up over time, so the short-term complication rate predicts the type and risk of long-term complications.

The biggest open question is whether cryotherapy offers good cancer control. Given the lack of clinical trials, we know little about the long-term success rate of this treatment. While both the European and the American Urological Associations consider cryotherapy as an alternative treatment for localized prostate cancer, I believe that the long-term risks and benefits still make it less attractive than radiation therapy (external beam or seed implants) or surgery.

In the few trials that have been published, cryotherapy failed to offer good cure rates when compared with modern, high-dose IMRT radiation or radical prostatectomy. In a review of over 2,000 men who received cryotherapy, the probability of a positive biopsy after treatment ranged from 1 to 20 percent. The probability of being free of cancer at one year after treatment (using PSA as a measure) was 63 to 75 percent.[3]

Cryotherapy fared better in two studies of men with locally advanced T3 or T4 cancers, when compared with radiation. In both groups, hormone therapy was used for 4 to 6 months before treatment. But in these trials, the radiation dose was much lower than the levels we recommend today.[4]

In the early days of cryotherapy, the urethra was often damaged by the ice ball. After treatment, sloughing of the damaged tissues was common, requiring a catheter for as long as six weeks or a TURP to alleviate urinary obstruction. Today, doctors performing cryotherapy use a urethral warmer to protect the urinary channel. This has markedly reduced the sloughing problem, though it still occurs in 2 to 5 percent of patients.

Unfortunately, protecting the urethra may increase the risk of leaving cancer behind. Sixty-five percent of prostate cancers occur within 5 mm of this urinary channel.[5] In addition, 93 percent of patients have cancer at the apex (bottom) of the gland, which is a difficult area to treat with cryotherapy. Because of these limitations, the treatment should not be used in men with prostates larger than 40 grams.

Both normal and malignant prostate cells are remarkably resilient. From biopsy results and elevations in PSA, we know that many normal and some cancer cells persist after freezing. Since normal prostate cells typically remain, new cancers may develop in the gland years later.

There is considerable debate about the right measure of success after cryotherapy. Unlike surgery, where the PSA becomes undetectable and a subsequent rise signals that the cancer has recurred, with cryotherapy, some normal prostate tissue persists, making both the PSA and the biopsy results difficult to interpret. Proponents argue for the use of the ASTRO or Phoenix definitions (PSA nadir plus 2 ng/ml) of cancer recurrence that are used after radiation. But using these measures underestimates the failure rate and can markedly delay the realization that the cancer has not been destroyed, and we can miss a second chance to cure the disease.[6]

Because of its limited efficacy, optimal candidates for cryotherapy should have a cancer of limited size (clinical stage T1 or T2), PSA less than 20 ng/ml, Gleason score 6 or less, and a prostate gland less than 40 grams in size. Cryotherapy is best used in older men (65 and older) since the long-term results are unknown.[7]

Salvage Cryotherapy: While freezing offers little advantage for someone newly diagnosed with prostate cancer, it has developed a niche for the treatment of recurrence after radiation or surgery, for which we have few attractive alternatives. With local recurrence of cancer after radiation, cryotherapy is somewhat effective and has fewer complications than salvage radical prostatectomy. In one study, 83 percent of patients had a detectable PSA, but using the definition of recurrence that is currently accepted for radiation therapy, 55 percent showed no progression of their cancer after five years, and in 67 percent the biopsy showed no cancer. Most men receive hormone therapy in conjunction with cryotherapy, so it has been difficult to judge the relative beneficial contributions of each treatment to the success rate.

In salvage cryotherapy, complication rates are high. Over 4 percent of men having salvage cryotherapy develop urinary incontinence, and over 1 percent have a rectal fistula (hole). Loss of erections is universal, and sex drive is eliminated if hormones are added.[8]

When compared with radical prostatectomy for cancers that recurred after radiation, cryotherapy was less likely than surgery to cure the cancer or to prolong survival.[9]

HEATING THE PROSTATE (THERMOTHERAPY)

Thermal therapies, which use various energy sources and delivery methods to effectively cook target tissues, are experimental and not yet approved for use in medical practice in the U.S. outside a formal clinical trial. In Europe, these treatments have been used for the past decade.

High-intensity focused ultrasound (HIFU) destroys tissue with the extreme heat generated by high-energy ultrasound waves. The procedure requires regional (spinal or epidural) anesthesia. A probe inserted in the rectum contains two ultrasound transducers, one to image the prostate and identify the target and another to send out the destructive thermal energy. The lining of the rectum is protected from overheating with a cold water balloon.

HIFU was first used in the prostate to treat BPH (see Chapter 5, BPH [Benign Prostatic Hyperplasia]) by eliminating excess tissue to relieve blockage in the urinary passage. The results were not particularly good. Symptoms recurred in about half of the men treated this way within four years, and they then had to be treated with a TURP, so the technique has largely fallen out of favor.

For prostate cancer, HIFU has attracted considerable recent interest in Europe, where brachytherapy and cryotherapy are not widely used to treat the disease. These techniques all share the attraction of being "minimally invasive" and convenient. Treatment can be completed in one session, but it does require general or spinal anesthesia and takes several hours. It is logistically simpler than external beam radiation, which requires repeated trips to the radiation center over two months. And it is immediately less invasive than surgery.[10]

HIFU may eventually have a role in treating relatively small, favorable prostate cancers, especially in elderly men who do not want radiation or surgery. The treatment focuses intense, destructive thermal energy in a tiny cylinder of tissue, measuring about 2 to 3 by 10 to 15 millimeters. By lining up these cylinders on the ultrasound image of the prostate, the surgeon can program the computer-driven machine to treat the cancer.

Just how effective is HIFU in eradicating cancer? This is difficult to tell, since few case series have been published, and there are no randomized trials as yet. Patients have not been followed long enough to tell whether the treatment really destroyed the cancer or if the slow-growing cancer was just "laying low" for a while. After HIFU, a biopsy of the prostate converts to negative in about 75 to 90 percent of the cases, but PSA levels rarely become unmeasurable, as they regularly do after surgery. A favorable response, which occurs in about a quarter of patients, occurs when the PSA declines to less than 0.2 ng/ml and a repeat biopsy is negative for cancer. A recent review found that follow-up after HIFU tended to be short, providing little information about long-term survival.[11] Six to 23 percent of men had a positive biopsy within the first six months, and cancer had recurred, as measured by a rising PSA, in 16 to 31 percent. The best long-term study we have included 163 patients treated at a European center who were followed for at least three years. Ninety-three percent had a negative biopsy. In 86 percent, the PSA dropped to less than 1. But by five years after treatment, 34 percent of men had recurrent cancer or needed further treatment with surgery, radiation, or hormones.[12]

When used for small early cancers (clinical stage T1c or T2a, Gleason 2 to 6, PSA levels less than 10), the short-term results seem adequate. For larger or more aggressive cancers, the failure rate (i.e. chances of a recurrence of cancer) is high. The treatment is not generally used if the prostate is larger than 40 to 50 grams, because the HIFU beam cannot reach the whole prostate gland.

Most experts in the field agree that HIFU should be used only in men who have a short life expectancy or a serious medical condition that precludes surgery, or for patients who refuse surgery or radiation. At MSKCC, we are conducting a study of HIFU. The protocol excludes patients under 60, and requires a prostate smaller than 40 grams containing a low-risk cancer. For such men, short-term results of HIFU seem adequate. We do not yet know the risks involved in salvage surgery or radiation for cancer that recurs after this treatment.

Since the heated prostatic tissue swells after the procedure and then sloughs into the urethra, the risk of urinary blockage after HIFU is fairly high. Men typically require a urinary catheter or a superpubic tube (through the skin of the abdomen into the bladder) for one to two weeks after the procedure, unless a TURP is performed at the same time. (See Chapter 5, BPH [Benign Prostatic Hyperplasia]). Complications include acute urinary retention in about half the patients. About 1 in 4 men develops a urethral stricture or bladder neck contracture requiring dilation or a TURP. In a number of reported series, the risk of some urinary incontinence generally ranged from 7 to 25 percent. The most serious and dangerous complication is a fistula (opening) between the rectum and the urinary tract, which occurs in 0.7 to 3.2 percent of patients and could require a colostomy. Fortunately, fistulas have become rare when the procedure is performed by an experienced surgeon. Approximately 20 to 66 percent of patients lose their erections after treatment. Most recent series report a 43 percent incidence of long-term ED.[13]

The complication rate is much higher when HIFU is used for men who have failed radiation therapy. Used in this "salvage" setting, the risk of rectourethral fistula ranges from 7 to 16 percent. Seven to 50 percent of men given salvage HIFU develop urinary incontinence. Severe urinary obstruction or strictures occur in over one third of patients. HIFU should be used with caution in men previously irradiated, and should be performed only by highly experienced surgeons.[14]

Ultrasound-guided HIFU is being tested in the United States in an

NOTE: A U.S. company is currently recruiting patients to be treated with HIFU in Canada, Mexico, or the Dominican Republic. Though this is not illegal, conflict of interest is inescapable. Doctors recommending this approach administer and charge for the patient's care before and after treatment. But because it is done out of the country, the procedure is not eligible for insurance reimbursement. Be sure that your treatment choice is not being driven by the financial interests of your doctor.

NOTE: The problem with cryotherapy and HIFU is anatomy. Cancer almost always lies adjacent to the capsule of the prostate (see illustration on page 10), and the rectum, urinary sphincter, and erectile nerves lie just a few millimeters away. Heat or freezing damages these exquisitely sensitive structures. These energy sources are not nearly precise enough to destroy all prostate tissue and all cancer within the gland without permanent damage to erections, if not urinary and bowel function. It is easy to make a treatment safe by backing away from thoroughly destroying the cancer. And it is easy to destroy the cancer if you do not care about side effects. What is truly difficult is to destroy the cancer with little or no damage to normal nearby structures and few if any side effects.

FDA–approved study comparing results and complications with those of brachytherapy. In general, HIFU seems to result in a bit less ED though more urinary obstruction than cryotherapy, and seems to be about as effective. I find it difficult to imagine that cryotherapy or HIFU will ever assume a leading role in the treatment of prostate cancer. Technically, it will prove almost impossible to destroy all cancer within the prostate without unacceptable damage to the erectile nerves, which lie within millimeters of the capsule of the gland. Small, early cancers can be "treated" with almost anything and do well, as they do in a hands-off active surveillance program. Unless the entire gland is treated, neither cryotherapy nor HIFU is likely to prove effective for treating serious cancers.

With HIFU, the hope was that the column of heat could be controlled precisely, but if a small nerve fiber is heated to just 56 degrees C, well below the 80 degrees C of a column of HIFU, the nerve is permanently destroyed. For this reason, large prostate cancers, those lying close to the capsule of the gland (where prostate cancers typically arise), or those that are aggressive cannot be treated effectively with HIFU without destroying the erectile nerves. We cannot see these nerves on the ultrasound that guides HIFU treatment, so we do not know where they are.

PHOTODYNAMIC (LIGHT) THERAPY

An interesting and novel approach to the treatment of localized cancers is **photodynamic therapy**. Let me disclose at the outset that I have been paid to advise a company, Steba Biotechnology, that is studying this method.

Photodynamic therapy has been around for decades, stirring little serious interest in the medical community. Recently, however, scientists have developed a new, more powerful chemical derived from plant chlorophyll, nature's premier agent for converting light into energy. The photodynamic agent is administered intravenously. Then, a laser light source is inserted into the prostate, activating the chemical to destroy the cancer along with its blood supply.[15] Initial experiments in Europe and Canada have been favorable. Large areas of prostate tissue can clearly be destroyed, and there has been surprisingly little effect on urinary function, even when the entire gland is treated. With more limited treatments directed at only part of the prostate, there appears to be no harm to erectile function, but the experience to date is too limited to say for sure. Since this treatment does not work by heating or freezing, it's possible that this may be a more effective way to treat the entire prostate or to treat close to the neurovascular bundles or the sphincter without the harm caused by cryotherapy or HIFU. Exactly how effective and safe photodynamic therapy will be remains to be proven by good clinical trials, which are now under way in Europe, Great Britain, and the U.S.

FOCAL THERAPY OF PROSTATE CANCER

Not long ago, I saw a healthy 50-year-old man, I'll call him David, who was married and sexually active. On biopsy, he'd been found to have 1 mm of Gleason 3 + 3 in 1 of 12 biopsy cores. His tumor was not palpable on DRE. His prostate cancer was very favorable and posed no present risk to his life or health. He and I wrestled with whether to put him on a program of active surveillance at such a young age. What if his cancer proved to be more aggressive than it appeared? Even if we had assessed his tumor accurately, given his long remaining life expectancy, there was always the risk that his cancer might progress. On the other hand, if he had surgery or radiation treatment for this tiny, innocent-seeming tumor, he might have troubling side effects.

David couldn't deal with the idea of living with an untreated cancer, and he opted to have surgery. When we removed his prostate, the initial pathology found no tumor at all. On reexamination, the pathologist found one tiny area of Gleason 6 cancer. One third of men over 50 have such clusters of cancer cells in their prostates. Few are ever bothered by them, and many live out their lives without even knowing that the cells exist.

This patient had early return of erections, but he developed Peyronie's disease, a painful curvature in his penis. He became depressed and his marriage suffered. This experience made me think there had to be a better alternative than radical treatment for a tiny cancer that poses little risk. And I began to search for alternative approaches.

Nearly one third of the cancers that we operate on today prove to be small, favorable (indolent) cancers that would pose little threat to life or health if left alone for many years (see Chapter 13, Watchful Waiting [Active Surveillance]). We examined nearly 1,000 prostates removed surgically at Memorial Sloan-Kettering. Of those patients with a PSA level less than 10 ng/ml before surgery, 82 percent of the cancers were multifocal, but the largest focus of cancer represented the overwhelming bulk of the tumor. One to four additional microscopic foci of cancer were found in the prostate, but they were almost uniformly tiny, low-grade, and confined to the gland. In fact, they were no different from the cancers found on autopsy in a third of men over 50 who die of other causes. If we could get rid of the largest "index" tumor, we might be able to sharply reduce the chances that an aggressive cancer would develop later, making it much safer for a man to accept active surveillance and avoid radical surgery or radiation for the rest of his life.[16]

Why have doctors not embraced this previously? Traditionally, it has been difficult to know for certain how much cancer is in the prostate and where it lies. We have lacked the technology to destroy one small area of the gland precisely with little harm to surrounding tissues.

Today, with systematic "mapping" biopsies (see Chapter 9, Biopsy), we are able to identify the sector or region of the prostate where the principal focus of cancer lies and, more important, be sure there is not a large, high-grade cancer lying elsewhere in the prostate.[17] While modern MRI cannot see small tumors within the prostate, it can help rule out the presence of a large, more aggressive cancer that the initial biopsy might have missed, so a mapping biopsy, used in combination with MRI, can go a long way toward eliminating the worry that drives most doctors and many patients to elect radical therapy for even the smallest early cancer. Mapping biopsy plus MRI can help us locate and characterize prostate tumors with enough precision to make focal therapy rational.[18] Given modern technology, I believe it is reasonable to target therapy to the dominant focus of cancer within the prostate. If this main area can be eradicated, the tumor would be drastically reduced.

Focal therapy for prostate cancer is a new concept. It has not yet been adequately tested, and safe indications have yet to be sorted out. We do know that this approach is inadequate for men with an aggressive (Gleason score 7 or higher) or a large cancer (clinical stage T2b or greater). Focal therapy is probably inadequate for patients with more than 3 positive biopsy cores, men with any biopsy core containing more than 7 to 10 mm of cancer, or those with a PSA density greater than 0.15. (See Chapter 10, Understanding Your Cancer.) In these men, focal therapy is unlikely to have a sufficient effect, and it may mislead patients into believing that their cancer has been treated adequately.

Focal therapy is an exciting possibility that may give men a way out of the frustrating dilemma of doing nothing about their cancer (watchful waiting) or enduring radical therapy. At this point, focal therapy should be considered "investigational," to be performed only with the informed consent of the patient in a clinical trial.

Some doctors are using cryotherapy to treat one lobe (half) of the prostate in men with unilateral cancer. They argue that this allows them to avoid the ED that is so common after freezing the whole gland.[19] But cryotherapy is a blunt tool, and treating half the gland almost certainly destroys the nerve on that side. If they ever have to go back and treat the other side, which is likely given that prostate cancer often recurs after cryotherapy, the level of ED could be as high as it is when cryotherapy is used on the whole gland. To date, we lack clinical trials, ongoing follow-up, and a standard protocol for cryotherapy on half the prostate. As a result we don't know how often these cancers will recur or how sexual function will be in the long term.[20]

Technologies that may prove to have the necessary precision and power to "zap" a small focal cancer, while leaving the nerves and urinary sphincter intact, are on the horizon. The most promising are MRI-guided HIFU[21] and photodynamic therapy,[22] described above.

THE BOTTOM LINE

Focal therapy is intriguing and deserves serious study. As yet, there is no good evidence that treating specific areas of cancer within the prostate can alter the long-term course of the disease. Other untreated clusters of cancer cells may continue to grow and spread. For men with very small cancers, however, the promise of controlling the disease with few if any side effects is extremely attractive. If it proves possible to destroy these tiny tumors with ease and safety, and the treatments can be repeated as new cancer clusters are detected, many men may be able to avoid the risks of radical surgery or radiation therapy as well as the anxiety of living with an untreated cancer.

GENE THERAPY AND ONCOLYTIC VIRUSES

In the 1990s, the research team that Tim Thompson and I led at Baylor College of Medicine in Houston conducted the first successful clinical trial of so-called "suicide" gene therapy for prostate cancer. The idea is to inject a Trojan horse in the form of a virus that infiltrates the cancer cells and leaves behind a gene called **thymidine kinase**, or **TK**. Later, we administer an antiviral drug called ganciclovir. The genetically altered cells render the drug far more lethal, and the cancer is destroyed. In several subsequent studies, viruses have been used successfully to introduce suicide genes or to attack cancer cells directly.

Gene therapy by local injection appears to be safe. None of the feared consequences—viruses migrating to other parts of the body and wreaking harm, permanently infecting and destroying the normal gland, or getting into sperm and being transmitted to offspring—has occurred. Unfortunately, the approach has shown limited effectiveness because of the difficulty involved in getting the virus into all of the cancer cells. Development of viral gene therapy has been hindered by its prohibitive cost, the worry about unforeseen consequences of using viruses, and the limited promise of financial reward, which makes the research unattractive to pharmaceutical companies. The pursuit of this treatment has been relegated to the few university laboratories able to afford the research and development costs but appears to be poised for a commercial rebirth. Recently, a group led by one of the original team of inventors I worked with at Baylor received a federal grant for a clinical trial that will test the benefits of adenoviral gene therapy given before radiation versus radiation alone for the treatment of intermediate-risk prostate cancer.[23]

Most studies to date have tested gene therapy in patients with local recurrences of prostate cancer after radiation therapy. The treatment may yet play a major role when radiation or surgery fails to control a localized prostate cancer, or for very small cancers. Another exciting possibility is that local gene therapy may stimulate generalized immunity to prostate cancer, ridding the body of microscopic metastases that otherwise cannot be controlled.

THE FUTURE

At Harvard and MIT in the laboratory of Robert Langer, an expert in nanotechnology, scientists have produced nanoparticles one hundred times smaller than a red blood cell. These minuscule particles are coated to make them unrecognizable to the immune system. And they have a dissolvable shell. It may be possible to insert a drug such as Taxotere, the main chemotherapeutic drug used for prostate cancer, into these nanoparticles. On the surface, researchers place molecules called aptamers, which are coded to seek out and stick to the surface of prostate cancer cells. In experiments with mice, this technique has been shown to make prostate cancers melt away.[24] Hopefully, it might prove effective in human tumors as well, for direct injection into the prostate or into a vein to fight metastases anywhere in the body.

Steba Biotechnology is developing photodynamic therapy for focal ablation of selected prostate cancers. And General Electric, in association with InSightec, an Israeli company, is finalizing a version of HIFU that can be guided and monitored in real time by magnetic resonance imaging and thermography (temperature monitoring) capable of discerning a change in tissue temperature of 1 degree C. These new technologies promise to open the door for trials of focal therapy for prostate cancer.

IN SUMMARY

New treatments for localized prostate cancer are constantly being developed and tested. While some of these novel approaches may become standard practice in the future, they do not have a demonstrated track record of cancer cure as yet, and their long-term risks are uncertain. Be wary of extravagant, unproven claims, and remember that many new therapies that promise to cure cancer with no side effects have come and gone. Most are effective at eliminating only small cancers that probably did not need to be treated, and come up far short of curing serious, life-threatening malignancies.

17

◾

Urinary Side Effects

READ THIS CHAPTER TO LEARN:

- Why do prostate diseases and their treatments affect urinary function?
- What urinary problems can radiation, radical prostatectomy, and other treatments cause?
- What can be done about urinary side effects?

Urination should be a routine bodily function, but for many men the prostate throws up a major roadblock to that routine. The upper portion of the urethra, the conduit that channels urine from the bladder to the outside, runs directly through the gland. Benign or malignant prostate overgrowth can narrow the passageway, triggering a variety of urinary problems. Symptoms can range in severity from a minor slowing of the urinary stream to a sudden, complete inability to urinate. Acute urinary retention is a medical emergency that requires immediate relief to avoid serious bladder or kidney damage.

Because of the hand-in-glove relationship between the urinary channel and the prostate, treatments for prostate diseases, including surgery and radiation, all carry a risk of urinary side effects. Imagine trying to repair the Lincoln Tunnel without affecting the traffic running through it. Urinary problems can take the form of **obstructive voiding symptoms** (slow stream, hesitancy, intermittency, waking at night to urinate), **irritative voiding symptoms** (frequency, urgency, blood in the urine, burning), or urinary **incontinence** (leaking, loss of urinary control).

URINATION AFTER RADICAL PROSTATECTOMY

To cure prostate cancer surgically, we remove the entire gland, the seminal vesicles, and the bladder neck, which runs into and is virtually indistinguishable from the adjacent prostate. Sparing the bladder neck increases the risk of leaving cancer behind. Nevertheless, some surgeons do so in the misguided belief that this is necessary to preserve urinary continence.

The bladder neck contains the **internal urinary sphincter**, a sturdy muscular trapdoor that keeps urine from escaping until you're ready to void. After radical prostatectomy, the **external** (or **outer**) **urinary sphincter**, which normally acts as a second line of defense against accidental leakage, must assume the entire responsibility for keeping you dry.

Typically, the body makes this adjustment uneventfully on its own, though the time it takes to regain full urinary control varies widely. Any leakage that occurs until the transfer of function is completed can usually be managed with the use of small pads that might require changing anywhere from one to several times a day.

NOTE: These pads are specifically designed for this purpose in men and come in a variety of styles. They can be purchased by mail order, online, or in drugstores. (See Resources.)

INCONTINENCE

Though prostate cancer commonly evokes an image of severe incontinence and patients often worry that they'll have to use adult diapers or wear a catheter and leg bag, such serious leakage is rare following competent surgery to remove the gland. In the hands of the typical surgeon in this country, about 7 percent of radical prostatectomy patients report troublesome incontinence.[1] For those operated on by expert surgeons, any long-term urinary control problem—including minor leakage—is uncommon.[2] Some of my patients are dry as soon as the catheter is removed, and more than half stop needing pads within a few days. By six weeks after surgery, 90 percent achieve social continence, meaning that urinary leakage has ceased altogether or lessened to the point that it has little or no impact on normal activities. Sixty percent of these men are sufficiently dry to stop wearing pads altogether, and the rest use one or two pads to contain minimal leakage. By 6 months, 80 percent are completely dry, and by 12 months, 93 percent. One year after radical prostatectomy, only 1 percent of men I see continue to have leakage troublesome enough to warrant treatment, and 5 to 7 percent wear a small pad when they go to work or exercise. In general, this holds true for patients of highly experienced surgeons nationwide.[3]

Studies show that recovery after surgery depends to a great extent on the experience of the surgeon.[4] On average in the United States, the return to full urinary control after radical prostatectomy takes six weeks to three months, and about 7 percent of patients report moderate or severe distress from leakage two years later. When compared with the results of top surgeons, this represents double the time to regaining full control and a four- to eight-fold greater risk of lasting incontinence. The presumption that "minimally invasive" laparoscopic or robotic surgery reduces the risk of urinary problems is unfounded. In fact, in our studies, men recover continence sooner after open surgery.[5] When choosing a doctor, keep in mind that the quality of your care can have a major impact on your quality of life.

How Much Leakage Constitutes Incontinence?

Though it's common for people to equate the term "urinary incontinence" with the complete lack of bladder control seen in infants, in fact, the generally accepted definition of *severe* incontinence after prostate-cancer treatment is leaking 2 or more tablespoons of urine per day *and* being moderately to severely bothered by it as measured by a questionnaire.[5] The response to leaking urine is highly subjective. Some men find it intolerable to lose a single drop, while others are not particularly troubled by the need to use a few small, unobtrusive pads per day to keep their clothing dry.

When weighing the risk of side effects, keep in mind that doctors may differ enormously in what they mean when they report their results. If you see one surgeon who sets his incontinence rate at 30 percent and another who claims only a 1 percent incidence, they could be describing entirely different outcomes. The former doctor might be telling you about every patient who leaks even a small amount of urine for a short time after surgery, while the latter only counts patients as incontinent if they have severe, intractable leakage that persists for years. Be sure to ask physicians you consult to define their terms.

NOTE: Most men live a full, active life, even though they wear only one pad per day. Nevertheless, quality of life questionnaires indicate that these men perceive the pad as a detriment.[6]

Who Is at Risk for Incontinence?

Age plays a significant role. Men over 65 have more difficulty regaining urinary control, and after age 70, the problems tend to be even greater. Older men may be more susceptible to incontinence because of benign enlargement of the prostate, preexisting bladder outlet obstruction, or the reduced muscle mass that typically accompanies advancing age. Men also vary in the length of their external urinary sphincter muscle. A longer muscle will function more effectively than a short one. There are two ways to determine the length of the sphincter. One is a bit invasive—passing a special catheter through the penis during urodynamic testing and measuring the urethral pressure profile. The other is to estimate the length from an MRI of the prostate.[7] Urethral sphincter length plays no apparent role in urinary control before radical prostatectomy, but afterward, when the sphincter is the only source of control, a short sphincter (less than 10 mm) is strongly associated with a longer time to gain control and a greater risk of persistent incontinence.[8]

Men whose erectile nerves are damaged or removed to cure their cancers during radical prostatectomy experience greater problems with urinary control. Having these nerves intact appears to play a role in normal voiding—an important reason to have nerve-sparing surgery where possible, even if sexual function is not a concern.

Urinary incontinence is much more likely in men who develop a stricture and those who do not have a water-tight anastomosis (i.e. they leak urine through the drain site after the operation). (See page 385.) But your risk of incontinence is not affected by an enlarged prostate, a previous TURP, symptoms of prostatitis, your weight, or the size of your cancer.

Leaking Urine During Sex

Some men recover erections while they are still experiencing lapses in urinary control. Worries about losing urine while with a partner during intercourse or orgasm can inhibit sexual activity and hamper recovery of erectile function. In most cases, the problem clears up on its own. Some men find emptying their bladder immediately before sexual relations or using penile constriction rings very helpful both to reduce leakage and to enhance erections.[9] Many types of rings are available from online pharmacies and stores that sell sexual aids. You may need to experiment to find the one that works best for you. Definitely discuss this and any other postoperative concerns with your doctor. Open communication with your sexual partner is also a good idea. Something you view as a major issue may not concern your partner. Also, rest assured that urine is sterile, and a little leakage is harmless.

NOTE: When it comes to sensitive, private concerns about urinary and sexual function, many men are tempted to "grin and bear it," but this won't get the problems solved. Today, treatments exist for most side effects.

What Can You Do About Early Problems with Urinary Incontinence?

In patients who continue to experience some leakage more than six weeks after surgery, the problem is typically minor, requiring the use of no more than one to two pads per day, and it usually resolves over time on its own. Pelvic floor (Kegel) exercises, discussed in greater detail in Treating Persistent Incontinence on page 394, can help. Some men have **stress urinary incontinence (SUI)** after surgery and lose urine only when they stand up, sneeze, cough, or bend, or when they engage in strenuous physical activity, such as swinging a golf club, jogging, or lifting weights. Paradoxically, some highly conditioned athletes only have a problem when they're relaxed. Early on, it's not uncommon for men to lose urine when they are tired or have been drinking alcohol, both of which relax the sphincter muscle. Some men urinate at night, during deep sleep, without realizing it, so even if you experience no leakage during the day, a protective pad on the mattress may be a good idea for the first month or two.

For the first six weeks or so after surgery, extra vigilance can help you avoid any embarrassment. If you're scheduled to be in busy social situations or in the spotlight, such as an actor onstage, a lawyer presenting to a jury, or a public speaker delivering a speech, it's wise to empty your bladder beforehand and wear a pad.

Fortunately, most of these issues clear up without intervention. By a year after surgery, only 5 to 10 percent of men I see continue to need a pad. If you experience persistent, severe incontinence (most often this occurs in men who had urinary problems prior to surgery), it's a good idea to have a detailed evaluation by a urologist who specializes in lower urinary tract function, a field known as **urodynamics**. Thorough **uro-dynamic testing** can rule out possible contributory causes such as an unstable bladder or urethral stricture and ensure that you'll get the most appropriate treatment. (See Treating Persistent Incontinence, on page 394.)

> NOTE: Radical prostatectomy alters your anatomy. By making some minor adjustments, you may be able to reduce or even avoid urinary leakage. Simple actions like emptying your bladder more frequently might improve your urinary control. Be aware of factors, such as fatigue, that increase your probability of losing urine. In situations where you are likely to drink alcohol or engage in strenuous physical activities that test your ability to stay dry, you may want to wear a pad as a precaution.

STRICTURES

Since the urethra runs through the prostate, it must be severed and then reconnected when the prostate is removed. The cut ends are sewn back together in an end-to-end connection called an anastomosis. If excessive scar tissue forms at this juncture, the urethra narrows and urinary flow slows severely. We call this scarring a **urethral stricture**. Patients with strictures may appear to recover continence early because the scarring acts as a natural dam, but since strictures get in the way of normal void-ing, these men have a higher incidence of incontinence in the long run.

A **stricture** generally develops at four to six weeks after surgery. The urinary stream gradually slows, becoming weaker, and some men have to strain to urinate. Voiding may be incomplete, with urine left in the blad-der, which can lead to overflow incontinence. The urinary reservoir is always at or near capacity, so the slightest increase in abdominal pressure causes spillover.

Treatment of simple, early strictures involves passing a flexible or metal catheter called a "sound" through the urethra to stretch the constricted area. If the scarring is too thick or too firm, a doctor can visualize the urethra through a scope and incise the stricture in a procedure called an **internal urethrotomy** to relieve the blockage. In certain cases, scarring is in a location that impedes the sphincter mechanism. If treating the stricture requires cutting, the sphincter could be damaged.

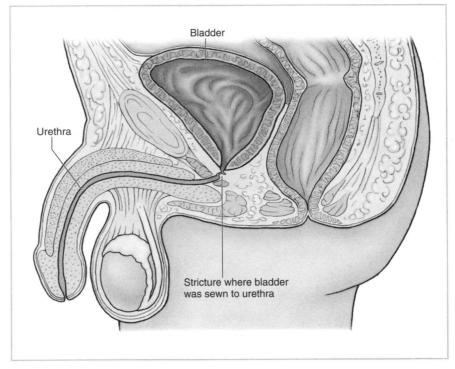

Scarring at the site where the bladder is sewn to the urethra can form a urethral stricture, blocking the urinary channel and causing symptoms.

NOTE: The national average incidence of strictures after radical prostatectomy is 10 to 20 percent. For experienced surgeons, less than 1 percent of patients develop the problem.[10] Strictures are less common after laparoscopic and robotically assisted prostatectomy, but the skill and experience of the surgeon are the major factors in stricture formation.

A special case, and a bit troublesome, is the development of a stricture at the very tip of the penis (**meatal stenosis**). This is a narrowing at the end of the urethra that can create a very fine, high-velocity urinary stream or a spray, which men find troublesome. This is caused not by the surgery, but by the catheter, which is necessary to drain the bladder until the reconnection between the bladder and the urethra heals. Some men are born with a narrow opening, and the passage of the catheter can cause a little crack or trauma. When the catheter is removed, that area can scar and cause a meatal stenosis. If it's minimal, it can be treated with gentle dilation. If the problem is severe, plastic surgery may be required. The best way to for a surgeon to prevent a stricture is gentle handling when the catheter is initially placed and the use of a smaller, 18F catheter to drain the bladder after the operation. A stricture at the tip of the penis occurs in only one out of every two or three hundred men.

OTHER URINARY SIDE EFFECTS OF SURGERY

In rare instances (2 in 1,000) surgery causes a ureteral obstruction. One of the slender tubes (ureters) that lead from the kidneys to the bladder gets damaged or caught in a suture. This might cause flank pain, but it can also be symptom-free, where the only warning is an increased blood creatinine level that signals a possible reduction in kidney function. To avoid kidney damage, surgery must be done to relieve the obstruction. Also rare is a urinary fistula, where the bladder and urethra are not rejoined properly and urine leaks out. This can cause scarring and increase the risk of incontinence. Experienced surgeons know how to avoid both of these problems.

IMPORTANCE OF SURGICAL SKILL AND TECHNIQUE

Outcomes vary widely, depending on precisely how a radical prostatectomy is performed. Surgeons differ in fine details of the procedure, and that can make a major difference in the incidence and severity of side effects.

But even among the busiest surgeons, results can be all over the lot. Our study of men 65 and over found that incontinence rates a year or more after radical prostatectomy ranged from 1 percent to a whopping 50 percent, depending on surgical know-how and technique.[11] For example, it's important to avoid shortening the external urinary sphincter, which is called upon to take over the job of holding back urine after the internal sphincter is removed during radical prostatectomy. Highly experienced surgeons are more likely to know this and incorporate it in their standard procedure. Doctors who perform radical prostatectomy infrequently may fail to consider important nuances that can make a major difference in results. Make sure you know your surgeon's track record and put yourself in the care of someone with a demonstrated capacity to avoid serious side effects such as urinary incontinence.

> NOTE: Incontinence is far more common when the prostate is removed in a so-called **salvage radical prostatectomy**, when a man's prostate cancer recurs after external beam therapy, brachytherapy, HIFU or cryotherapy. These treatments often inflict incidental damage on the external urinary sphincter, which must take charge of urinary control after the prostate and the inner sphincter are removed. Salvage surgery leaves two men in four incontinent, one in four severely enough to require surgical correction. (See Treating Persistent Incontinence, on page 394.)

URINARY SIDE EFFECTS
OF RADIATION

In treating prostate cancer, radiation therapists face a delicate balancing act. The challenge is to deliver enough radiation to kill the cancer without inflicting unacceptable damage on healthy innocent bystanders like the erectile nerves, the bowel, and the urinary tract. Lower radiation doses cause less injury to neighboring structures, but they also increase the chances that the cancer will recur. Higher doses raise the probability of cancer cure, but that comes with a greater risk of collateral damage.

The problem is compounded by the fact that some organs are far more susceptible to the effects of radiation than others. Destroying prostate tissue requires a hefty dose that would severely harm more vulnerable surrounding structures, including the bladder and urethra.

Although external beam radiation and seed implants leave some men with urinary problems, the incidence of short-term urinary incontinence is far less than after surgery. A major risk of brachytherapy is urinary obstruction, sometimes leading to complete retention and requiring a catheter or a TURP for relief.

After radiation—more commonly with brachytherapy than external beam radiation—there is also an immediate risk of frequency, urgency, and urge incontinence that tends to clear up on its own within six to twelve months after treatment. Later, with both external beam radiation and seed implants, irritative symptoms and some strictures may develop. With brachytherapy, there tend to be more obstructive symptoms early on and more irritative symptoms later.

EXTERNAL BEAM THERAPY

Radiation of any kind causes inflammation and irritation. During the typical nine- to ten-week course of external beam therapy, the lining of the urethra may sustain damage and cease to provide an effective barrier to urine. This can cause bleeding, irritation, and pain. Depending on the target area or "field" of radiation, a patient may develop an inflammation of the urethra (radiation urethritis) or, if the bladder is exposed, **radiation cystitis**. Both of these conditions cause urinary frequency, urgency, burning, pain, and the need to get up during the night to urinate. During external beam therapy, 10 to 20 percent of men develop these symptoms of irritation. Typically, the problems appear after four to six weeks of treatment, continue to worsen for one to three months after therapy is completed, and then resolve by six months to a year.[12]

Until symptoms clear up, an analgesic such as phenazopyridine (Pyridium) taken orally, may soothe the pain, though it will also turn your urine bright orange. Anticholinergics, such as tolterodine (Detrol or Detrol LA) and oxybutynin (Ditropan), reset the bladder's trigger point, quieting the signals that prompt the frantic urge to urinate. Some men undergoing radiation find it difficult to void because of inflammation and swelling, and alpha blockers, such as tamsulosin (Flomax), terazosin (Cardura), and alfuzosin (Uroxatral), which relax smooth muscles in the bladder neck and prostate, help to alleviate the problem.

In the long term, radiation can cause ulceration in the sensitive lining of the urethra and consequent bleeding and pain. Blood vessels in the field may become abnormal and more prone to bleed spontaneously. Conventional radiotherapy targets a box-shaped area, and the bladder receives a great deal of incidental injury. About 7 percent of patients given conventional radiation experience severe bleeding, strictures, radiation cystitis, or bladder contractures requiring hospitalization. Problems with serious bleeding, requiring transfusion or, in the worst cases, removal of the bladder, are far less common with modern radiation therapy involving 3-D conformal technology or, better yet, IMRT. Still, 1 to 3 percent of patients experience serious bleeding from radiation. Using modern techniques such as IMRT, serious problems are far less common, but we still see troublesome irritative symptoms such as urgency and frequency. Fifteen percent of men develop late urinary problems, up to five years after treatment, that are bothersome and require treatment, but are not severe or life-threatening. With any external beam radiation, there is a 3 percent risk of a serious stricture in patients who have had a TURP, so TURP is often considered a contraindication for radiation.

BRACHYTHERAPY

The procedure involves the placement of dozens or even a hundred or more radioactive seeds through multiple needles inserted in the prostate. The implant causes swelling in the gland that can obstruct urinary flow. In severe cases, a patient is suddenly unable to urinate (acute urinary obstruction). For this reason brachytherapy is ill-advised for men with moderate to severe obstructive voiding symptoms or with a large prostate (greater than 60 grams). The risk of acute retention is often associated with a man's score on the IPSS (International Prostate Symptom Score; see page 75). Men whose symptom score is less than 10 have only a 2 percent risk of acute urinary retention. With a symptom score above 20, the risk rises to 30 percent. (See Chapter 5, BPH [Benign Prostatic Hyperplasia].)[13]

> NOTE: Prostate size is measured by ultrasound at the time of a prostate biopsy and should be included in your biopsy report.

Treating acute urinary retention may necessitate prolonged use of a Foley catheter through the penis, a suprapubic tube inserted into the bladder through the lower abdomen, or an emergency TURP to remove obstructing tissue. In any man, a TURP after radiotherapy increases the risk of urinary incontinence.

Typically, the severity of urinary obstruction can be gauged from the patient's responses on the IPSS (see page 75). Still, since it's possible to have obstruction without symptoms, the best way to determine whether seed implants are appropriate is to have a urinary flow test and measure the amount of urine left in the bladder after urinating (post-void residual urine). If a question remains about the degree of urinary obstruction, urodynamic studies can help to provide an answer. To avoid the risk of acute retention, all brachytherapy patients typically take alpha-blocking drugs before the implant and continue to take them for several months afterward.

As damage from the implanted seeds accumulates, other urinary problems can develop. Radiation can damage the sensitive lining of the urethra, leaving the area raw and highly sensitive, like a scraped knee. Without this protective lining, urine passing through the urethra causes inflammation, burning, and pain.

Brachytherapy is associated with symptoms of lower urinary tract irritation, including frequency, urgency, and burning, painful urination, waking at night to urinate (sometimes as often as every hour), or urge incontinence. In more than half of patients receiving seed implants, these symptoms are severe enough to require medications such as alpha blockers. These drugs provide relief for two thirds of men, but are ineffective in the remainder. Urinary symptoms persist for an average of two years in 20 percent of men after brachytherapy, but they can take as long as six to seven years to clear up. On average, two years after brachytherapy, men describe overall urinary function as troublesome and worse than before treatment.[14]

Complications from brachytherapy depend on the skill of the radiation oncologist in placing the seeds optimally. Dr. Michael Zelefsky, a brachytherapy expert at MSKCC, has shortened the time course of irritative symptoms to a mean of six to eight months and reduced long-term symptoms by using three-dimensional, real-time treatment planning during seed implantation.[15]

In less than 1 percent of cases, bleeding around the needle sites after the implant is serious enough to require catheterization to wash out the blood clots in the bladder. Long-term urinary bleeding (**hematuria**) after radiation is more common with external beam therapy, though 1 to 3 percent of men receiving modern brachytherapy develop blood in the urine from radiation urethritis or radiation damage to blood vessels in the area.

> NOTE: Despite a commonly held belief to the contrary, drinking cranberry juice or taking vitamin C does nothing to alleviate these symptoms. Such home remedies cannot change the pH of urine.

COMBINATION EXTERNAL BEAM RADIATION AND BRACHYTHERAPY

In the past, when seed implants were given in combination with external beam radiation, the risk of serious urinary side effects, including obstruction, irritative voiding symptoms, and bleeding, was greater than when either form of radiation was given alone. With modern techniques, carefully controlling seed placement, and carefully planning external radiation with IMRT, the results are better, but the urinary side effects are still greater for combination therapy than when a single treatment is used. All the problems described above for external beam radiation and for brachytherapy are more common with combined radiotherapy.[16]

Adding hormone therapy to radiation does not increase urinary side effects. On the contrary, by shrinking the prostate, hormone therapy relieves obstruction and reduces the risk of sudden urinary blockage.

URINARY SIDE EFFECTS OF OTHER LOCAL TREATMENTS

Cryotherapy causes more urinary problems than radiation and about the same long-term risk of incontinence as radical prostatectomy. Freezing is designed to kill both normal and malignant prostate tissue. As the dead tissue sloughs off, it can block the urinary channel. Some patients require drainage with a catheter or suprapubic tube (through the base of the abdomen) for three to six weeks after cryotherapy. Urinary frequency, urgency, pain, and a weak stream may persist for months.[17] Some patients need a TURP to remove the dead, obstructing tissue. In the long run, about 3 to 7 percent of patients complain of persistent incontinence. The most devastating complication of cryotherapy is a rectourethral fistula—a hole between the rectum and urinary tract that requires a colostomy to divert feces away from the damaged site. Fortunately, this occurs rarely. The risk is greater in the hands of inexperienced cryosurgeons.

Ultrasound-guided **high-intensity focused ultrasound (US-HIFU)** is not yet approved for treatment of prostate cancer in this country, but it has been widely used in Europe and is currently undergoing trials for approval in the U.S. The procedure has been associated with mild to moderate urinary incontinence in 1 to 19 percent of patients and bladder neck stenosis (blockage), requiring intervention in 4 to 27 percent.

Bladder outlet obstruction requiring surgical intervention occurs in up to one third of men who do not have a TURP at the time of HIFU and in 6 percent of men who have a TURP. In the best reported series, mild stress urinary incontinence affects 6 percent of men and 2 percent have moderate stress incontinence.[18]

WILL AVOIDING TREATMENT PREVENT URINARY PROBLEMS?

In the short term, avoiding treatment does mean you avoid the risk of urinary complications. But while a small, favorable cancer can be safely monitored in a careful program of active surveillance, a serious aggressive tumor will eventually enlarge, blocking the urinary channel and invading the urinary sphincter. In a Swedish study comparing radical prostatectomy and traditional watchful waiting (i.e. doing nothing until the cancer caused symptoms), the untreated patients experienced far more urinary problems. Surgery patients had a greater incidence of urine leakage in the short run, but watchful-waiting patients had far more urinary obstruction requiring invasive treatments, and their urinary quality of life was substantially worse. An unchecked serious cancer can also grow into the bladder, obstructing the ureters that drain the kidneys.

TREATING PERSISTENT INCONTINENCE

The best-case scenario is to avoid the problem. A major cause of incontinence after radical prostatectomy is a shortened external sphincter. Highly skilled, experienced surgeons know how to leave this critical mechanism with sufficient length to function properly and minimize the risk of leakage. A doctor's record of results should reflect this know-how.

If you're going to have surgery, seek someone whose patients rarely have serious trouble with long-term urinary control.

Because they run an increased risk of incontinence, older men, especially those over 70, are often better served by radiation therapy than by radical prostatectomy. Nevertheless, some older men who are anxious to have the cancer removed opt to have surgery anyway. If this applies to you, make sure you fully understand the nature and extent of potential problems. If you are seriously troubled by the risk of incontinence, ask your doctor to estimate the length of your external sphincter on an MRI of your prostate. A very short sphincter (< 10 mm) may mean a greater risk of incontinence.[19]

Incontinence after radiation can best be avoided by making sure you receive treatment with high-quality, state-of-the-art equipment using IMRT. A highly skilled radiation oncologist knows how to target the appropriate field, while minimizing injury to the urethra and bladder. Seed implants are not a good idea if you have a large prostate or symptoms of bladder outlet obstruction.

PELVIC FLOOR (KEGEL) EXERCISES

In 1932, a New York obstetrician named Joshua W. Davies theorized that women troubled by incontinence after childbirth could regain control by strengthening the muscles used to interrupt the urinary stream. Davies recommended that his patients contract these pelvic floor muscles voluntarily several times a day, but many women found it difficult or impossible to isolate them. They did the exercises incorrectly, squeezing abdominal, thigh, or buttocks muscles instead. The effort proved useless and, in some cases, actually made the incontinence worse.

A breakthrough occurred in the mid-1940s, when Arnold Kegel, a Los Angeles gynecologist, invented the world's first biofeedback device: the Kegel perineometer. A probe placed in the vagina was connected to a gauge that registered successful contractions of the target muscles. Though this invention and the pioneering discovery of biofeedback won

Kegel little recognition, his name continues to be widely associated with simple isometric exercises that may help to restore urinary control in men and women.[20]After radical prostatectomy, Kegel exercises can be used to strengthen the muscles that act like scaffolding to support the urethra.[21]

To isolate the correct muscles, try stopping and starting the urinary stream several times. Be sure to keep your thigh, abdominal, and gluteus muscles relaxed. If you have difficulty doing this on your own or are unsure that you're doing it correctly, your doctor can refer you for biofeedback training. A probe is placed in the anal canal, and a gauge indicates when you're stimulating the right muscles.

Kegel exercises should not be performed while the catheter is in place. After it's removed, wait a day or two to see if you actually leak. Many men never need Kegel exercises. If you do have leakage, try forcefully contracting the pelvic floor muscles and holding the contraction for five to ten seconds, and then relax for thirty seconds before squeezing again. By doing ten repetitions every morning, afternoon, and evening, you may strengthen the supporting muscles sufficiently to reduce urinary leakage. As with any physical conditioning, the process could take weeks or even months.

> NOTE: One in four to five men does these exercises improperly, so biofeedback training is a good idea if the leakage is not subsiding.
>
> NOTE: While doing Kegel exercises may help and should not cause any harm, overdoing them is inadvisable. You could fatigue the muscles and exacerbate the problem.

IDENTIFYING AND TREATING SECONDARY CAUSES

If incontinence persists, you should discuss it with your doctor. A secondary cause might be the culprit. **Urinary tract** infections can compromise urinary control. They are easy to diagnose and treat with antibiotics.

Another possible secondary cause for incontinence is a urethral stricture. Scar tissue narrows the urinary channel and can make it difficult to empty the bladder completely (see page 385). Urine left in the bladder after voiding, also known as post-void residual urine (PVR), sets you up to leak with any increase in intra-abdominal pressure, as occurs when you bend, lift, sneeze, or cough. Your doctor can check for strictures by examining the urethra through a cystoscope inserted in the penis. The presence of post-void residual urine can be determined by an abdominal sonogram. A urinary flow test can point to the existence of a stricture or other obstructions that impede normal voiding and increase problems with urinary control.

MEDICATIONS

Though no drugs have been FDA-approved as yet for the treatment of stress incontinence, tricyclic antidepressants are sometimes prescribed to treat incontinence, because they can relax the bladder muscle and stimulate the muscular urinary sphincter. Another antidepressant, duloxetine, is awaiting FDA approval for the treatment of stress incontinence.

Drugs for radiation cystitis and urethritis are targeted to the symptoms. If radiation causes urinary frequency, anticholinergics such as tolterodine (Detrol) or oxybutynin (Ditropan) are prescribed. When pain is the primary symptom, the preferred medications are anti-inflammatories or urinary anesthetics such as phenazopyridine (Pyridium).

BULKING AGENTS

Beefing up the urinary sphincter can increase its resistance to urinary flow. Originally, Teflon suspended in an aqueous solution was used for this purpose, but the substance tended to migrate to other areas of the body. Currently, two bulking agents, Durasphere and Contigen, are FDA-approved to treat incontinence.

Contigen, derived from bovine collagen, causes allergic reactions in

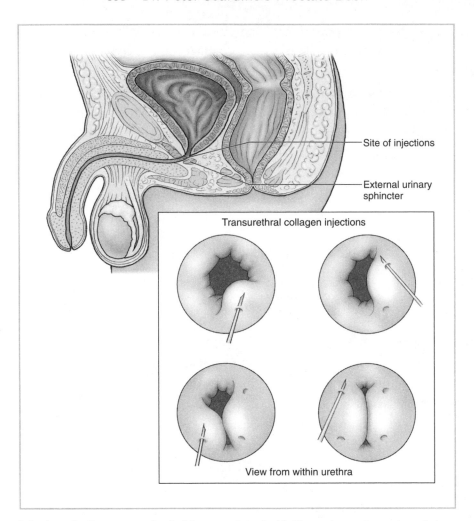

Injection of collagen or another bulking agent into the bladder neck to reduce urinary leakage after radical prostatectomy.

about 3 percent of patients, so an allergy test must be conducted four weeks prior to treatment. Durasphere, made of tiny carbon-coated beads, does not provoke allergic responses, but, like Contigen, it has limited effectiveness, and with both substances, calibrating the correct amount to implant can be tricky. Too little material will fail to stop the leak; too much may result in a total inability to urinate. Finding the "just right" amount can be hit or miss. Fifty percent of patients improve with bulking agents, but it often takes four to five expensive injections to achieve a satisfactory outcome. Also, results are not permanent or even durable, lasting only a few years. Consequently, the use of bulking agents for incontinence in men has largely dropped out of favor.[22]

Both agents carry a risk of infection, bleeding, and urinary retention. In rare instances, the leakage gets much worse after the injections. Other bulking materials are in current development with an eye toward offering improved durability, safety, and effectiveness.

SLING PROCEDURES

Though they are a relatively new way to treat incontinence after radical prostatectomy, **sling procedures** have been used in thousands of women. Stress urinary incontinence—losing urine with strenuous activity, coughing, sneezing, etc.—is far more common in women than men. In women, when the problem does not respond to medication or exercises, a sling operation is the corrective procedure of choice. The simplest sling used in men after radical prostatectomy is a silicone model made by American Medical Systems. Held in place by screws that are fixed to the pelvic bone, the sling compresses the urethra below the sphincter just enough to keep the patient dry. The operation is a fairly simple, one-day surgery procedure, but so far, the results have been a bit disappointing. Too many men will develop infection, erosion, or break down over time. While sling implantations are still being performed, enthusiasm for them has diminished and there is greater reliance on the artificial sphincter.[23]

ARTIFICIAL SPHINCTER

For patients with severe incontinence that doesn't respond to exercises or medications, an artificial sphincter can provide excellent relief. Ninety-five percent of people who have the device implanted see considerable improvement, though they still may have to wear one or two small pads per day.[24]

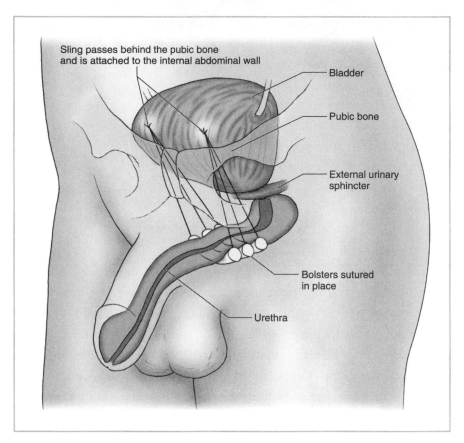

Sling passes behind the pubic bone
and is attached to the internal abdominal wall

Bladder

Pubic bone

External urinary
sphincter

Bolsters sutured
in place

Urethra

One type of sling or suspension operation to treat stress urinary incontinence after radical prostatectomy.

Surgery to implant an artificial sphincter is not trivial. The procedure is sometimes done on an outpatient basis, but an overnight hospital stay may be required. Patients continue to leak for six weeks afterward, since the implant cannot be activated until the area heals.

Complications include infection that could necessitate long-term antibiotics or require that the device be removed or replaced. An artificial sphincter can erode the urethra, causing infection and necessitating removal. Every year, 3 to 5 percent of men experience mechanical failure or erosion and need to have further surgery to replace or remove the device. Still, 95 percent of patients are very satisfied with this treatment.

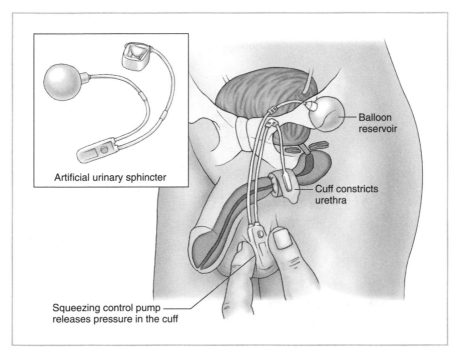

Surgical implantation of an artificial urinary sphincter is the most effective procedure for treating severe, persistent stress urinary incontinence.

All in all, the artificial sphincter sets the gold standard for effective treatment of severe urinary incontinence.

IN SUMMARY

Prostate cancer and all treatments for the disease carry a risk of urinary complications. Many men do not suffer urinary side effects or do so only for a short time. For those with persistent, troubling symptoms, we have several highly satisfactory means to solve the problem.

18

Sexual Side Effects

READ THIS CHAPTER TO LEARN:

- How do erections work, and what causes erectile dysfunction?
- What are the sexual side effects of prostate cancer treatments?
- What can be done about erectile dysfunction?

The first time a drug was shown to be effective for cancer was in the early 1940s, when hormone therapy was used to treat men with metastatic prostate cancer. Once the testicles were removed or female hormones were administered, the cancer responded dramatically. This spectacular improvement came at a cost. In addition to other troubling symptoms (see Chapter 21, Treating Advanced Prostate Cancer), patients on hormone therapy suffered a loss of libido and erections. This led to the common and persistent assumption that treating prostate cancer always meant the end of sexual function.

Not long ago, that view was fairly accurate. Until the development of nerve-sparing surgery in the early 1980s, a loss of erections was seen as the price men had to pay to get their prostates out (though some patients, inexplicably, confounded their doctors' expectations and regained sexual function after radical prostatectomy).

In the 1960s, radiation became the preferred treatment choice for prostate cancer because it was thought to have no sexual side effects. That assessment proved to be unrealistically optimistic. During treatment and soon after radiation, sexual function appeared to be unchanged, but as damaging effects accumulated, patients often found that their erections steadily diminished. Because many of these men were not followed regularly after treatment, researchers were slow to recognize the negative sexual effects of radiation. When patients did report erectile loss over time, doctors often chalked it up to a normal consequence of aging.

WHY THINGS CHANGED

In the pre-PSA era, many prostate cancers went undetected until they were advanced and incurable. Sexual concerns took a distant backseat to keeping men alive. Before PSA testing, the disease was typically diagnosed in older men, whose sexual function had already declined, making it more difficult to restore satisfactory erections after treatment. Given the average patient's age, sexual function was not seen as a major issue (though that supposition is often incorrect). Until the FDA approved sildenafil (Viagra) in 1996, we had no simple, reliable means to promote the early recovery of erections after cancer treatment and preserve sexual health.

Thankfully, things have changed. We now detect most prostate cancers while they are relatively small, contained, and curable. The median age at diagnosis has declined steadily from 71 in 1995 to 68 in 2008, and the average age at radical prostatectomy is 58. An ever-increasing number of prostate cancers are now diagnosed before age 60, so we see the disease much more commonly in healthy, vital men for whom sexual function is of major importance. Advances in radiation and surgery have reduced the incidence of sexual side effects, and a variety of highly effective therapies can alleviate, or even reverse, the problems that occur. After treatment, most prostate cancer patients can look forward to resuming an active, satisfying sex life.

ERECTILE DYSFUNCTION (ED)

Erectile dysfunction (ED) refers to the inability to produce and maintain erections satisfactory for sexual relations. In professional parlance, the term is now generally preferred over "impotence," though the meaning of both terms is largely synonymous.

Note that the definition of ED uses the term "satisfactory," highlighting the fact that only *you* can be the judge of whether your sexual abilities are adequate to suit your needs. For some men, sex is not an issue. To others, sexual performance is so crucial that they rank it above survival on a questionnaire to assess their priorities.

NORMAL ERECTIONS

The penis has two large erection chambers—the **corpora cavernosa**—and one small chamber surrounding the urethra—the **corpus spongiosum**—filled with spongy erectile tissue (**corporal sinusoids**). Triggered by direct genital stimulation, psychological arousal, or REM (dream) sleep, a number of nerves and hormones relax the smooth muscle in the blood vessels of these three chambers, allowing a rapid inflow of blood. Under sufficient pressure, the penile veins are compressed, causing a valve-like effect, which traps blood in the penis and keeps it rigid until orgasm occurs or the stimulus that caused the erection stops. The same hydraulic principle applies when you inflate a bicycle tire. To make the tire rigid, you have to force in sufficient air and then keep it contained under pressure. A leaky valve would make it impossible to maintain rigidity, and the tire would quickly go flat.

Many men who cannot achieve erections can still experience the pleasure and release of orgasm, and after radical prostatectomy, erection

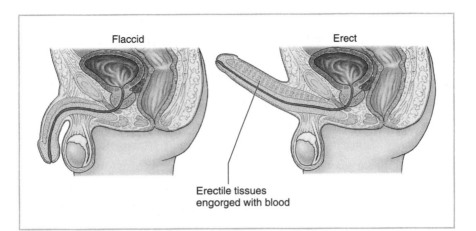

Flaccid Erect

Erectile tissues
engorged with blood

A view of the flaccid and the erect penis from the side.

> NOTE: *Orgasm, erection, and ejaculation are separate, independent functions.* Erections require good blood flow and intact nervous impulses to the penis. Ejaculation relies on fluid production by an intact prostate and seminal vesicles followed by nerve and muscle action to force the fluid out. Orgasm is a psychophysiological event, requiring nothing beyond a healthy, well-functioning brain.

and orgasm can occur even though patients no longer ejaculate. (See Chapter 2, Normal Male Function.)

WHAT CAUSES ED?

An erection is a marvel of engineering that hinges on a series of intricate, interdependent events. As in a factory, damage to any aspect of the complex mechanism can cause the entire system to break down. Erectile problems can result from a single factor or have multiple causes. The problem may be psychological, physical, or, most commonly, both.[1]

PSYCHOLOGICAL CAUSES OF ED

Stress, anxiety, and depression are all common triggers for erectile dysfunction. While excitement and arousal are necessary for erections to occur, an extreme excess of either can overload the circuits and cause a shutdown. Under psychological siege, your body shifts into combat mode, pumping extra adrenaline that directs blood flow away from peripheral structures like the penis into core organs. This reaction serves people well in emergencies—if you were fleeing a foe or a fire, you'd need maximum heart and lung capacity and a fully alert brain, not a firm, reliable erection.

Unfortunately, this crucial survival mechanism can kick in and cause problems when no real or imminent danger exists. It's common for men to experience a loss of erections when they're worried about finances, relationships, or troubles on the job. Erectile failure can trigger a vicious cycle, causing performance anxiety, which leads to further erectile dysfunction, which intensifies the performance anxiety, and so on.

Losing a partner can also result in self-perpetuating erectile

---

NOTE: Men normally have an average of five erections per night, each lasting about thirty minutes and associated with REM (dream) sleep. Tests of **nocturnal penile tumescence (NPT)**, in which an elastic gauge linked to a monitor is placed around the penis, determine whether or not you're having these erections.

Until recently, if a man had normal erections during sleep, the problems he had while awake were thought to be psychological. We now know that this is not necessarily the case. Only 10 to 15 percent of ED is currently thought to have primarily emotional roots, though in as many as 85 percent of cases, a loss of erections will have a secondary psychological impact that makes matters worse.

dysfunction. "Widower's syndrome" refers to erectile problems caused by depression, performance anxiety, or guilt following the death of a spouse. The condition may lead men to retreat from social and sexual situations, which, naturally, exacerbates the problem.

Physical Causes of ED

Vascular Disorders

Vascular (blood vessel) disorders are the most common physical culprit, responsible for 10 to 20 percent of erectile dysfunction. Heart disease, hypertension and the drugs used to treat it, and high cholesterol with resultant hardening of the arteries all can impair circulation to the penis, making it impossible to fill the organ with enough blood to induce rigidity.

If blood flow is insufficient, the erection chambers may not exert sufficient pressure to compress the veins. The condition is tantamount to a loose drain plug in the bathtub. The blood runs out, and the erection cannot be sustained.

Nervous System (Neurogenic) Causes

Damage to the autonomic (involuntary) nervous system, which regulates dilation and contraction of the blood vessels that lead to the penis, can interrupt the electrical impulses required to trigger erections, causing the equivalent of a power outage. Multiple sclerosis, Parkinson's disease, and spinal-cord injury are common causes of neurogenic erectile loss, as is damage to the erectile nerves during surgery, radiation, freezing during cryotherapy, or heating during HIFU.

We have learned that heating any small nerve fibers, like the erectile nerves, to greater than 56 degrees centigrade will irreversibly damage these nerves. (Normal body temperature is 37 degrees centigrade.)[2] This has major implications for the feasibility of heat-related treatments such as HIFU to be able to destroy the cancer near or just beyond through the prostate capsule without inflicting severe damage on the adjacent erectile nerves.

Hormones

A deficiency or excess of thyroid hormone or an abnormal increase in the pituitary hormone prolactin can lead to a loss of erections. So can anabolic steroid abuse.

Hypogonadism (low testosterone), which can be congenital, caused by damaged testicles or from central nervous system diseases that affect the pituitary or hypothalamus glands, may retard sexual development, causing infertility and erectile dysfunction. While erections can sometimes occur despite a low testosterone level, a paucity of the hormone does cause a lack of libido and a general weakening of erections.

> NOTE: Be aware that "nutraceuticals" such as **DHEA**, which are often touted as having "miracle" sexual performance-boosting and anti-aging properties, are unregulated. Their safety and effectiveness have not been rigorously tested or proven. In addition, there is concern that these substances may cause serious side effects, including an increased risk of prostate cancer.

Diabetes

Diabetes causes both nerve and vascular damage, putting patients at high risk for erectile dysfunction.

Smoking

Though it has not been proven to be a direct cause of impotence, smoking increases the risk of cardiovascular diseases such as atherosclerosis, which impair erectile function. The risk of erectile dysfunction increases with the number of cigarettes smoked per day.

Alcohol and Drugs

In moderate doses, alcohol may help you relax and heighten your sex drive. But because alcohol acts as a powerful nerve inhibitor, heavy drinking markedly depresses erections. The same is true of recreational drugs, such as marijuana and heroin. Cocaine users also risk **priapism**, a persistent erection lasting four hours or more that can cause severe, permanent damage to the penis.[3] Chronic drug abuse can lead to permanent vascular and neurological damage and a consequent loss of erectile function.

A wide variety of medications, including antianxiety drugs, antidepressants, chemotherapeutic agents, drugs for heart disease and hypertension, and glaucoma treatments put men at risk for erectile dysfunction.

PROSTATE CANCER AND ED

Because the prostate lies so close to the erectile nerves and some of the small arteries that feed blood to the penis, all treatments for cancer in the gland carry a risk of sexual side effects.[4] (See illustration on page 10.) We know approximately where the nerves lie, but there is considerable variability from man to man. Also, we cannot visualize these nerves or small arteries before treatment. Prostate cancer typically arises just beneath the capsule of the prostate in the area overlying the neurovascular bundles. (See illustration on page 275.) It is a persistent challenge to find ways to treat the cancer without harming these nerves and arteries.

Your particular outcome after treatment will depend on your anatomy (i.e. the size and shape of your prostate and the proximity of nerves and arteries to the tumor in your prostate gland). Sexual side effects will also hinge on the nature of your cancer and the quality of care you receive. Larger, more aggressive tumors typically require more extensive treatments, increasing the probability that potency will be impaired. Awareness of the sensitivity of the erectile nerves to heat has changed the technique used by many open and robotic surgeons. Surgeons have learned to avoid electro-cautery of blood vessels which can damage nearby nerves. Highly skilled surgeons and radiation oncologists know how to minimize damage to erectile nerves and reduce the incidence of ED. Keep in mind that how well you are treated may have a greater impact on your outcome than which treatment you decide to have.

If you have a cancer that's small and favorable enough to monitor, you can avoid the sexual side effects by delaying treatment until and unless the tumor shows signs of progression. But if your cancer is serious, avoiding treatment in fear of sexual dysfunction is unwise, especially for a young, healthy man. Left alone, serious prostate cancer can penetrate the capsule of the gland and grow into the erectile nerves, causing a loss of erections. Should the cancer spread and metastasize, hormone therapy, which destroys libido and erectile function, would be necessary to slow progression of the disease and ease symptoms. You would lose the chance for a cure while still risking erectile dysfunction as well.

SEXUAL SIDE EFFECTS OF RADICAL PROSTATECTOMY

ERECTILE FUNCTION

Erections depend on triggering signals from the **cavernous (erectile) nerves**, which run along the prostate like string on a package. (See illustration on page 275.) During radical prostatectomy, surgeons using accepted modern techniques attempt to spare these nerves unless doing so would compromise cancer cure. Still, erectile nerves are exquisitely delicate. Even with a top-notch, nerve-sparing procedure, it's difficult to remove the gland without causing some temporary trauma to these fragile fibers. The nerves suffer the equivalent of a bad concussion, leaving them temporarily dazed and unresponsive. As a result, most men experience some loss of erectile function for the first few months following radical prostatectomy (though some are able to function right away).

During the healing process, inflammation and scarring around the nerves can deliver what amounts to a further blow that can interrupt or delay sexual recovery. Some men who regain erections early note a marked decline in the quality of erections after two or three months, putting them back at square one in the recuperative process.[5]

Two years after radical prostatectomy, about 45 (with nerve sparing) to 55 percent (without nerve sparing) of men report a loss of erections nationwide.[6] In an excellent recent study of sexual function before and after radical prostatectomy, 14 percent of men complained of poor erections before surgery. Two months after the operation, 88 percent had erectile dysfunction. Two years later, 58 percent still reported ED. Men who had nerve-sparing surgery were significantly more likely to recover erections than those with non–nerve-sparing prostatectomy. In this study, 44 percent of partners reported moderate or severe distress as a result of their partner's sexual problems. The chances of ED are greater in older men, those with higher-stage cancers, and those with a larger prostate.[7]

These results contrast with the outcomes from Centers of Excellence, where highly skilled surgeons perform nerve-sparing surgery in the vast majority of patients. At Memorial Sloan-Kettering, if we look at the typical 58-year-old man who had good sexual function before radical prostatectomy, 60 percent will recover normal erections by two years after surgery, though some of these men need a drug like sildenafil (Viagra) to do so. In 30 percent, erections sufficient for intercourse will require Viagra or a similar drug. Without the drug, erections will not be sufficient for relations. About 10 percent will not recover erections sufficient for intercourse, even with a pill. Overall, long-term recovery of erections depends on a patient's age, the quality of his erections before surgery, and the skill and experience of the surgeon.[8]

In some cases, one or both erectile nerve bundles must be removed to cure the cancer. Surgeons skilled in nerve grafting can insert a nerve from the ankle (sural nerve) or groin (genitofemoral nerve) between the cut ends of the lost erectile nerve. The sheath of the graft provides a conduit through which the cut nerves can regenerate. There is also now a synthetic nerve substitute that may preclude the need to harvest a normal nerve for grafting.[9] At Memorial Sloan-Kettering, in our patients with grafts, 33 percent of men who lost both nerves were able to recover erections, versus none without the graft. Replacing one lost nerve with a graft appears to increase recovery compared with those with no graft.[10] (See Chapter 14, Surgery.)

While the main artery that supplies blood to the penis (the pudendal artery) lies well away from the prostate, other important collateral arteries can be injured during radical prostatectomy. It is essential that these accessory arteries be identified and preserved during the operation to maximize the chances of recovery of erectile function.[11] Insufficient blood flow means the erectile chambers will not fill completely and the penis will not achieve full rigidity.

Some men have functional erections a few weeks after surgery, but typically recovery is a long, gradual process. The average patient takes four months to achieve an erection sufficient for intercourse. Older men, patients with diminished erections before the operation, and those with damage to or removal of a nerve will be slower to recover. Healing can continue for several years. One patient came to see me three and a half years after surgery, having long since given up hope of ever having sexual intercourse without drugs. "You can have all those medicines back," he said. "I'm *finally* back to normal."

LOSS OF EJACULATION

After radical prostatectomy, you can continue to enjoy normal sensation in the penis, experience normal desire, and have orgasms. Removing the gland means you will no longer ejaculate when you climax (dry orgasm). The response to this change varies. After surgery, some men experience heightened orgasms and some judge their climax to be less intense, but most men report no significant difference.

PAIN DURING ORGASM

For a time after surgery, 20 percent of men report pain in the penis, scrotum, or perineum during orgasm (**dysorgasmia**). Though this can be disturbing, it typically clears up over time without treatment.[12]

PENIS SIZE AND SHAPE

Removing the prostate does not pull the penis into your body and make it shorter. During radical prostatectomy, the penis and urethra are never dislodged. When the prostate is removed, the bladder is brought down and sewn to the urethra. The urethra *is not* pulled up with an effect like a retracted hose.

Still, some men observe that their penis seems smaller or shorter after surgery. I'm aware of three reasons for this—two misleading and one real. If there is intense scarring between the lower part of the abdominal incision and the penis, as the scar retracts, the penis may be pulled toward the pubic bone and appear shorter. This can be prevented by careful placement of sutures. Alternatively, after the operation, some men gain weight for a variety of reasons, including sexual frustration. Fatty deposits over the pubic area can cover part of the penis, making it appear smaller. In both instances, there is no actual shortening, though the penis looks shorter to the patient. When erection occurs, the penis fills out and functions normally.

Penile shortening is a real concern, and it has been reported in as many as one in five men. In one study, the loss was as much as 1 inch on average after radical prostatectomy.[13] In other reported trials, using a comprehensive evaluation of penile size and girth, there was no change following bilateral nerve sparing in men who had good recovery of erections.[14] Severe damage to erectile nerves may cause a loss of penile length or girth. This makes sense, as penile size—in both the flaccid and erect state—depends mostly on blood flow. The penis is like a balloon, stretching and enlarging with increased blood. Since blood flow is controlled by the erectile nerves, the penis is likely to be smaller until nerves recover and blood flow returns to baseline levels. This has been shown in animal studies and in limited trials in prostate cancer patients. Penile shortening is related to age, the quality of erections before radical prostatectomy, and to the degree of nerve sparing and the quality of erections after surgery. Men under age 60 with excellent nerve sparing and return of erectile function after prostatectomy rarely see a change in penile size.[15]

Profound and long-lasting nerve damage may lead to atrophy of the delicate vascular channels of the penis, and the walls of the erectile bodies can become hard and inelastic (fibrotic). Fibrous tissue does not expand when the penis fills with blood, so the organ remains shorter and erections may not be as firm or as thick. In men with persistent erectile dysfunction after surgery, about 40 percent will have this fibrosis. The problem is rare in men who recover erections early.

In 8 to 11 percent of prostate cancer patients following surgery, large blocks of fibrous tissue form along the walls of the erectile bodies, mimicking the hard plaques of **Peyronie's disease**. This condition ranges in severity from small, inconsequential areas of thickening to a serious, painful bend in the shaft that can make intercourse impossible. Some men report curvature of the penis with erections, or a penis that is rigid near the body but softer near the tip.

These changes are uncommon but are certainly troublesome when they occur. Fibrosis after radical prostatectomy is an area of intense research. Men in the prostate cancer age group can develop Peyronie's disease spontaneously. There have been no studies of penile fibrosis after external radiation or seed implants, even though these treatments can cause impotence in 40 to 56 percent of patients over five years after treatment. We don't know whether hormone therapy, either alone or in combination with surgery or radiation, makes fibrosis worse or prevents it.

How Great Is the Risk of ED After Surgery?

In the care of the average surgeon nationwide, about 40 to 45 percent of men who were fully functional before the operation recover workable erections by two years after radical prostatectomy. Surgeons with special expertise in nerve sparing report a 75 to 90 percent potency rate. Here again, the skill of the surgeon can make an enormous difference in how well you're likely to fare. Rates of ED vary, however, with the age of the patient and the quality of his erections before the operation, as well as with the degree of preservation of the neurovascular bundles.

PENILE REHABILITATION

Many doctors urge prostate cancer patients to use any effective means to have regular, frequent erections as soon as possible after surgery.[16] This may promote recovery of erectile function and reduce the risk of fibrosis (Peyronie's disease). There is very good data from animal studies that damage to erectile nerves leads to atrophy of blood vessels and fibrosis in the penis and that these changes can be minimized or prevented by the use of PDE-5 inhibitors, such as sildenafil (Viagra). In humans, there is evidence that with serious nerve damage, similar changes can be seen in the penis over six months. Whether these changes can be prevented in humans with oral medications, injections, or vacuum devices has not been convincingly demonstrated. Several uncontrolled clinical trials support the concept of "use it or lose it." Men who are sexually active seem to end up with better erection. Two small randomized trials—one using Viagra and one with injections—suggested that **penile rehabilitation** works. But there has also been a large, prospective, randomized trial of Levitra (vardenafil), given on demand or in a regular nightly dose versus placebo. After the medication course, everything was stopped for two months and the subjects' sexual function was evaluated. This study found no difference between the group that was given daily erection-enhancing drugs and the men who took the medicine only when needed for sexual activity.[17] More intensive research is needed to confirm whether penile rehabilitation really promotes recovery of erections.

INFERTILITY

After radical prostatectomy, you will no longer ejaculate. If fathering children is a current or potential future issue, you should bank sperm before the operation. Plan on making at least six to ten deposits, spaced several days apart.

If you haven't banked sperm and later wish you had, they can sometimes be harvested directly from the testicles in a simple procedure involving a small biopsy-like needle under local anesthetic. Using a method called **intracytoplasmic sperm injection (ICSI)**, a single sperm is then injected into an ovum in the lab. Pregnancy results in about 65 percent of cases.

WHAT PUTS MEN AT RISK FOR SEXUAL PROBLEMS AFTER SURGERY?

Recovery of erections after radical prostatectomy depends on your age, the quality of your erections before the operation, the degree of preservation of the nerves during the procedure, and how skillfully the surgery is performed. Men with diabetes, high cholesterol, hypertension, or coronary artery disease as well as cigarette smokers all have some intrinsic lowering of blood flow to the penis that will make recovering erections less likely after radical prostatectomy. A larger cancer that extends into a neurovascular bundle may risk incomplete resection, in order to spare a nerve. The judgment and skill to negotiate between the cancer and the nerve a few millimeters away challenges the most experienced surgeons.

Men under 60 years old and those with good erectile function before surgery are more likely to recover full potency afterward. If you have weak or unreliable erections prior to the operation, they *will not* be better afterward.

If both nerves are spared, your chances for sexual recovery will be greater than if one nerve is removed or severely damaged. All things considered, removing one nerve reduces the chance of erectile recovery by half. When I deliberately excise both erectile nerves to control cancer, none of my patients has recovered erections unless a nerve graft procedure was performed.

NOTE: Dr. John Mulhall, a sexual medicine specialist at MSKCC, encourages patients not to give up if the surgeon reports that he had to remove both nerves. In Mulhall's experience, 15 percent of such men are able to achieve good erections with the help of sildenafil or similar drugs.[18] Erectile nerves are a large group (plexus), not a single fiber. Sometimes, less experienced surgeons leave a portion of the nerve behind inadvertently, so a trial with an erection-inducing drug is a good idea.

SEXUAL SIDE EFFECTS OF RADIATION

The effect of radiation on erections can begin soon after treatment, but the full extent of damage may not become evident until years later. Radiation causes a gradual loss of erections by injuring the blood vessels that provide crucial circulation to the penis. These blood vessels lie so close to the prostate they cannot be completely protected from exposure to damaging rays.

Hormone therapy is often given in conjunction with radiation therapy, particularly for men with a large prostate or a serious cancer. Hormone therapy adds substantially to ED. Even a short course of three to six months of hormones, when combined with radiation, leads to a much greater risk of erectile dysfunction years later.[19]

The chances that a man will have good erectile function after radiation therapy depends on his age, the quality of erections before radiation, the seriousness of the cancer, the size of the prostate, the specific nature of the therapy, whether hormone therapy is involved, and the skill of the specialist delivering the radiation. More aggressive disease requires higher-dose radiation to a wider field with more resultant damage.

The type of radiation given is crucial as well. Conventional therapy with a linear accelerator bombards a broader, box-shaped area with damaging rays. 3-D conformal therapy narrows the field, but the blood supply to the penis is still exposed to the full dose. In brachytherapy (seed implants), the precision of the implant will affect how much incidental damage is inflicted on crucial blood vessels.

Overall, radiation therapy causes a loss of erectile function at the rate of about 10 percent per year for the first five years. One year after radiation treatment, 10 percent of men will experience a loss of erections; by five years, half of men treated with radiation will have ED.[20] The loss seems to continue after five years, and that would be consistent with what we know about the late effects of radiation, but there is too little data to be sure.

There is considerable debate about whether sexual function is better preserved with brachytherapy than with external beam radiation. Patients treated with seed implants tend to be younger with lower-stage disease and smaller prostates than those men who receive external beam radiation, and that could account for the impression that brachytherapy inflicts less harm on sexual function. In the early days of brachytherapy, radiation doses delivered were largely too low to damage erectile function (though they were also too low to damage the cancer). One large study comparing modern higher-dose brachytherapy with external beam radiation found that seed implants were more likely to cause problems with erectile function, even when neither group received hormone therapy in conjunction with the radiation.[21] Another good study found that brachytherapy has about the same effect on erectile function as high-dose 3-D conformal radiation with IMRT.[22]

After radiation, the severity of ED increases gradually, and fewer and fewer men continue to respond to ED medications. The effectiveness of Levitra, Cialis, or Viagra after radiation is better for younger men, patients who did not receive hormone therapy, and those treated with a lower radiation dose.

INFERTILITY

Following radiation, men are generally infertile because of damage to the prostate and the seminal vesicles. Scarring in the prostate and seminal vesicles results in decreased volume of ejaculatory fluid and obstruction of the ducts that allow the semen to get out. It would be rare for a man to be able to father a child after treatment. While radiation to the prostate should not be considered a guaranteed method of birth control, if fathering children in the future is important to you, it would be wise to bank sperm before treatment begins. (See page 415.)

SEXUAL SIDE EFFECTS OF HORMONE THERAPY

Prostate cancer relies on male hormones to grow and spread. Blocking these hormones can slow progression of the disease or shrink the cancer to facilitate treatment.

Removing the testicles will stop testosterone production, and some patients with advanced prostate cancer still opt for this approach. Drugs called **LHRH agonists** shut down testicular function and reduce testosterone to the same level achieved by surgical castration. **Antiandrogens** block the effects of testosterone on hormone-responsive cells but leave blood levels of testosterone intact. **Estrogens** (female hormones) lower testosterone levels by blocking the natural secretion of hormone-stimulating substances by the brain. In treating advanced prostate cancer, a combination of these drugs is sometimes given to produce a **complete androgen blockade**.

Any therapy that markedly reduces blood testosterone levels—surgical castration, LHRH agonists, or estrogens—will have a profound effect on libido and erections. Over a period of weeks or months, 80 to 90 percent of men report a loss of interest in sexual activity and an inability to get or maintain an erection. Along with the other effects of androgen deprivation (see Chapter 21, Treating Advanced Prostate Cancer), most men notice atrophy of the testicles and decreased size of the penis. Estrogens, antiandrogens (e.g., bicalutamide), and 5 alpha-reductase inhibitors (finasteride, dutasteride) may also cause swollen, tender, and painful breasts.

Some experts believe that the resultant low hormonal levels cause permanent scarring of the erectile tissues. Administering hormone therapy intermittently might minimize damage. Once the drugs succeed in driving down the PSA, a patient may be taken off therapy for a while, during which time testosterone levels rebound and sexual function is

Testosterone Replacement Therapy After Prostate Cancer Treatment

Sometimes men with low testosterone levels are diagnosed with prostate cancer and treated with radiation or surgery. Some of these patients ask if it's safe to go back on hormone replacement therapy they were receiving before they were diagnosed. This issue is controversial since replacing testosterone may allow their prostate cancers to grow, so doctors have been reluctant to administer hormone replacement, even to men with troublesome symptoms of low testosterone, including decreased libido, poor erections, hot flashes, decreased muscle mass, decreased energy, and osteoporosis.

An argument in favor of hormone replacement therapy in this setting is that a typical man with normal testosterone levels before treatment for prostate cancer will continue to have normal levels after treatment (except for men who are given androgen deprivation therapy to control their cancers). Why then would it be more dangerous to give testosterone to a man unable to make adequate amounts on **his** own? If the prostate cancer is cured, testosterone will not make it come back. If it is not cured, it would **eventually** come back as a hormone refractory cancer that would be difficult to treat. Since PSA is so accurate in identifying recurrent cancer, we have been comfortable replacing testosterone in men who continue to have low levels of this male hormone along with troublesome symptoms and no evidence of prostate cancer a year after treatment.[24]

regained. If your treatment involves hormone therapy, you may want to discuss the possibility of intermittent therapy with your doctor. The negative effect on sexual function is one reason to delay hormone therapy as long as possible.[23] Monitoring PSA is such an effective way to gauge the course of the cancer that at Memorial Sloan-Kettering, we generally recommend delaying hormone treatment until the PSA is rising so fast that problems from the cancer are imminent. (See Chapter 20, Rising PSA After Surgery, Radiation, or Other Therapy.) Hormone therapy should definitely be started before metastases appear.

PREVENTING AND TREATING ED

There has been great interest in administering **neuroprotective agents** before radical prostatectomy to prevent the diminished function that results from trauma to the exquisitely delicate erectile nerves during surgery, but two randomized prospective clinical trials have tested two different (though similar acting) neuroprotective drugs, without success. At present, no FDA-approved or proven effective neuroprotective drugs are available.

The primary goal of treatment for ED is to restore spontaneous, functional erections as soon as possible after radical prostatectomy and to maintain functional erections in the long run after radiation treatment.

ORAL MEDICATIONS

The first-line treatment for erectile dysfunction is the family of erection-inducing medications that include sildenafil (Viagra), vardenafil (Levitra), and tadalafil (Cialis), all of which act to relax smooth muscles in the penis. This encourages blood flow, allowing the penis to become firmer and remain so longer. These drugs work by blocking the enzyme phosphodiesterase-5 and are therefore also known as PDE-5 inhibitors.[25] All boast an 80 to 90 percent or greater response rate. For most men, these drugs can be used daily with no ill effects, but two to three times per week is what most prescription drug programs cover.

Remember, these pills are a catalyst, not a catapult, and they do not act as aphrodisiacs. Physical stimulation or psychological arousal is necessary to induce an erection once the medication takes effect. In the absence of stimulation, the penis remains flaccid. An erection is maintained only as long as the sexual stimulus persists.

Because food reduces absorption of sildenafil by 30 percent, it's important to take the drug on an empty stomach. (Vardenafil absorption can be slowed by a high fat meal, and tadalafil is not affected by food intake.) For most men, that means waiting two hours after a meal or thirty minutes before eating to take sildenafil. Normally, this drug takes sixty to ninety minutes to work. If you take it on an empty stomach, a glass of ice water may speed the effect. Men with diabetes, whose digestion may take longer, should wait three hours after eating. Given that heavy drinking can interfere with erections, you should minimize alcohol consumption when trying these drugs.

Sildenafil and vardenafil provide about a six-hour window of

NOTE: If you are on any form of nitrates or nitroglycerin, including recreational drugs containing nitrates, such as "poppers," you *must not* take PDE-5 inhibitors. These medications can interact dangerously, causing a profound drop in blood pressure that could lead to sudden death.

Makers of vardenafil and tadalafil also caution against using those medications if you are taking alpha blockers for hypertension or benign prostate enlargement, if you've had a recent stroke or heart attack and have low or uncontrolled high blood pressure, or if you have a rare irregularity in your heart rhythm, known as a Q-T prolongation. If so, you should consult your cardiologist before starting one of the erection-promoting drugs.

opportunity for erectile function, though in some men, effects last up to twelve hours. Tadalafil acts for twenty-four to thirty-six hours, so a low daily dose, 5 mg/day, would allow men to be ready for sexual encounters whenever the mood strikes.

Some men fail to respond to these drugs. Others experience unacceptable side effects, which may include headache, facial flushing, nasal stuffiness, heartburn, and in the case of sildenafil, distortions in the perception of the color blue. Less common is a hung-over feeling the next day. Be especially aware of severe muscle aches or cramps with any of these drugs. Stop them immediately and talk to your doctor.

INJECTIONS

Ninety percent of men with erectile dysfunction who do not respond to or can't tolerate oral medications have good results with direct injection of an erection-inducing drug into the penis. The drug takes five minutes to work, and results last for twenty to ninety minutes. Though some men are squeamish about injecting themselves, the therapy uses a tiny 29-gauge needle (29 would fit in an inch), and causes no more discomfort than a mosquito bite. With training, most patients get past their aversion to the needle and find this therapy highly satisfactory. If it seems preferable, your partner can be trained to administer the medication for you.

Caverject, which works for 65 percent of men, is the only FDA-approved injectable medication for erectile dysfunction. It comes prepackaged in a syringe with a drug called alprostadil, which causes blood vessels in the penis to dilate, permitting blood to rush in and fill the erection chambers, causing rigidity.[26] On the downside, the drug can cause burning penile pain when used in the first few months after radical prostatectomy. For 90 percent of men, **trimix**, a mixture of papaverine, phentolamine, and alprostadil, provides good workable erections with far less risk of the burning sensation because it only contains a small amount of alprostadil. **Bimix** is available if there is a reason to remove alprostadil from the formula. The combination is not commercially available and

must be compounded by your pharmacy or hospital. A four-month supply costs about $200 to $250, and it may not be covered by insurance.
These formularies are highly effective and less likely to cause pain in the
early postoperative period, so we prefer to use them.

Side Effects of Injections

Alternating the injection site minimizes the risk of fibrosis or scarring
from the needles, which is extremely rare. The most serious potential
problem is **priapism**, a persistent erection lasting more than four hours
that can damage the penis, but with adequate instruction and training
this can be avoided.

> NOTE: After nerve-sparing radical prostatectomy, men are exquisitely
> sensitive to these drugs, so they should be tried in very low doses under
> medical supervision. The dose should be increased gradually as toler-
> ance improves. Be sure your doctor is aware that the standard dose is
> not appropriate after this surgery and that administering too much of
> the medicine could cause pain or even priapism, a dangerous erection
> lasting more than four hours.

> NOTE: If your erection lasts for more than three hours, call your doc-
> tor or go to the nearest emergency room right away! The erection
> can usually be reversed with an injection of a vasoconstrictor like
> phenylephrine.

SUPPOSITORIES

For some men who do not do well with oral medications and cannot deal with injections, the **MUSE (medicated urethral system
for erection)** provides a satisfactory alternative. The treatment involves

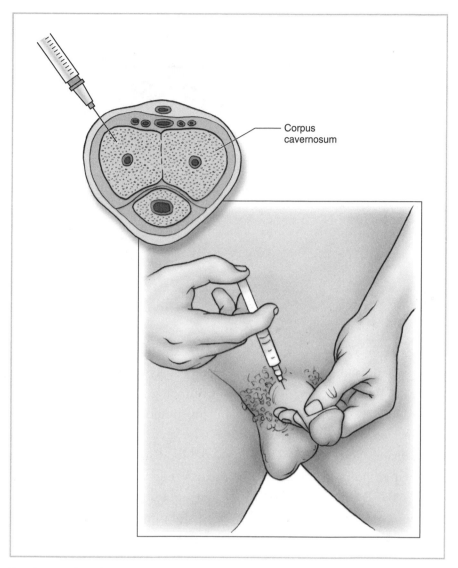

Erections can be achieved by injecting drugs that dilate blood vessels into an erectile chamber (corpus cavernosum). Note that the site of the injection should be near the body on the side of the penis.

insertion of a small pellet containing alprostadil into the urethra, through an applicator introduced into the tip of the penis.

The procedure can be awkward. Men must urinate first, insert the drug, and then massage the penis for ten to twenty minutes while standing, until an erection occurs. Results are inconsistent, and some men lose

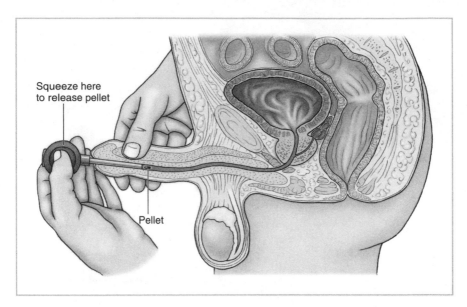

Squeeze here
to release pellet

Pellet

Insertion of a pellet of alprostadil (MUSE) to aid erections.

their erection when they lie down. The medication causes burning and penile pain in about 50 percent of cases, especially in the first few months after radical prostatectomy. Two percent of men get dizzy when they first use MUSE, and some faint, so initial trials should be done under medical supervision.[27] Nevertheless, MUSE, like oral medications and injections, dilates blood vessels. This increases blood supply to the penis and may help to promote healthy penile tissue. While not especially powerful alone, MUSE can be helpful for men with mild degrees of erectile dysfunction, and some men have been successful using MUSE in combination with oral medications.

CONSTRICTING RINGS

Erections that are not quite stiff or durable enough for intercourse can be bolstered by using a **constricting ring** or band like the one that comes with the VED (see page 427). The adjustable or elastic band is lubricated and then placed around the base of the penis before arousal. This helps to retain blood in the penis after an erection is achieved, while not

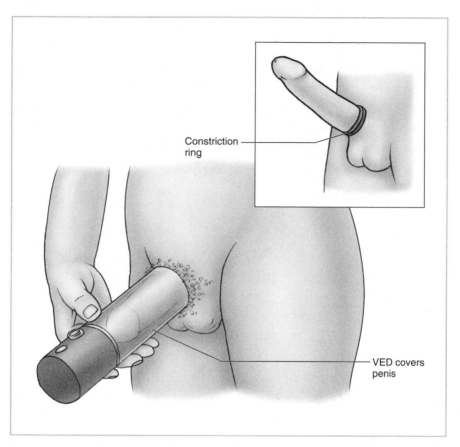

Constriction
ring

VED covers
penis

A vacuum erection devide (VED) with a constriction ring is a simple way to achieve a firm, work-able erection.

interfering with the overall circulation or arterial inflow. These bands are inexpensive and readily available, and they have been underutilized in men who have some difficulty maintaining full erections after surgery or radiation.

Vacuum Erection Devices (VEDs)

A tube is placed over the penis and an erection is induced by pump-ing out the air in the tube to create a vacuum. A rubber ring placed at the base of the penis maintains rigidity. **Vacuum erection devices (VEDs)** do not produce an actual physiological erection and therefore don't promote the circulation of fresh, oxygenated blood. Consequently, they may not help avoid fibrosis after radical prostatectomy.

VEDs are simple to use, and they come with an instructional videotape, but the apparatus is cumbersome. The resulting erections are rigid and lasting, but the penis remains 1 degree F below body temperature, so it registers as cold and looks rather blue. Nevertheless, some men prefer these relatively simple devices to oral medications or injections.

Penile Implants (Prostheses)

For men who can't use oral medications, suppositories, or injections, and are not satisfied with bands or VEDs, **penile implants** can be an excellent means to restore functional erections.[28]

The prostheses can be semirigid or inflatable. Semirigid devices are simpler to implant and have a lower risk of mechanical failure, but they do not provide normal-looking erections and, since they remain semirigid all the time, can be difficult to conceal under clothing and could make showering in a locker room awkward.

With inflatable implants, erectile chambers are surgically implanted in the penis. There are two different types: a two-piece device and a three-piece device. The two-piece device has a pump in the scrotum which forces the fluid in these chambers to move forward, causing rigidity. To reverse the process, a man bends the penis at mid-shaft to release the fluid, and the erection subsides. In the three-piece device, the scrotal pump forces fluid into the erectile chambers from a reservoir in the abdomen to which it returns after sexual activity is completed. It is deflated by pressure on the release valve. The non-erect penis appears nearly normal. Generally, the three-piece device provides a fuller erection at maximum inflation.

Implants do involve surgery and anesthesia. Two to 3 percent of men will have postoperative infections, and 15 percent experience mechanical or other failure requiring a second surgery to repair or replace the device. The procedure is permanent, but, like a hip prosthesis, once implanted, the device becomes part of your body and you have no conscious awareness that it is in place. Some of the happiest men I see are those who truly needed and were enormously satisfied with an implanted penile prosthesis.

NOTE: Since it can take two to three years to recover erections completely after radical prostatectomy, men should postpone permanent interventions like penile implants until their level of recovery is clear. Partial erections may continue to improve gradually. If a man has no hint of erections eighteen to twenty-four months after surgery, he's unlikely to ever recover workable erections. At that point, an implant, even though it requires surgery, is worth careful consideration.

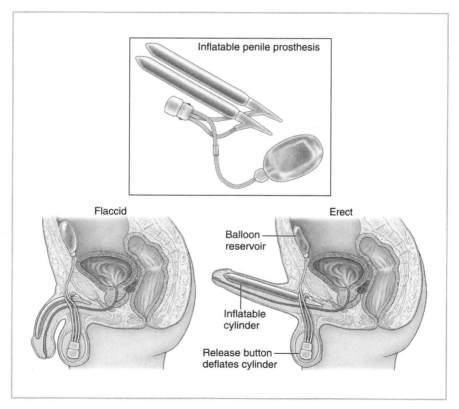

The three-part inflatable penile prosthesis shown in flaccid and erect states after it is implanted.

THE FUTURE

Prostate cancer doctors continue to seek improved techniques to better treat the cancer while minimizing side effects. Surgeons are constantly refining nerve-sparing procedures to reduce trauma to the delicate erectile nerves. Newer forms of radiation therapy, such as a single-dose (hypofractionation) may prove less damaging to sexual function. Conformal techniques for brachytherapy may reduce the incidence of sexual side effects. Testing for genetic predisposition to radiation injury may help identify men at high risk of erectile dysfunction and other side effects of radiation therapy, steering them toward an alternative treatment. While robotic surgery has not proved to be the panacea for sexual complications of surgery, as was initially advertised, refinements in both open and robotic surgery are being pursued with improved cure rates and reduced side effects in mind. The development of focal therapy for small prostate tumors shows promise as a way to minimize the effects of treatment on sexual function.

While the data from early trials of neuroprotective drugs was disappointing, the concept of neuroprotection has been clearly established in laboratory studies. Future trials may identify the best drug or combination of drugs, given systemically or even applied directly to the nerves during surgery, that could reduce the loss of function that results from handling these nerves.

We will continue to test the concept of penile rehabilitation. Recent clinical trials of this "Use it or lose it" approach have been disappointing, but since the idea has such a firm scientific basis in animal models, it needs to be explored further. Today, we have no drug to reverse reduced libido, but this is another fertile area for scientific research.

IN SUMMARY

Prostate cancer and treatments for the disease can cause erectile dysfunction. Many men recover good sexual function after radical prostatectomy, though this can be gradual and in some cases takes years. Following radiation, problems with erectile function appear slowly but increase in frequency and severity over time, as damage from the treatment accumulates. Fortunately, we have excellent means to deal with ED after radiation and surgery, and most men are able to resume a satisfactory sex life after treatment for prostate cancer. Hormone therapy presents a larger problem, causing a loss of libido and erections and exacerbating the damaging effects of radiation.

19

■

Bowel Side Effects

READ THIS CHAPTER TO LEARN:

- How can treatments for prostate cancer affect bowel function?
- Which prostate cancer therapies carry a risk of bowel side effects?
- What can be done about bowel problems when they occur?

Mention prostate cancer, and other than the prospect of dying of the disease, the thing patients worry about most is a loss of erections or urinary control. Though problems with bowel function can have a greater impact on quality of life than urinary incontinence or impotence, men with this disease are typically unconcerned about these side effects. In fact, most patients (and many physicians) have no idea that the risk of such problems exists.

This general lack of awareness is unfortunate though certainly understandable. The effects of prostate cancer treatments on gastrointestinal function have been sparsely investigated and scarcely mentioned in literature in the field. For the most part, the problem has been simply, inexplicably ignored. Bowel side effects have been treated like the metaphorical elephant in the room that no one talks about, as if that magically might make it cease to exist. Unfortunately, for the men affected by bowel problems, this particular elephant looms undeniably real and very large indeed.

The rear of the prostate sits mere millimeters from the anterior (front) rectal wall. (See illustration on page 6.) Given this anatomical coincidence and the fact that the prostate is buried deep in the pelvis and otherwise extremely hard to reach, doctors who specialize in diagnosing and treating prostate diseases have come to rely on the lower end of the bowel, also known as the rectum, as the equivalent of an access road or service entrance to the gland. To conduct a DRE, a doctor places a gloved finger in the rectum and examines the rear of the prostate for abnormalities. The needles used for prostate biopsies, along with the ultrasound that guides them, are inserted through the rectum. Transrectal ultrasound can also be used to gauge the size and shape of the prostate and may show the shadow of a large cancer in the gland—both pieces of information significant for diagnosis and treatment planning. Endorectal MRI, another sophisticated imaging technique, allows us to visualize the prostate and may help to gauge the location and seriousness of cancers in the prostate, seminal vesicles, and pelvic lymph nodes.

Being so close to the prostate renders the rectum both useful in cancer treatments and vulnerable to their effects. When we conduct a search-and-destroy mission to eradicate cancer in the prostate, bowel function can be an accidental casualty.

DOES RADICAL PROSTATECTOMY AFFECT BOWEL FUNCTION?

To remove the prostate during a radical prostatectomy, the rear of the gland must be peeled away from the rectum. In doing so, there's always a risk that the surgeon will nick or even perforate the rectal wall. Fortunately, these small tears occur rarely (about 1 in 300 cases), and when they do and are recognized during the operation, they can be irrigated with antibiotic solution and uneventfully repaired. A course of intravenous antibiotics will prevent infection from fecal contamination. An unrecognized injury, while very rare, poses a greater problem. A serious abscess could develop, requiring surgical drainage and a temporary colostomy, meaning the colon is diverted to the outside through the abdomen until the wound heals, at which point the colostomy can be closed and normal function restored. This almost never happens in the hands of experienced surgeons.

Today, laparoscopic and robotically assisted laparoscopic prostatectomy are becoming more popular, but the rate of rectal and other intestinal injuries is higher (0.5 to 1.5 percent) than with the open procedure (0.5 percent).[1] Just as with open surgery, the damage can be repaired without consequence if it is recognized during the operation, but an injury that goes unrecognized can cause a catastrophic problem.

A few surgeons still prefer the perineal approach (between the scrotum and rectum) to radical prostatectomy. Though the rectum is more easily visible with this method, rectal injuries are more common than with the retropubic approach (through the abdomen). Among other disadvantages of perineal prostatectomy, since the prostate is approached through the rectal sphincter, fecal incontinence (some soiling) has been reported in 1 of 6 men in the first three months after surgery. In 1 of 30 men, this problem persists for over a year.[2]

Removing the prostate with any type of surgery leaves a space into which the rectum can expand. This can lead to a temporary decrease in rectal tone and an increased vulnerability to constipation. Most surgeons recommend a clear liquid diet for twenty-four hours before radical prostatectomy and a Fleet enema the evening before or morning of the operation. For about six weeks after surgery, until things return to normal, it's important to avoid constipation by drinking plenty of water, eating food rich in fiber, and getting adequate exercise. Simple stool softeners such as docusate (Colace) or Metamucil, taken by mouth twice a day for six weeks after surgery, will help to keep you from having to strain to move your bowels. Doing so could damage your incision and increase the risk of a blood clot moving to your lungs.

While it usually takes four to five days after a radical prostatectomy before your first bowel movement and a week or two to resume normal regularity, most men notice no other changes in their bowel habits after surgery. In fact, surgery is the least likely of all the standard treatments for localized prostate cancer to cause bowel problems. Patients with serious, chronic, intestinal conditions, such as Crohn's disease or ulcerative colitis, and those who have had rectal reconstruction or resection for any reason, are better candidates for surgery than radiotherapy because of the sensitivity of the intestine to the damaging effects of radiation. If you have severe hemorrhoids or irritable bowel syndrome, surgery is also a better option than radiation, but this is a recommendation, not an absolute contraindication.

> NOTE: For the first few weeks after a radical prostatectomy, you *should not* use enemas, which could risk perforating the rectal wall. Rectal suppositories, on the other hand, pose no danger and are used commonly after the operation to encourage recovery of bowel function.

BOWEL SIDE EFFECTS OF RADIATION

To effectively treat prostate cancer, radiation oncologists must bombard the entire gland with damaging rays. In doing so, it's impossible to spare the rectum completely from radiation exposure and injury. To make matters worse, the rectal wall is far more susceptible to radiation damage than the prostate gland.

All normal cells in the human body are programmed to grow for a time, die off, and then replace themselves. Radiation works by destroying blood vessels and by damaging the genetic blueprint (DNA) that cells rely on to reproduce, and a sufficient dose shuts the replication process down completely. As a result, the faster cells turn over, the more quickly and dramatically they register radiation's destructive effects and the injury to blood vessels makes healing slow and difficult. Radiation sensitivity varies from organ to organ, depending on the speed of that turnover and the number of delicate blood vessels in the organ. Prostate cells are analogous to the brick house in the tale of the three little pigs—very difficult to destroy. Because they turn over so rapidly, cells lining the rectal wall are the straw house equivalent, highly vulnerable to external assaults.

Key predictors of radiation side effects are bowel troubles before the treatment, the strength of the dose, and the area of the rectal wall hit by that dose. Anything over 50 Gy risks damage to the rectum, and modern treatment for prostate cancer involves a dose of at least 75.6 Gy. Still, bowel symptoms rarely occur unless a significant portion of the rectal wall receives that much radiation.[3] When radiation fields are extended to include the seminal vesicles (which they usually are) or the pelvic lymph nodes (which varies from center to center and depends on the seriousness of your cancer), a larger area of the rectum is exposed to radiation. In the first few months during or after radiation, 10 to 15 percent of all radiation patients develop symptoms of acute **proctitis** (inflammation of the rectum), which can cause diarrhea, frequent passage of mucus (tenesmus), and rectal bleeding that requires men to use tampons or pads. In men with prior bowel problems, these numbers could be much higher.

While conformal radiation with IMRT targets the prostate more precisely and avoids damage to the rectal wall, conventional radiation exposes more of the bowel to damage. As radiation injury accumulates after conventional treatment, other troubling and more intractable bowel side effects can appear. Radiation damage and resultant exposure to bacteria can lead to erosion or ulceration of the anterior rectal wall, causing painful bowel movements and bleeding. One study found that a year after conventional radiation, 26 percent of patients were troubled by intestinal cramps, 38 percent reported moderate to severe flatulence, 17 percent suffered with chronic diarrhea, 12 percent experienced persistent rectal bleeding or mucus discharge, and 30 percent had rectal pain. In another investigation, 35 percent of men reported problems with bowel urgency a year after external beam radiation.[4]

Radiation damage can reduce the effectiveness of the anal sphincter, decrease rectal capacity, or increase sensitivity in the lining of the rectal wall. Some patients develop **fecal incontinence** as a result, and some men are unable to control the expulsion of gas. Radiation damage can also exacerbate hemorrhoids, which can bleed and cause pain. Overall, with conventional radiation about 10 to 15 percent of radiation patients have problems with liquid or solid soiling, though one study found the incidence to be as high as one man in four. These problems can lead to major alterations in lifestyle, seriously hindering social interactions and triggering depression.

With modern radiation techniques such as IMRT, and with higher quality brachytherapy implants in recent years, the risk of bowel complications is much less. For example, in a survey of patients from the University of Michigan, 8 percent reported an overall problem with bowel habits three years after external beam radiation and 13 percent complain about problems after six years. For brachytherapy, bowel problems improved over time: 17 percent had bowel problems two years after the implant, while only 10 percent reported problems at six years. This compares with 3 to 4 percent who had bowel problems after radical prostatectomy, the same as an age-matched control group.[5]

The best study of the effects of radiation on bowel function before and after radiation therapy, found that 9 to 16 percent of men reported moderate or severe distress from bowel symptoms beginning two months after radiation, and 9 percent reported distress related to rectal urgency, frequency, pain, fecal incontinence, or rectal bleeding a year or more after IMRT or brachytherapy.[6] With IMRT, it is possible to give very high doses of radiation with a low risk of rectal complications.

Complications can be reduced by meticulous attention to the delivery of radiation. For example, Dr. Michael Zelefsky from MSKCC reported that only 3 percent of patients treated with 81 Gy developed troublesome bowel complications. The problems were severe in less than 1 percent.[7]

Dietary changes, such as increasing bulk and fluids, can relieve constipation, as can stool softeners, while over-the-counter medications like loperamide (Imodium) may alleviate diarrhea. Bleeding used to be common, but thankfully, it is rare now and typically clears up on its own. Fewer than 1 in 1,000 men has bleeding severe enough to require transfusion. The risk of rectal bleeding is higher in frequent aspirin users. Often, colonoscopy is recommended to diagnose the source of bleeding in men who have been irradiated for prostate cancer. If the bleeding stems from

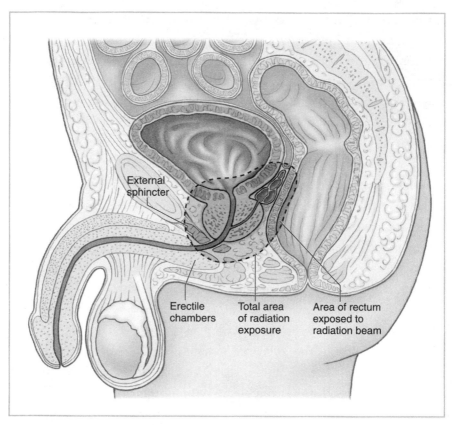

External
sphincter

Erectile
chambers

Total area
of radiation
exposure

Area of rectum
exposed to
radiation beam

Area exposed to the full dose of radiation during external beam radiation therapy for prostate cancer. Note that some part of the rectal wall receives a full dose of radiation.

the anterior rectal wall that lies next to the prostate, the area should not be biopsied. Taking a biopsy from a heavily irradiated bowel can lead to a rectal urinary fistula (hole) that could require a colostomy.

BOWEL EFFECTS OF
OTHER TREATMENTS

Other techniques for treating prostate cancer, such as cryotherapy and HIFU (see Chapter 16, Focal and Other "Local" Therapies), aim to destroy the prostate without surgical removal. These approaches carry a risk of injury to the nearby bowel.[8] The most serious is a fistula (hole) between the rectum and the urinary tract that results from extreme tissue damage. Rectourethral fistulas have been reported in up to 2 percent of patients treated with cryotherapy or HIFU. Typically, they occur when doctors are learning the procedure. With sufficient experience, surgeons should rarely cause a fistula. They should be avoidable completely, except in the most complicated cases (i.e. men with an unusually large prostate or prior radiation to the area). There is a real risk of rectal injury when HIFU or cryotherapy is used as a salvage technique when prostate cancer recurs after radiation.[9]

REDUCING THE RISK

The incidence and severity of gastrointestinal problems is highly related to the type of treatment you get. With conventional external beam therapy that irradiates a box-shaped area around the prostate, about 30 percent of men develop serious proctitis (rectal inflammation). 3-D conformal therapy reduces the incidence to 14 percent, and only 2 percent of those who receive 3-D conformal therapy with IMRT develop bowel frequency, urgency, tenesmus, or bleeding. For men who opt for modern seed implants, 3 percent experience severe rectal inflammation early on, and 10 to 15 percent develop moderate irritative bowel symptoms, such as flatulence, urgency, bleeding, and cramps. Severe bleeding, requiring multiple cauterizations, occurs in 2 to 3 percent of men who receive conventional radiation, occasionally leading to a colostomy. With seed implants or 3-D conformal radiation with IMRT, serious bleeding requiring such drastic measures is very rare.

With all types of radiation, side effects increase in direct proportion to the size of the dose and—more important—the area of the rectum that's included in the field. If more than 25 percent of the rectal wall is exposed to radiation, the risk of side effects goes up markedly. For this reason, computer-assisted treatment planning is essential to limit the side effects of radiation therapy. In some cases, the particular relationship of the rectal wall to the prostate and seminal vesicles makes it impossible to deliver an adequate dose of radiation to the cancer without risking damage to the rectum. Prudent radiotherapists refer such patients to a surgeon.

To avoid bowel problems, many men receive a short course of reversible hormone therapy with LHRH agonists and/or antiandrogens to shrink the prostate before radiation, reducing the size of the field and the area of the rectum that will be bombarded by damaging X-rays. However, reducing testosterone with hormone therapy through a course of radiation exacerbates problems with erectile function in the short and long term. Even a short, temporary course of hormones can substantially increase the chances of erectile dysfunction in the short run, and the problem may prove to be permanent.

Certain medical conditions place you at greater risk for serious bowel problems after radiation. Men with bleeding problems and those who require permanent anticoagulation are not good candidates for external beam therapy or seed implants because of the risk of rectal bleeding. Most radiation therapists will not treat men with these conditions, but some will consider doing so, depending on the severity of the disease, whether it has necessitated surgical procedures, and how well it is controlled by medication. Because of the risks of severely exacerbating the illness, patients with Crohn's disease or ulcerative colitis should not receive radiation. Ataxia telangiectasia, a rare genetic disorder, is another absolute contraindication to radiation, since the cells in the intestinal wall cannot repair the damage inflicted by even low doses of radiation.

Combination therapies, including brachytherapy with external beam radiation, may increase the risk of bowel problems. So does treatment with outmoded technology, such as a conventional linear accelerator. If you decide to have brachytherapy or external beam radiation, make sure you're treated by a highly experienced radiation oncologist at a facility that offers state-of-the-art equipment. There is no evidence to date that the risk of bowel injury is lower with proton beam radiation than with IMRT.

CAN YOU PREVENT BOWEL PROBLEMS BY AVOIDING TREATMENT?

Prostate cancer rarely grows around the rectum or blocks the intestinal tract. But if your cancer is serious enough or you are young enough to require treatment and you are concerned about the gastrointestinal effects of radiation, you should consider having surgery instead. Even men with previous rectal surgery, such as total removal of the colon (colectomy) with the small bowel connected to the rectum (ileorectal anastomosis), can have a radical prostatectomy safely. If your age, health, or the extent of your cancer excludes surgery as an option, and radiation is the right treatment choice, consider taking hormone therapy to reduce the area of rectal wall that will be exposed. In the final analysis, the risk of bowel problems can best be minimized by seeking optimal treatment from highly skilled and experienced experts.

THE FUTURE

Studies are under way to determine whether novel radioprotective agents can prevent damage to rectal tissues from external beam therapy or seed implants. As we learn more about the way radiation therapy works to destroy cancers, we may discover drugs that promote cancer eradication or protect normal tissue.

IMRT was a major advancement in radiation therapy that substantially reduced side effects and increased cure rates for prostate cancer. Gastroenterologists at Memorial Sloan-Kettering Cancer Center report far fewer serious bowel complications of prostate cancer radiation today than they saw fifteen years ago, before IMRT was developed. This technique continues to be refined as we explore the optimal dose for each type of prostate cancer and study ways to combine high-dose radiotherapy with hormone therapy more effectively. In the future, image-guided radiotherapy (IGRT) and delivering radiation in higher doses per day over fewer days (hypofractionation) may further reduce the risk of bowel injuries.

IN SUMMARY

Though it is rarely discussed and little known, treatment for prostate cancer can alter or impair bowel function. For several weeks after surgery, men must avoid constipation. After radiation, some men suffer bowel inflammation, urgency, bleeding, and fecal incontinence. These problems can be troubling and difficult to manage.

20

Rising PSA After Surgery, Radiation, or Other Therapy

READ THIS CHAPTER TO LEARN:

- Why do some prostate cancers recur?
- How do you know if a recurrence is local or distant?
- Does a rising PSA always mean cancer?
- What can be done if the PSA rises after treatment?

While modern surgery and radiation are highly effective against prostate cancer, 20 to 30 percent of patients will eventually have a recurrence of the disease that is first evidenced by a PSA that fails to fall after treatment, remains measurable, or begins to rise. In fact, each year in the United States, 50,000 men with prostate cancer develop a rising PSA after treatment. If the cause is a recurrence in the local prostate area, salvage radiation (after surgery) or salvage prostatectomy (after radiation) offers a second chance to cure the disease. Once you have been treated for prostate cancer, you need to measure your PSA regularly for the rest of your life, since cancers have been known to recur years, or even decades, after the initial treatment. PSA is a remarkably accurate indicator of the presence of cancer after treatment and signals a problem many years before metastases would appear or symptoms would develop.

Why does cancer recur after the prostate is treated? Local treatments cannot cure cancers that have already spread, and even the best modern tests (bone scans, MRIs) are incapable of detecting tiny clusters of cancer cells that may have spread elsewhere in the body before the tumor in the prostate was treated. The local tumor may also send out microscopic roots into the surrounding tissue that can be missed at the time of surgery and can regrow over time. Sometimes, even when the tumor is locally contained, the surgeon may fail to remove all the cancer (positive surgical margins) or mistakenly leave some normal prostate tissue behind (benign surgical margins). In the first case, the tumor would eventually grow again. In the second instance, the remaining prostate tissue or a new cancer that develops within it might grow. Any of these situations could cause the PSA to rise.

Treatments like radiation, HIFU, and cryotherapy leave the gland in place. Any prostate tissue that remains undestroyed continues to produce PSA, which is why most men have a detectable PSA after these forms of therapy. If all the cancer cells are not killed, the tumor will recur and the PSA level will rise. Even if the original cancer is eradicated completely, a new cancer could develop within the gland at some future time.

NOTE: After treatment, patients always ask what they can do to prevent a recurrence. Men wonder about the effectiveness of diets or supplements, but to date, nothing—including Vitamin E and selenium, which were thought to be promising—has proven useful. The best we can recommend is a heart-healthy diet, high in fruits and vegetables, with little red meat, and regular exercise to maintain a healthy weight. We also counsel men to have regular checkups so recurrences can be treated early. The earlier a return of the cancer is detected, the more treatment options there are, and the more likely it is that such "secondary" treatment will prevent metastases and prolong life.[1]

DOES A RISING PSA ALWAYS MEAN CANCER?

PSA tests can be a source of intense, or even debilitating, anxiety. After surgery, radiation, cryotherapy, or HIFU, many men anticipate the test with dread and await the outcome like the verdict in a capital case. Occasionally, an elevation in the PSA represents nothing more than a laboratory error, a benign condition, or meaningless background noise. One study showed that less than half of men who at some point had a PSA that registered 0.2 or higher after surgery ever experienced a genuine rising PSA over time.[2] After radiation, PSA levels tend to fluctuate for the first few years, sometimes for no apparent reason. (See PSA Bounce, on page 453.)

Even when the PSA is genuinely rising because of cancer, it suggests trouble on the distant horizon, *not* an imminent threat. PSA levels rise an average of 6 to 8 years before any cancer would be detected by physical examination, bone scans, or other tests. A cancer recurrence may be contained in the prostate area and curable with further (**salvage**) treatment. Sometimes the PSA rises so slowly (suggesting that the cancer is growing very slowly as well) that no treatment is needed for many years. In an older man with a limited life expectancy, further treatment may never be required. The disease may not cause any problems in his lifetime.

> NOTE: Once you are treated for a cancer thought to be located within or around the prostate, the only test you need to check on the status of the cancer is the PSA. Patients with breast cancer must have regularly scheduled CT scans and bone scans to see if the cancer has recurred. PSA is far more accurate than scans and is the only test regularly required after prostate cancer treatment. If your PSA is undetectable after surgery, or low and stable after radiation, cryotherapy, or HIFU, no other tests are needed.

HOW LOW SHOULD THE PSA LEVEL BE AFTER RADICAL PROSTATECTOMY?

After the prostate is surgically removed, your PSA should become undetectable. By taking out the gland, we destroy the PSA factory, and no more of the antigen is produced. Residual PSA is flushed from the bloodstream in a few weeks, eliminating the final inventory.

This creates a peculiar conundrum. It's impossible to measure something that does not exist. Proving there is no PSA is like trying to demonstrate as a certainty that there is no arsenic in the drinking water. How do we know we looked everywhere? Couldn't there have been a few PSA molecules that we failed to detect among the trillions in the tube? The best a laboratory can do is report that, in the sample they studied, the PSA was found to be less than some very low, arbitrary number they predetermine in an attempt to avoid reporting insignificant background noise. In our lab at Memorial Sloan-Kettering Cancer Center, the threshold for a detectable PSA is 0.05. Any result below that level is reported as "less than 0.05" and is equivalent to "no measurable PSA." Other facilities set the threshold much higher, at 0.1 to 0.2.

Ultrasensitive PSA assays have been available for some time and are gaining broader acceptance.[3] They can measure as low as 0.001, but most of the labs using these measures would not consider a PSA to be positive unless it is above 0.003. The benefits of measuring such low levels are debatable. The lower you set the threshold, the more false positives you get. But some studies suggest that you may be able to detect, and therefore treat, recurrences early, or at the very least be reassured that the prostate cancer has really been cured.

The problem with relying on such low levels is the varying quality of tests for PSA and the laboratories running them. With the standard assay (0.05 is the lower limit of detectability) in two or three of every hundred tests, a reported elevation turns out to be false. The problem could be laboratory error or some other innocent artifact. If, after treatment, you have fifty or more PSA tests over the years, chances are that one or more of them will show a spurious elevation. To confirm that a positive result is genuine, repeat the test in a few weeks and recheck the value in a different lab. It is essential to confirm that the PSA is measurable and rising before you consider any further therapy.

HOW LOW SHOULD THE PSA LEVEL GO AFTER RADIATION, CRYOTHERAPY, OR HIFU?

After brachytherapy, external beam radiation, cryotherapy, or HIFU, the PSA rarely becomes undetectable as it does after radical prostatectomy, and it can be difficult to determine the cause of a rising PSA. The prostate is not removed as it is with surgery. Any detectable PSA may be coming from benign overgrowth or inflammation of normal prostate tissue, not necessarily from cancer.

As seed implants or external beam radiation kills cancer cells, the PSA slowly declines until it reaches its lowest level, which we refer to as the **PSA nadir**. During the course of radiation, the PSA may actually rise at first and not begin to fall until six months after the treatment course is finished. The average time it takes to reach PSA nadir is eighteen months, but it can take as long as three years. Ideally, we want that lowest number to be 0.5 or less. The nadir is predictive of how you're likely to fare. The lower the PSA goes, the smaller the chance that your cancer will recur.

The American Society for Therapeutic Radiology and Oncology (ASTRO) defines radiation failure as a PSA that rises 2 ng/ml above the PSA nadir.[4] This is the definition that most accurately predicted which patients would eventually develop metastases, troublesome local recurrence, or die from prostate cancer. It is not a very good definition, however, if you are eager to learn whether your cancer has been completely destroyed. Using this definition, it's possible to ignore a tumor recurrence for a very long time and miss a second chance for a cure. Ideally, the PSA should fall to a very low level and stay there. If it begins to rise from the lowest point, is higher than 1, and the rise is confirmed by two further increases, even if they're not consecutive, I'd advise you to meet with your radiation oncologist, medical oncologist, or urologist to consider the next steps.

The purpose of the three-peak rule is to make sure the PSA increase is genuine. But if your level begins to rise above the nadir, I believe it's prudent to wait three months—not six—to repeat the test with an eye to further assessment and possible treatment if you see three new peaks. Don't be falsely reassured if the peaks are not consecutive. This was an arbitrary criterion for recurrent cancer in the earliest ASTRO definition. What you should be concerned about is why the PSA level keeps getting higher, whether the peaks are consecutive or not.

After cryotherapy or HIFU, the PSA almost always remains detectable, and the treatment is considered successful if the nadir is low (less than 0.5 ng/ml). The remaining PSA indicates that either some normal tissue or some cancer was not destroyed. A rising PSA after cryotherapy or HIFU, confirmed on at least two occasions, is ominous, and means that a consultation with the treating physician, or even better, a second opinion from a urologist, is in order. Ask if you need a biopsy to determine if the cancer has regrown. Early detection of recurrent cancer is the key to successful treatment.

NOTE: Don't be put off by your doctor if he insists that a rising PSA is meaningless unless it fits the formal ASTRO or Phoenix definitions. Those were developed for statisticians to analyze how well a given treatment worked in a clinical trial or case series. Your concern is whether your cancer is growing back, and a rising PSA is an early warning sign of recurrence.

WHAT IF THE PSA LEVEL BEGINS TO RISE?

There is no need to panic. Even if cancer is the cause of the PSA elevation, you could enjoy many, many years with no symptoms of recurrence, often without any further treatment. Your doctor can help you evaluate how long a horizon remains until the next level of trouble, and what course of action makes sense. Try not to let worries about what may happen down the road stand in the way of enjoying the present.

The first order of business is to repeat the test. You'll want to make sure the elevation is not a fluke. To be significant, your PSA must be both reliably measurable and unequivocally rising.

RISING PSA AFTER SURGERY

After radical prostatectomy, the PSA should be undetectable and any measurable level probably means that the cancer has recurred. Rarely, the PSA fails to drop to undetectable levels after surgery. But even when it does, the PSA can start rising again and become detectable months or years later. But if a man is ever to develop a rising PSA, it is more likely to happen in the first few years. As time passes with an undetectable PSA, the chances of recurrence decrease. While I have seen PSAs become elevated eight to ten years after radical prostatectomy, it is extremely rare when the PSA is less than 0.05 five years after the operation. Despite this, I advise men to have a PSA test every six months for the first five years and every year thereafter for the rest of their lives as long as they are healthy and would have treatment if the cancer recurred. If the PSA level becomes detectable, it should be followed closely (every two to three months) to confirm the rise and how fast it is increasing.

Properly done, radical prostatectomy should remove the entire gland. There should be no benign prostatic tissue left in the patient. Unfortunately, that does not always happen. Residual prostatic tissue, if it is benign, may cause no health risk at all. But if it begins to grow or becomes inflamed, the PSA can become detectable and continue to rise, causing considerable consternation for the patient and his doctor, since the apparently benign tissue might harbor a focus of cancer that can be difficult to diagnose.[5]

In the vast majority of cases, if the PSA is monitored regularly, a rising level can be recognized when it is still low, 0.1 or 0.2 ng/ml. At this point, examinations and scans rarely detect any abnormal areas. The cancer is simply too small. While it is important to go through the right diagnostic evaluation (we add an endorectal MRI to the physical examination and bone scan), the next step is to see a radiation oncologist and begin salvage external beam irradiation to the prostate bed as soon as possible. Regardless of the features of your cancer, the interval after the operation before the PSA became detectable, or the rate of rise in the PSA, the single most important factor in determining the success of salvage radiation is your PSA level when you begin. The best results are in men with a PSA less than 0.5. If the PSA is over 2, the results are poor.[6]

In the past, we made a serious mistake thinking that local recurrence of cancer after radical prostatectomy was rare. In fact, in the Swedish randomized trial of prostatectomy versus watchful waiting, 1 in 5 men developed biopsy-proven local regrowth of cancer within eight to ten years.[7] Adjuvant radiation given to high-risk patients early after prostatectomy prolongs survival by an average of two years.[8] Even when given to men whose PSA is rising, radiation leads to longer life and less risk of metastases.

Doctors used to believe that men with high Gleason (8 to 10), seminal vesicle invasion, lymph node metastases, or a short PSA doubling time (less than ten months) almost certainly had metastases and would gain nothing from salvage radiation. Today, the opposite is true. If your PSA begins to rise after prostatectomy, confirm the test, consult your doctor, have a complete evaluation, and then start radiation therapy as soon as possible, certainly before the PSA reaches 0.5.[9]

NOTE: PSA is such a sensitive indicator of recurrent cancer that we typically detect the problem 12 to 18 months after surgery.

After radiation therapy, PSA levels are harder to interpret, and we typically do not appreciate that the cancer has come back for 5 to 6 years. Consequently, secondary treatment for cancer is much more likely to be effective and prevent later metastases after surgery than after radiation.

RISING PSA AFTER RADIATION, CRYOTHERAPY, OR HIFU

Because the prostate is still in place after radiation, cryotherapy, or HIFU, it can be a real challenge to prove that a rising PSA indicates a cancer recurrence. Radiation kills cancer cells gradually, so a biopsy is not considered reliable until two to three years after radiation therapy. Cancer cells found in a biopsy done earlier could be lethally irradiated, though not yet dead. Radiotherapists often recommend waiting two and a half years for the full effects of treatment to kick in, but generally an expert pathologist can tell at two years whether there is a radiation effect. If undamaged cancer cells remain at this point, they are unlikely to disappear.

If the PSA begins to rise at two to two and a half years after radiation therapy, the cancer has likely recurred. A bone scan or CT scan rarely shows any sign of metastases before the PSA reaches 20. We have found that an MRI of the prostate can be helpful in detecting local recurrence of cancer within the prostate after radiation, especially if a comparable MRI was done before therapy, and we can compare the results.[10] Cancers tend to recur in the same location in the prostate where they started. I always prescribe this sophisticated imaging study before doing a biopsy of the prostate in this situation. The results help guide where I will place the biopsy needles and how I should treat the cancer if it has recurred.

If a biopsy is negative, and we find no cancer in the prostate, we would continue to follow the PSA and plot its doubling time. A biopsy is not perfect and may miss a growing cancer, so it should be repeated once or twice if the PSA continues to rise and if you are a candidate for salvage radical prostatectomy. If repeated biopsies fail to find cancer, the next step would be hormone therapy. Most doctors recommend withholding hormonal manipulations until the PSA becomes quite high (over 20) or begins to rise very rapidly (PSA doubling time less than a year). Periodic bone scans and CT scans should be done to search for sites of metastases. Hormone therapy should begin before or at the earliest appearance of metastatic sites.

Unlike radiation, both cryotherapy and HIFU kill cancer cells immediately, if at all. Three to six months after cryotherapy or HIFU, the PSA should reach a nadir of less than 0.5 and remain there. A confirmed rising PSA later on raises a strong suspicion that the tumor was not completely destroyed and a biopsy is indicated. Unlike after radiation, there is no problem interpreting a biopsy after cryotherapy or HIFU.

With any of these treatments, cancer can recur years, even decades later. Even if the cancer does not regrow, a new cancer can develop in the prostate. Just as we recommend after surgery, men should have PSA checked every six months for five years and then once a year for the rest of their lives.

NOTE: If the PSA dips only slightly after radiation, cryotherapy, or HIFU and then begins to rise, it's wise to do an early biopsy. Some men receive grossly inadequate treatment and some men have resistant tumors. If the cancer has not spread, there remains a chance that it can be cured with salvage local treatment.

NOTE: PSA can fluctuate for no reason from month to month by as much as 30 percent for men who still have the gland in place after radiation therapy, cryotherapy, or HIFU, so you're bound to see some meaningless ups and downs. After surgery, the PSA should become undetectable and remain so.

PSA Bounce

Though the reason remains unclear, in 30 to 40 percent of brachytherapy patients and 5 to 15 percent of men who have received external beam therapy (without hormones), the PSA level falls to its nadir, goes up for a while, and then falls again without any additional treatment. This PSA "bounce" tends to occur within the first three years. The level can rise long and steadily enough to meet the old ASTRO definition of a radiation failure (three consecutive rises from the nadir) but it rarely rises more than 2 ng/ml above the nadir, which would meet the new Phoenix definition of recurrence. Any rise within the first three years after radiation should be taken seriously. If the rise is rapid and persistent, a biopsy of the prostate and an evaluation for metastases should be done. Because a biopsy is tricky to interpret within the first two to three years, I would be cautious about intervening with salvage therapy too quickly. If the cause is a bounce, the PSA should begin to decrease within six to twelve months. If not, and the biopsy at three years confirms active cancer in the prostate, you should consider salvage therapy.[11]

Rising PSA When Hormones Are Used with Radiation, Cryotherapy, or HIFU

Hormone therapy is often used before treatment to shrink the prostate and the tumor, decreasing the risk of collateral damage for men with a large prostate and improving the chances of cure for a large, aggressive cancer. Depriving the prostate and the cancer of androgens also reduces the PSA level dramatically. Once the hormones are stopped, the testosterone level rebounds and the PSA goes up—almost everyone has a PSA bounce.

PSA levels should be monitored carefully over the first three years after radiation, which kills cancer slowly. The radiation effect on PSA should kick in, counteracting the rise as the hormone effect ends, and the PSA level should begin to decline by eighteen to twenty-four months. If not, an evaluation for recurrent cancer would be wise.

There is no such delayed effect after HIFU or cryotherapy. The cancer should be destroyed immediately, and a rise in PSA after hormones are stopped should be small. A PSA that rises over 1 to 2 indicates the need for a biopsy and complete evaluation.

HOW DANGEROUS IS A RISING PSA?

If your PSA begins to rise, it is natural to worry, but the level of threat depends on your PSA level and the rate at which it is rising. In general, the PSA indicates the extent of the cancer and the rate of rise reflects how quickly the tumor is growing.

PSA DOUBLING TIME

The rate at which your PSA rises is a critical indicator. The longer it takes for the PSA to double, the longer the time before metastases might appear. One year is the typical cutoff. If the PSA doubles in less time, the cancer is more serious, with a greater chance of metastases, while a doubling time longer than a year suggests local recurrence. Doubling times less than three months are ominous indicators of early metastases and shorter survival.[12] Nevertheless, changes in PSA are only one indicator, not an absolute determinant of whether further therapy is warranted. Your doctor should consider all factors—the absolute level of PSA, its rate of rise, the results of a physical examination and scans for metastases, and the original stage and grade of your cancer—in deciding on the timing and nature of any further treatment.

Doubling time is a complex and dynamic measure. You cannot plot the slope correctly by simply looking at your first and most recent test results. To get an accurate picture of how rapidly your PSA is rising, you should accumulate all of your available scores and use a doubling calculator such as the one you can find online at www.MSKCC.org.

Remember that PSA doubling time does not necessarily remain constant. It should be recalculated from time to time to gauge the effects of treatment or any change in the rate of tumor growth.

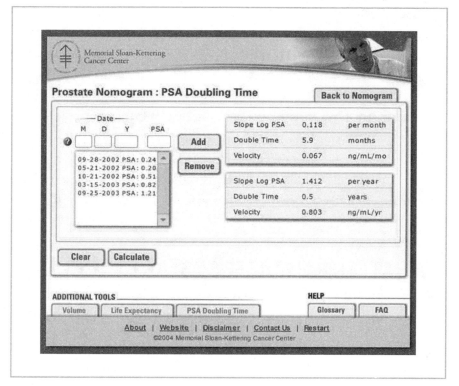

PSA doubling time calculator available online on the Memorial Sloan-Kettering Cancer Center website.

NOTE: Combining the PSA doubling time, the time from treatment to the first rise, and the information from your pathology report or the original characteristics of your tumor improves our ability to assess whether a recurrence is local or distant and to estimate your prognosis. A useful exercise for men who initially had surgery is to go to the nomograms on the MSKCC website and calculate the probability that your cancer would respond to local radiotherapy. (Visit www.MSKCC .org and search for "salvage radiotherapy nomogram.")[13]

Time to First Rise

The longer your PSA remained undetectable after surgery before it began to rise, the greater the chances that the recurrence is local rather than metastatic. If surgery (or cryotherapy or HIFU) failed to remove all the local tumor, your PSA may never become undetectable, but you still could respond to radiation therapy. The time until your PSA first begins to rise is a factor, but not a particularly powerful one, in determining your prognosis and your chances of responding to local salvage therapy.

WHAT FURTHER TESTS ARE NEEDED IF THE PSA BEGINS TO RISE?

An annual digital rectal exam (DRE) should be part of the standard monitoring after any therapy for prostate cancer. If the doctor feels a suspicious area on DRE, a biopsy of the suspect tissue is indicated. Cancer regrows in the prostate bed (the area left behind after surgery) with disturbing frequency. In several studies, cancer was detected on biopsy in a whopping 40 percent of patients who had a rising PSA after radical prostatectomy. I have sometimes been surprised and dismayed to find an obvious residual segment of the prostate or the entire seminal vesicles left behind by surgeons after a so-called "radical" prostatectomy (which should remove the entire gland and the seminal vesicles).

The location of a cancer recurrence is hard to pin down. Biopsies of the prostate area after the gland is removed only detect about half of existing cancers, so a negative result does not rule out the possibility that the tumor has recurred locally. In this situation, an endorectal MRI may be illuminating. Using MRI after surgery, Drs. Hedvig Hricak and Howard Scher at our hospital found signs of tumor recurrence in or around the urethra or bladder neck—areas difficult to appreciate with DRE alone—with surprising frequency. As an added benefit, the MRI allowed a good look at pelvic lymph nodes and pelvic bones, frequent sites of cancer spread. These endorectal MRIs even found areas of cancer in some men with very low PSA levels.[14]

It's rare for bone scans, CT scans, or MRI to find any evidence of metastases if the PSA is less than 10. In fact, such tests are unlikely to detect metastases until a man's PSA rises over 20. At lower levels, these imaging tests are unlikely to show any abnormality. To predict the likelihood of a positive bone scan, we've developed a nomogram that combines the PSA level, PSA doubling time, the time since surgery, and other relevant factors.[15] (Visit www.MSKCC.org and search for "positive bone scan nomogram.")

A number of cutting-edge investigational tools show promise in allowing us to identify areas of metastatic spread. **Monoclonal antibodies** are substances produced in the laboratory that can track down and bind with cancer cells. Essentially, these are detective molecules that locate and attach to the suspect tumor cells with the equivalent of chemical handcuffs. While the first generation of these scans (**ProstaScint**) has not produced consistently reliable results, a new form of monoclonal antibody, developed by Neil Bander of Weill Cornell Medical College, appears to be safer and better able to detect tiny amounts of prostate cancer.[16]

TREATING A RISING PSA AFTER SURGERY

ACTIVE MONITORING

If your PSA begins to rise, one possibility is to continue to monitor the situation regularly, postponing treatment until you're sure it is necessary. Every treatment carries some risk of side effects. If your PSA is low and doubling very slowly, and your cancer was favorable at the time of surgery, it may be ten or even twenty years before you face the likelihood of symptoms from local growth or metastases. Depending on your age, general health, lifestyle, and personal preferences, periodic checkups may be all you need. The key tests to monitor the cancer are

the PSA doubling time and the absolute level of PSA. The Memorial
Sloan-Kettering Cancer Center nomograms (visit www.MSKCC.org
and search for "prostate nomograms") can help you and your doctor
predict the chances of success with salvage radiation therapy if you have
a rising PSA after surgery.

Of course, the main goal is to keep the cancer under control, hopefully for the rest of your life. The best thing to do is watch closely and be
ready to institute treatment if and when it becomes necessary.

Is there anything else you can do while you're monitoring? A heart-
healthy diet and regular exercise program may be helpful and will keep

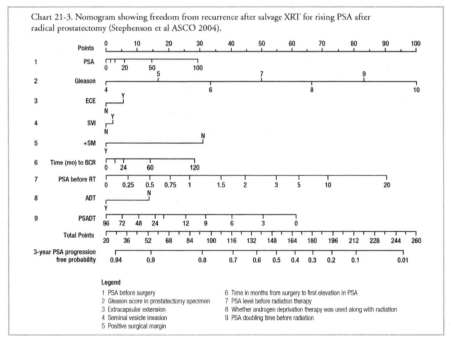

Chart 21-3. Nomogram showing freedom from recurrence after salvage XRT for rising PSA after radical prostatectomy (Stephenson et al ASCO 2004).

Nomogram to predict chances of a favorable response to radiation for men with a rising PSA after surgery. To use the nomogram, drop a line straight down from the "points" line to the value of each factor (PSA, tumor stage, etc.) to determine the points for each factor. Add the sum of points for each, then drop a line from the "Total Points" line to determine the "predictive value" or probability that the cancer is indolent.*

*Source: Modified from A. J. Stephenson, and K. M. Slawin, "The Value of Radiotherapy for the Treatment of Recurrent Prostate Cancer After Radical Prostatectomy." *Nature Clinical Practice Urology* 1, no. 2 (2004): 90–96.

you in the best shape to tolerate treatment when and if it is needed. One study found that a rigorous regimen of diet, exercise, and stress management caused a small reduction in PSA levels as compared with men with prostate cancer who made no such lifestyle changes.[17] Whether this will translate into improved survival rates remains to be seen.

SALVAGE RADIATION

If the recurrent tumor is restricted to the prostate area, radiation offers a second chance for a cure. In fact, radiation is the only available therapy that can cure a patient with a rising PSA after radical prostatectomy. Keep in mind that the window of opportunity is limited. If the PSA rises above 2, the odds for a cure decline significantly.[18] The best chance for success is to have the radiation before your PSA reaches 0.5, though the earlier the better. While any man may respond well to radiation, the chances are better if the PSA doubling time is greater than ten months, the surgical margin was positive (meaning some cancer was likely left behind), and the Gleason score was less than 8. (For nomograms showing the chances of success, visit www.MSKCC.org and search for "salvage radiation nomograms.")

Radiation after radical prostatectomy does have a downside. Lacking a clear map of where the tumor lies, the radiation therapist cannot take advantage of precise, modern, conformal techniques and must target the general area instead. Consequently, the side effects are higher for any given dose. There is a real chance that **salvage radiation** to treat a recurrence will impair erections, and 3 percent of previously dry patients treated with this approach will develop some degree of urinary incontinence. That number is even higher in men who are still having stress incontinence after radical prostatectomy. If possible, it's best to wait until urinary continence has been regained and stabilized after surgery before beginning salvage radiation. This is feasible as long as the PSA remains low.

Because more of the bladder and more of the rectum are included in the targeted field, the incidence of **radiation proctitis** (bowel irritation) and **cystitis** (bladder irritation) is as great as if you were getting full-fledged radiotherapy to treat a primary cancer.[19] This is true even though the dose is lower for salvage radiation (typically 70 Gy). If you have a low, slowly rising PSA and no nodule that the doctor can feel on DRE, along with a negative ultrasound or MRI, at MSKCC we recommend that the salvage dose should be about 70 Gy. If a definite area of cancer can be located by biopsy or MRI, we recommend adding hormone therapy in the form of LHRH or antiandrogens to the treatment program, and targeting a high dose of radiation to the nodule. The increased possibility of long-term cure justifies the added risk of erectile dysfunction and other side effects from hormone therapy. One uncertainty is whether the radiation should be extended to cover the pelvic lymph nodes. We generally do not, because of the increased risks, unless the cancer was poorly differentiated (Gleason 9 to 10), there was extensive seminal vesicle invasion, or the lymph node dissection at the time of prostatectomy showed metastases.

TREATING A RISING PSA AFTER RADIATION

WATCHFUL WAITING

Doing nothing beyond continuing to monitor the PSA is a reasonable approach, especially for older men, those with significant health problems aside from prostate cancer, and patients unwilling to risk the side effects of available treatment options. This approach is especially attractive if a biopsy of the prostate turns up no local cancer, the PSA is low, and the PSA doubling time is longer than a year.

SALVAGE RADICAL PROSTATECTOMY OR ABLATIVE THERAPY (HIFU, CRYOTHERAPY)

Removing the prostate after primary radiation treatment may cure the cancer if it is still locally contained. In our experience at MSKCC, 50 percent of patients remained cancer-free ten years after salvage surgery, and 35 percent still show no sign of recurrence at fifteen years.[20] Because this is a risky, technically-challenging procedure, it should be attempted *only* by highly skilled, experienced surgeons. Fortunately, today, in the hands of expert surgeons, the operation and the time it takes to recover are no different from a standard radical prostatectomy.

Before considering salvage surgery, it's important to be certain that your PSA rise really signifies a cancer recurrence and not an innocent artifact or a PSA bounce. Careful interpretation of the biopsy is critical as well. Radiation can cause cells to look abnormal, and an inexperienced pathologist might have trouble distinguishing these innocent changes from cancer.

If the cancer has spread beyond the local area, removing the prostate will not cure it. In evaluating whether a patient is a good candidate for salvage surgery, I take a look at the original Gleason grade, stage, and PSA to judge whether the cancer was initially curable. If the original PSA was over 20 and the Gleason sum was over 7, and the cancer was extensive (clinical T3 or T4), the chance of curing the original tumor with surgery was low then and it is not likely to be curable now. If after radiation therapy the PSA is now above 4, there is detectable invasion into the seminal vesicles or spread to the lymph nodes, or the biopsy shows extensive, high-grade cancer in most of the cores (Gleason 8 through 10), the cancer is probably not curable and an operation to remove the gland might not be appropriate.

If the cancer is more favorable and potentially curable with salvage surgery, the next question is whether you are otherwise healthy and have a long enough life expectancy to justify the operation. Salvage radical prostatectomy may make sense if you have a life expectancy greater than ten years. For older men or those in poor health, hormone therapy will likely keep the cancer in check for many years.

Even in the best of hands, the incidence of side effects—especially incontinence and erectile dysfunction—is considerably higher with a salvage operation than it is for radical prostatectomy on a gland that has not been irradiated. Still, given the best modern techniques, this procedure has become increasingly successful and less hazardous. Rectal injuries are rare (no more than 1 to 2 percent), and dramatic bowel damage no longer occurs. In the last twenty years, I have not seen a patient who required a colostomy after this operation. Recovery of urinary continence tends to be slow, and only half of men regain normal function. In 20 percent, incontinence is severe enough to require an artificial sphincter, which is usually effective in restoring urinary control. The risk of a urinary stricture at the anastomosis between the bladder and urethra is 25 percent, and men who develop a stricture are more likely to have trouble regaining continence. After salvage radical prostatectomy, most men (84 percent) do not recover spontaneous sexual function, even with oral medications like sildenafil. Most patients who are candidates for salvage prostatectomy already have severe ED from the radiation. In addition, in order to cure the cancer, we generally have to remove the erectile nerves. Nerve-sparing is possible in some patients who still have normal erectile function, but only if the cancer recurrence is found early. Because of radiation damage, the results of nerve grafts with salvage prostatectomy have not been as promising as they have been in men who have not had radiation treatment, and we no longer recommend them.[21]

Radical prostatectomy can be performed after attempted ablation with HIFU or cryotherapy. While technically challenging, the complications are generally fewer than after radiation. The urinary sphincter is usually intact, so incontinence is much less of a problem. Recovery of erections is possible but not as common as after standard radical prostatectomy. Rectal injuries should be rare in the hands of an experienced surgeon.

CRYOTHERAPY

For cancer that recurs in the prostate area after radiation, freezing the gland is a reasonable option. Cryotherapy is less invasive than salvage radical prostatectomy and carries a lower risk of incontinence. Ten to 15 percent of cryotherapy patients develop serious urinary control problems, as opposed to half of men after salvage surgery. Impotence, however, is common, and nearly all men lose erections after cryotherapy. Also, though the incontinence rate is lower, the procedure does cause other bothersome urinary complications. Freezing kills the gland, and the dead tissue sloughs off into the urethra, where it can cause a blockage. This may require the use of a suprapubic catheter (a tube placed through the lower abdomen into the bladder) or a Foley catheter (a tube through the penis into the bladder) for up to six weeks.

With cryotherapy, you can be out of the hospital the same day, and catastrophic complications are rare in experienced hands. Unfortunately, the cure rate is not impressive. Most men convert to a negative biopsy in the short term after the gland is frozen, but many will later develop a rising PSA, indicating a recurrence of the tumor, which too often grows back within the prostate. Almost all patients resort to hormone therapy within a few years.

Other recently developed local therapies include **high-intensity focused ultrasound (HIFU)** and **photodynamic therapy (PDT)**. HIFU effectively cooks tumor cells with heat generated by sound waves. PDT directly destroys blood vessels and tumor cells using light. Though it's too early to determine long-term results, both approaches seem to inhibit the local growth of cancer with reasonable safety that is comparable to cryotherapy. Serious complications, including rectal injuries, can occur, however, and complete destruction of all tumor within the prostate remains uncertain. There have been too few clinical trials of either of these to judge how effective they really are.

THE FUTURE

Many men wonder if we're likely to develop a better test than PSA for monitoring cancer recurrence after treatment. But PSA is so closely coupled with the essential biology of prostate cancer, it would be hard to beat as a diagnostic tool. While the value of changes in PSA, such as doubling time and velocity, are questionable before initial treatment, they are powerful predictive tools that accurately reflect the growth of cancer after surgery, radiation, cryotherapy, or HIFU.

What About Investigational Treatments?

Many approaches are being investigated for treating locally recurrent prostate cancer. Scientists are studying radiation therapy using a single high dose to see if it is better able to destroy cancer with fewer side effects. Also under development are drugs that either sensitize cells to radiation treatment or protect normal tissue from radiation damage.

If your cancer has recurred within the prostate after radiotherapy, cryotherapy, or HIFU, a wide variety of innovative approaches are being tried. Since we have no standard treatment for recurrence in these settings, the time is ripe for clinical trials of new ideas. Researchers are developing nanoparticles capable of carrying drugs or biologic agents that destroy prostate cancer directly to the gland. Nanoparticles that target prostate cancer cells have been dramatically effective in laboratory mice. Clinical trials will be required to determine if they're safe and effective in men. Also under investigation is gene therapy and the use of oncolytic viruses (viruses capable of infiltrating and killing cancer cells). Immunotherapy, which enhances the body's own immune response or unblocks the clever barriers that prostate cancer develops to shield itself against the immune system, is also very promising.

Many patients are reluctant to participate in clinical trials. When considering such studies, keep in mind that care received by people involved in trials of new treatment methods is often better than standard care. Entering such a trial may give you access to treatments that would otherwise be unavailable. (See page 239 for more on clinical trials.)

IN SUMMARY

PSA is a remarkably effective indicator of how prostate cancer develops, grows and responds to treatment. After surgery to remove the gland, the PSA should become and remain undetectable. A rising PSA is an early warning that the cancer has recurred, opening the door for further curative treatment. After radiation, cryotherapy, or HIFU, PSA levels are more difficult to interpret and recurrences take longer to detect, so cure rates for secondary, salvage therapy are lower than for radiation given after radical prostatectomy.

Changes in PSA levels after initial treatment signal how the disease is progressing, and the rate of change (velocity or doubling time) is a powerful indicator of prognosis. In most cases, a rising PSA results from local recurrence of the cancer. If discovered early and treated effectively, the cancer can still be cured.

At present, radiation is the best salvage treatment we have for a prostate tumor that recurs after surgery. Not only can radiation stop a rising PSA, it can prevent metastatic spread and prolong life. Salvage surgery can also be curative after radiation failure, but the side effects are higher than when surgery is used initially. Regardless of how your cancer was treated, follow PSA results regularly for the rest of your life. PSA is the best way to detect recurrence early and have a second chance of cure.

21

Treating Advanced
Prostate Cancer

READ THIS CHAPTER TO LEARN:

- What is advanced prostate cancer?
- Why is PSA still important?
- What are the different kinds of hormone therapy and when should treatment start?
- What can be done about prostate cancer that has metastasized?
- How can you judge clinical trials and experimental treatments?
- Is there a role for alternative and complementary therapies?
- What about pain management and end-of-life care?

Every year in this country, 25,000 to 30,000 men die of prostate cancer. Double that number die of this disease in the EU. In all developed nations, prostate cancer accounts for about 3 to 5 percent of male deaths (roughly 1 of every 30), and it is taking an increasing toll in the developing world as life expectancy increases. While many more men with early-stage prostate cancer are worried about how best to treat their cancer while minimizing the effect on quality of life, men with advanced prostate cancer are understandably more preoccupied with their survival.

Advanced prostate cancer includes patients with metastasis, those with a rising PSA when no further curative local therapy is feasible, and those with locally extensive cancers that cannot be controlled with local treatment directed to the tumor in the prostate. When metastases appear, they are most commonly found in bones, but prostate cancer can also metastasize to lymph nodes in the pelvis and abdomen as well as to other organs, including the liver, lungs, brain, and skin—almost anywhere.

The prostate depends on male hormones (androgens), produced by the testicles, to develop and grow. Prostate cells contain an androgen receptor (AR) that receives the hormone's signal and then instructs the cells to grow, divide, and behave like prostate cells. One of the prostate's key functions, controlled by the androgen receptor, is to produce PSA. Shut down male hormones and the androgen receptor stops working and PSA production grinds to a halt. This usually means that the cell has been lethally injured.

NOTE: Rarely, in the final stages of terminal prostate cancer, prostate cancer cells become so wild and so poorly differentiated that they stop producing PSA. This happens more often when the cells have been forced to grow in the absence of androgens for a long time. And in many prostate cancers, rare cells are found that produce little or no PSA.

In the vast majority of cases, PSA levels closely reflect the action of androgens, powerful growth stimulators of the cancer. PSA has long proven to be a remarkably effective way to detect prostate cancer, estimate its extent, and monitor its course over time. Using this simple blood test, we can assess the effectiveness of treatment, whether surgery, radiation, or other forms. After treatment, a rising PSA alerts us six to ten years before metastases would appear without further intervention. This gives us ample time to try a second, and hopefully curative, local treatment. If that fails to arrest the disease, we can move to systemic treatment while a patient is still years away from having problems or symptoms from local regrowth or metastatic cancer. The most powerful systemic treatment for prostate cancer is a hormonal manipulation called androgen deprivation therapy (ADT), designed to drastically lower the level of male hormones in the blood through medical or surgical castration.

In recent years, our understanding of advanced prostate cancer and its response to ADT has increased exponentially. When cancer begins to grow back in a man who has been on hormone therapy, we used to believe the cancer had become "hormone-refractory," or independent of male hormones. In recent years, we have learned that other mechanisms are involved. These cancers learn to survive despite minimal androgens by enhancing the activity of their androgen receptor, enabling it to continue to stimulate cell growth and produce PSA. In fact, the almost ubiquitous production of PSA by "hormone-refractory" cancers is the best evidence that the androgen receptor is flourishing in these cancers.

When prostate cancer is metastatic, the treatment focus shifts from cure to control. Our goal is to delay progression of the disease for as long as possible, prolong survival, and maintain the best possible quality of life. Medicine in this setting is closer to an art than a science, as we work to optimize the benefits of available treatments and minimize their risks. New drugs become available every year. Traditional hormone therapy works dramatically well for a time, and new, better means are being developed to block the production of male hormones and inhibit or destroy the androgen receptor. Many new targeted, molecular, and immunological therapies are being studied, and there is now clear proof that chemotherapy prolongs life.

NOTE: "Castration" refers to removal of the source of androgens, the male hormones. This can be accomplished medically, by injections of LHRH agonists like leuprolide or goserelin, or surgically, by removal of the testicles (orchiectomy). Castration does not mean removal of all male organs. The penis and scrotum are not removed in a surgical castration.

Medical (LHRH agonists) or surgical (removal of the testicles) castration drives blood levels of testosterone below 50 ng/dl. The effects of medical castration on prostate cancer can also be accomplished by giving antiandrogens such as bicalutamide (Casodex) that block the action of the androgen receptor in the cancer while allowing blood levels of androgens to remain normal.

In the past, further attempts to lower testosterone and control regrowth of prostate cancer after castration were aimed at the adrenal gland, which produces small amounts of androgens. Surgical removal of the pituitary or adrenal glands did produce favorable responses in some patients, which lasted an average of four to six months. While these drastic maneuvers sometimes relieved symptoms, patients lived no longer, and such approaches have been abandoned in favor of drugs that turn off androgen production or block the androgen receptor. Exciting new drugs are in development that completely stop the synthesis of androgens everywhere in the body, such as abiraterone, and more powerful antiandrogens to block activity of the androgen receptor, such as MDV3100 (see page 483).

NOTE: Advanced prostate cancer is a highly complex disease and requires the deft hand of a dedicated and experienced physician to guide a patient through the maze. While the disease is rarely curable at this stage, it can be kept under control for a prolonged period. To minimize the risk of crippling symptoms and to maximize time spent in a healthy, active life, I strongly advise men to find a doctor they trust who has the experience and wisdom to make this journey as smooth as possible. Whether the physician is the urologist who diagnosed the cancer originally, a knowledgeable internist, or a medical oncologist, be sure he or she has the patience to work with you, interest in the disease, and knowledge about the ever-changing treatments available. It is a particular advantage if your doctor actively participates in clinical trials, offering you a chance to receive the latest drugs and treatments as they are developed.

The modest response of "castration-resistant" prostate cancer to secondary hormonal manipulations led most experts to conclude that further attempts to arrest the growth of these cancers by lowering testosterone or blocking androgen action in the cancer cell would prove futile.

We now know—and the continued relevance of PSA should have told us—that the androgen axis is functioning quite well in these tumors. These cancers develop several crafty ways to cope with diminished androgens. The most common trick, discovered by Charles Sawyers, a cancer sleuth now at MSKCC, is to increase the amount of AR in each cell. Just by increasing the AR level threefold, the cells become hypersensitive to androgens and can thrive on the minute amount of androgens produced in the adrenals.[1] The cells develop the spongelike capacity to soak up androgens from the blood much more effectively than they do in a normal, androgen-rich environment,[2] and some prostate cancers even learn to synthesize androgens themselves.[3]

Cancer cells desperate for androgens can perform a few more spectacular feats. The androgen receptor can become promiscuous, with the ability to function in the absence of male hormones by responding to other hormones.[4] The clever androgen receptor is even capable of altering itself so that antiandrogen drugs like bicalutamide actually stimulate rather than block hormone development.[5] These new realizations about androgens and the androgen receptor have led to new drugs like abiraterone, which shuts down the enzymatic pathways and slows the synthesis of hormones. The search is on for new drugs that can inhibit male hormones more reliably and powerfully and for drugs that act directly against the androgen receptor.

TREATMENT OPTIONS

The choice and timing of treatment for men with advanced prostate cancer depends on the extent of the cancer, its rate of growth, and a patient's age, general health, and risk tolerance. Possibilities include watchful waiting, hormone therapy, radiation, chemotherapy, immunotherapy, and clinical trials of investigational agents.

WATCHFUL WAITING

This is a reasonable option, since there is no proven way to cure prostate cancer in this situation, and though a few trials have suggested that early hormone treatment may prolong survival, most studies show it does not. The goal is to keep prostate cancer from being the cause of your death and to keep you feeling well and symptom-free for as long as possible. If the only indication of recurrent cancer is a rising PSA, and there is no sign of metastatic spread, many physicians recommend careful monitoring with regular checks of the PSA level, postponing hormone treatment and its side effects for as long as possible. Annual bone scans and CT scans or MRIs of the abdomen and pelvis are reasonable studies that may alert us to the presence of metastatic deposits. The PSA level and its rate of rise (PSA velocity, PSA doubling time) are the best indicators of when to intervene.[6] Treatment can reasonably be postponed as long as you have no symptoms, imaging scans show no cancer, your PSA is less than 20, and the doubling time is greater than one year. (To calculate your PSA doubling time and estimate how many years before your bone scan is likely to show metastases, search www.MSKCC.org for "nomograms.") Many men with a slowly rising PSA will live out their lives with no signs or symptoms of prostate cancer and never require any treatment.

HORMONE THERAPY

In 1941, Charles Huggins made the groundbreaking discovery that prostate cancer required male hormones to grow and spread. By removing the testicles or administering the female hormone estrogen to block the production of testosterone, Huggins achieved dramatic regression of advanced prostate cancers. In a matter of days, men who had been bedridden with debilitating pain from bone metastases were able to resume their active lives. Since then, hormone therapy, depriving the cancer of a source of the male hormones that normally circulate in the bloodstream, has been the standard of care for men with symptoms of advanced prostate cancer.

Unfortunately, hormone therapy is palliative, not curative, and eventually, if you live long enough, the cancer learns to survive despite androgen withdrawal.

What Are the Different Types of Hormone Therapy?

Historically, the preferred means to withdraw male hormones was surgical castration. The testicles, which produce testosterone, were removed in an operation known as **orchiectomy**. By the mid-1980s, medications called LHRH agonists were developed that could block hormone production without surgical excision of the testicles. Today, few men opt for orchiectomy, which is irreversible and can exact a psychological toll. Proponents of surgical castration emphasize that the procedure is simple, less expensive than prolonged medication, and may avoid some side effects of drugs (though the side effects of androgen withdrawal are identical whether castration is accomplished medically or surgically). Those patients who choose to have their testicles removed can have the doctor implant silicone prostheses shaped like testicles at the time of surgery. Limited operations, such as subtotal orchiectomy, in which the pulp but not the capsule of the testicles is removed, have been discredited because they leave too much androgen-producing tissue behind.

In sufficient doses, LHRH agonists such as leuprolide (Lupron or Eligard), goserelin (Zoladex), triptorelin (Decapeptyl), or histrelin (Vantas) given as a long-acting injection every one to twelve months, shut down the pituitary signals that stimulate the testosterone-generating Leydig cells in the testes, bringing androgen output from these glands to a halt. At first, these drugs ironically boost testosterone production, but within two weeks the level typically falls below 30 ng/dl, compared with normal testosterone levels of about 300 to 800 ng/dl. For reasons that are poorly understood, serum testosterone falls but not to the desirable level below 30, in about 5 to 10 percent of patients.

Single Versus Combination Therapy

Another class of drugs was later developed to block the effects of any remaining androgens on the cancer cells. These so-called antiandrogens, such as flutamide (Eulexin), bicalutamide (Casodex), and nilutamide

(Nilandron), can be taken in conjunction with LHRH agonists to achieve what is known as a **complete** or **total androgen blockade**. Flutamide, which requires a dosing schedule of two pills, three times per day, causes troublesome diarrhea and is more cumbersome than the one-a-day bicalutamide or nilutamide. Antiandrogens have not been shown to offer any significant advantage when used in a man who has had an orchiectomy. Their main benefit seems to be averting the effects of the flare, or sudden rise in testosterone during the first two weeks after an LHRH agonist injection. After that, their effect is marginal. Years of study have shown that life expectancy is slightly prolonged when a complete androgen blockade, continued for years, is compared with LHRH agonists alone. Still, given their cost and side effects, the benefit of long-term use of antiandrogens in addition to LHRH agonists is debatable, and today, they are generally given only for seven to ten days before and for the first few weeks of LHRH therapy.

NOTE: Estrogens (female hormones). For a time, the female hormone estrogen, in the form of DES, was used in hormone therapy for prostate cancer. DES is an inexpensive pill that reduces testosterone and controls cancer as well as orchiectomy. But at maximally effective doses, DES proved dangerous, causing heart attacks, emboli, and strokes, and it is rarely recommended today. Whether a low dose, 1 to 3 milligrams per day, would be equally effective without these side effects has never been adequately tested. DES is not readily available in the U.S. Other estrogens that have been used for prostate cancer include estradiol and Premarin, both available in pill form.

SHOULD YOU TAKE HORMONE THERAPY?

To decide if hormone treatment is indicated, doctors generally consider a patient's age and health in light of the seriousness of his disease. For example, Tom J. is 72 years old with heart disease and diabetes. His cancer at the time of diagnosis was a low-risk Gleason 6, clinical stage T1c, and his PSA was 4.5 ng/ml. Three years after a radical prostatectomy, his PSA began to rise and is now 0.3 ng/ml, with a doubling time more than two years. In his case, hormone treatment may never prove necessary, and monitoring the disease is the most sensible approach. On the other hand, Ben B. is a vigorous 61-year-old with no serious health problems apart from prostate cancer. His PSA started to rise only a few months after radical prostatectomy, which was not surprising, given that his original tumor was a Gleason 8 with seminal vesicle invasion. Despite salvage radiation therapy, the PSA continued to rise rapidly, is now 12.6, with a doubling time less than six months, and a bone scan showed a metastatic lesion in his left hip. In Ben's case, it's time to begin hormone therapy.

WHAT ARE THE SIDE EFFECTS OF HORMONE THERAPY?

Ten years is a long time to deal with the side effects of androgen deprivation, which can include loss of libido and erectile function, hot flashes, decreased muscle mass, obesity, a tendency to diabetes, increased lipid levels, thinning of bones, breast enlargement and tenderness, anemia, and possibly, diminished mental acuity. The most serious consequences, however, are a substantial increased risk of a bone fracture[7] and of a major cardiovascular event such as a heart attack.[8]

STRATEGIES TO REDUCE THE SIDE EFFECTS OF HORMONE THERAPY

With the increasing recognition of the serious side effects of ADT, there have been many efforts to find ways to reduce these problems while retaining the benefits of hormone ablation. These include giving hormones late rather than early, the use of intermittent hormone therapy, and giving antiandrogens alone, which leaves circulating androgens intact.

Giving Hormones Late Rather Than Early

Experts have long disagreed about the value of early versus late hormone therapy. We even lack consensus about what constitutes "early" or "late," though generally, early treatment means starting hormones as soon as the PSA begins to rise after local therapy and no further curative local therapy is feasible, and late means beginning the therapy when metastases are present. There is general agreement that, in the absence of metastases, it's *not* necessary to begin hormone treatment at the very first sign of a rising PSA. If hormones are started early in the course of a rising PSA, the average time until metastases develop is eight to ten years.[9] The side effects of hormone therapy are troublesome in the short run, but in the long term they can have serious adverse health effects. Most experts also concur that waiting until a man has definite signs or symptoms of metastases is unwise.

Unfortunately, we have no crystal ball that can predict with certainty when metastases will appear. The best clue is the PSA level and the rate at which it changes over time.[10] A short PSA doubling time, less than six months, strongly predicts a shorter time until distant spread appears. There is no known medical benefit to starting hormonal therapy before the PSA level rises to twenty and doubling time is shorter than six months, although these criteria have never been tested in a clinical trial.

Most of the time, the decision to start hormone therapy earlier is driven more by the anxiety of the patient and/or his doctor than by any real danger from the cancer. Some doctors use a predictive model, i.e. nomogram, to estimate the likelihood that metastases will appear on a bone scan in the future.[11] The nomogram combines information from the PSA level and its changes over time along with the features of the original cancer (stage and grade) to estimate the probability that bone metastases will appear within eight years. By repeating the calculation at each visit, the doctor can estimate whether the risk is increasing. This is one of the most important decisions that a man with a rising PSA can make, and the choice should be made with the best available information. Hormone therapy will lower your PSA, but that doesn't necessarily mean that your health has improved. Be sure to communicate carefully with your physician to ensure that you understand and agree with his policy about hormone treatment and that your personal needs and preferences are taken into account.

Intermittent Hormone Therapy

Intermittent therapy was developed with the idea that it might be a more effective way to control cancer. The thought was that prostate cancer cells continuously deprived of androgens would learn how to become androgen-refractory sooner and that withdrawing hormones intermittently might prolong their effectiveness. To date, no randomized trial has confirmed prolonged survival with intermittent therapy, but the studies that have been done seem to demonstrate that survival is no shorter.[12] The other hope for this approach has been substantiated by the trials. When hormone therapy is given intermittently, men spend 30 to 50 percent of their remaining life off hormonal therapy, and the side effects are definitely less troublesome. As a consequence, some experts prefer intermittent hormone therapy. Patients are given hormone-suppressing drugs until the PSA drops to a specified level, e.g., less than 4 ng/ml, at which point they are taken off the medication. Testosterone production resumes, and side effects associated with its absence (including sexual dysfunction) can resolve. When the PSA rises to the previous baseline, hormone treatment begins again. Compared with continuous therapy, intermittent therapy does improve quality of life.

Once a man has definite signs of metastases, most experts agree, androgen deprivation should be continuous. The overall survival is three to five years, so the risk of intermittent therapy appears to be greater than the benefits. Intermittent therapy is most suitable for men who choose to start androgen deprivation early, with a rising PSA but no signs of metastases. Should these men start hormones or wait longer? PSA is such a powerful, effective warning system that overall quality of life might be better, and the months of life spent without the side effects of hormones longer, if we simply postpone ADT until the PSA is rapidly rising and reaches 20 or so or there are other signs of impending trouble.

NOTE: All hormone treatments for prostate cancer result in infertility. Without adequate testosterone, sperm production stops. (This does not mean that you should cease using birth control as soon as you begin hormone therapy. Before doing so, you should be evaluated to ensure that you're no longer fertile.)

NOTE: Men vary widely in tolerance of hormone therapy. Side effects range in severity and, though common, are not universal or inevitable.

Antiandrogens Alone

Antiandrogens have been used alone for the treatment of prostate cancer because they block the action of the androgen receptor and the effects of androgens on prostate cancer cells without lowering male hormones circulating in the bloodstream. Using this approach, many more men retain their libido and erectile function, and some of the long-term effects of ADT are less severe. Two regimens have been compared. One is Casodex (bicalutamide) at a dose of 150 mg (the usual dose is 50 mg per day) versus combination therapy with an LHRH agonist. For men with locally advanced prostate cancer, survival appears to be similar. For men with metastatic cancer, survival was longer for those given LHRH than it was for men who took antiandrogens alone.[13] In large studies, bicalutamide has been tested against placebo to see if it might reduce cancer recurrence and improve survival after radiation or surgery. So far, those studies have shown a longer time until recurrence with ADT after local treatment, but no difference in survival.[14]

CAUTION: In men with low-risk cancers, those given bicalutamide rather than a placebo had a *shorter* survival. High-dose bicalutamide is contraindicated for men with low-risk prostate cancer.

In the United States, high-dose bicalutamide alone is not FDA-approved for the treatment of prostate cancer. There have been some clinical trials combining the standard 50 mg dose with a 5 alpha-reductase inhibitor (finasteride or dutasteride) to take advantage of the antiandrogen's ability to block the androgen receptor and the ability of 5 alpha-reductase inhibitors to reduce the conversion of testosterone to the far more powerful male hormone DHT in the hope that the combined effect would be greater, while still preserving sexual function. This approach is effective, but it has never been tested in a properly controlled trial to compare it with LHRH agonist alone. This combination is reasonable for men with a rising PSA, but it probably should not be used for those with metastatic disease.[15]

My advice is to delay ADT as long as possible and work closely with an experienced physician to monitor your PSA, bone scans, and other appropriate imaging studies. Once you start hormones, it is reasonable to take them intermittently if you have never had metastases, but it's best to stick with androgen deprivation continuously if you have metastatic spread of your disease.

Preventing and Treating Side Effects of Hormone Therapy

Bone loss and fractures: With androgen deprivation, men's bones respond as women's do after menopause. Gradually, the bones lose minerals, become thin, and osteoporosis results. A consequential increased risk of fracture begins within the first year of ADT and continues to increase as long as androgen deprivation continues. By five years after androgen deprivation begins, the chance of a fracture, which can have devastating consequences in older people, increases five-fold.[16] The rapid decrease in bone mineral density can be measured with a simple test called bone densitometry. Bone loss can be prevented and even reversed with the use of drugs called bisphosphonates, which are most effective when taken intravenously. Bisphosphonates bind to calcium carbonate in the bones and prevent the breakdown of bones by osteoclasts (cells that continuously remodel bone). Bisphosphonates, and more recently a new antibody, denosumab, as well as the selective estrogen-receptor modulators (SERM) raloxifen and toremifen, have been shown to preserve bone strength in men on ADT.[17] Thus far, only denosumab has been proven to reduce the risk of fractures.

Bisphosphonates, however, are not risk-free. One rare but extremely troublesome side effect is osteonecrosis of the jaw, when the lower jaw-bone around the teeth dies and the teeth fall out. This condition makes it impossible to implant new teeth and opens a site for infection. The binding of bisphosphanates to bone is almost permanent, so it's nearly impossible to reverse side effects. Because of the inconvenience and expense of intravenous administration and the small risk of serious side effects, some doctors recommend using vitamin D and calcium supplements instead. While these have long been used in an attempt to reduce side effects of osteoporosis in women, their benefits are unproven. If you are found to have an increased risk of fracture before ADT, you should consider taking bisphosphonates. Once you're on androgen deprivation therapy, you should have your bone density measured periodically and consider these drugs if the density declines.

Regular activity and exercise are important in maintaining bone strength, particularly for men on ADT. An exercise regime that promotes balance, coordination, and strength can reduce the risk of a fall that could lead to a fracture. In older people, fractures can result in serious health consequences, or even death.

In addition to reducing fractures, bisphosphonates have also been studied in breast and other cancers, to reduce the risk of metastases to bones. Bisphosphonates make bones harder and less vulnerable to infiltration by tumor cells. This approach has been shown to work in breast cancer, but as of now, the data in prostate cancer is less conclusive.[18] If you are at high risk of developing metastases, you may want to discuss the use of bisphosphonates with your doctor.

Cardiovascular: It has long been known that administering high-dose estrogens to men with prostate cancer, though effective as a hormone treatment, substantially increases cardiovascular risks. Estrogen can cause blood clotting, increase lipid (fat) levels, and lead to a higher death rate from cardiovascular incidents. Previously, we had thought that withdrawal of androgens by orchiectomy or LHRH agonists was safe, but recent analyses of men treated with long-term androgen deprivation have uncovered an increased risk of cardiovascular events, stroke, and death from cardiovascular disease, estimated at 1 percent for every year a man is on ADT.[19] Whether these risks can be mitigated by traditional methods, such as statins, exercise, diet, and control of blood pressure, is uncertain. Patients who require ADT would do well to consult their physicians, especially if they have cardiovascular disease risk factors, and should monitor their blood pressure and cholesterol levels and intervene aggressively to lower their risk factors.

Other Adverse Effects: Early on, most men on ADT notice hot flashes: a sudden increase in temperature, sweating, and facial flushing. In 20 percent of men, these symptoms are extremely troublesome, but the problem usually diminishes over time without treatment. For those with persistent, severe, bothersome hot flashes, several drugs provide symptomatic relief. These include progesterone (e.g., Megace), low-dose estrogens (e.g., estradiol), and calcium channel blockers (e.g., verapamil). Each of these drugs has potential side effects, and you should discuss them with your primary care physician as well as your oncologist.

While some men on androgen deprivation therapy complain about depression, reduced energy, and/or diminished cognitive function, studies of these problems have been limited by a lack of matched controls, and there is too little evidence about their frequency and severity. If you, your family, or your physician notices excess moodiness, feelings of depression, or other emotional changes, it would be wise to consult with a mental health practitioner, especially one who deals often with cancer patients. Mood disorders are highly treatable today. Left untreated, they can lead to serious consequences, including suicide.

WHEN HORMONE THERAPY
STOPS WORKING

Depriving a prostate tumor of androgens works only for a time. Eventually, cancer cells learn how to thrive in an environment where the male hormone level in the bloodstream has been drastically reduced and become relatively "hormone refractory." Though the mechanism is not clear, one theory holds that a small fraction of the cells in every cancer (possibly prostate cancer stem cells) are programmed paradoxically to flourish in the absence of male hormones. Another suggests that withdrawing androgens induces some cancer cells to learn to live without these hormones, finding alternative ways to survive and grow. Recent research has improved our understanding of the variety of mechanisms prostate cancer uses to thrive despite ADT. This hinges on the way male hormones work inside the prostate cancer cell. Testosterone, the most important male hormone in the bloodstream, is actively taken up by prostate cancer cells and converted to the far more potent dihydrotestosterone (DHT) by the enzyme 5 alpha-reductase. DHT, T, and other androgens bind directly to the androgen receptor molecule (AR) within the cell. When AR is bound, it migrates into the cell nucleus and turns on the genetic code to produce other "androgen response" genes, which help the cells to survive, grow, and reproduce. PSA is one of the most prominent genes under the control of AR, which explains why PSA levels are still present when a prostate cancer recurs after hormone therapy. For many years, it was thought that such prostate cancers were completely resistant to further hormonal manipulation. In fact an elevated PSA is clear evidence that AR remains viable and active.

One startling revelation was the finding that, with ADT, androgen levels within normal and malignant prostate tissues fall much less than than blood levels. Prostate cells are remarkably equipped to soak up androgens. While blood levels of testosterone fall 90 percent or more with medical or surgical castration, levels in the prostate fall only 50 percent and often remain high enough to stimulate the AR.[20] In addition, the AR employs a variety of adaptive measures to function despite a low testosterone environment. It is able to multiply, allowing it to respond to tiny amounts of androgens produced by the adrenal gland or, amazingly, by the cancer itself. The AR can become "promiscuous," capable of responding to other than male hormones and, paradoxically, to drugs that normally inhibit AR, like bicalutamide or steroids, which closely resemble androgens. Another possibility is an outlaw AR that can act on its own.[21]

As a result, today the treatment of prostate cancer that recurs after initial ADT is directed principally to the androgen axis. New drugs are available to block the production of male hormones from any source. More powerful antiandrogens are now available to block AR, and drugs that destroy the androgen receptor are being tested in clinical trials. And blockage or destruction of the AR is being combined with other drugs that target activated growth pathways in prostate cancer.

SECOND-LINE HORMONE THERAPY

When a prostate cancer shows clear signs of progression despite ADT— usually with a rising PSA but sometimes with the appearance of metastases—further hormonal manipulations often work. The side effects are low and the success rate is reasonable. For example, if a man has been taking an antiandrogen alone (or with finasteride or dutasteride), we would add an LHRH agonist. If he is on an LHRH agonist, we would add an antiandrogen such as bicalutamide. If the patient is already on both drugs, we would stop the antiandrogen, hoping to induce the favorable "androgen withdrawal syndrome." Withdrawing antiandrogens generally takes take a few weeks to work, and in the case of bicalutamide, the effects can take as long as two months. Either approach will reduce PSA levels in about 40 percent of men for an average of three to six months with little additional risk of side effects.[22]

If adding or stopping an antiandrogen fails to work, other equally effective hormonal manipulations are the usual next step. These include switching from an antiandrogen like bicalutamide to adrenal-blocking drugs such as ketoconazole (Nizoral) or aminoglutethimide. Sometimes, corticosteroids (hydrocortisone, prednisone, or dexamethazone) are effective, and they are often given in conjunction with adrenal-blocking drugs to prevent adrenal insufficiency. Years ago, we often used high-dose estrogens (estradiol, estramustine phosphate) as second- or third-line agents, though they increase the risk of blood clots and adverse cardiovascular events.

New Antiandrogens

An emerging new class of antiandrogens is based on the three-dimensional structure of the androgen receptor molecule. The drugs are designed to block the site at which male hormones bind with the AR. They may prove to be more powerful than conventional antiandrogen drugs, with fewer side effects.

The first in this new class of hormonal agents is being developed by Medivation, a biotechnology company. Currently known as MDV3100, this extremely promising drug has proven to be many times more powerful than bicalutamide when tested in laboratory animals.[23] Early results of clinical trials in men whose cancers no longer respond to standard hormonal therapy have also been promising. The drug is well tolerated, though some patients have experienced seizures at very high doses. Lower doses are effective in reducing PSA levels in most patients, sometimes dramatically. Whether this will translate into longer survival remains to be seen. A Phase III randomized trial is under way.

Drugs That Block the Production of Androgens

Androgens, like other steroid hormones, are synthesized in the body through a multistep process that depends on key enzymes called CYP17. Powerful new inhibitors of these enzymes have recently been discovered that completely shut off production of androgens by any cell in the body, normal or malignant. The first drug in this class, abiraterone, was discovered at the Institute of Cancer Research in London, developed by Cougar Pharmaceuticals, and will be marketed by Johnson & Johnson.[24] Taken by mouth, abiraterone shuts down androgen production not only by the adrenal glands but within the cancer cells, and dramatically lowers the blood levels of androgen compared with the levels present after standard ADT. Because it allows excess production of other adrenal steroids, the major side effects of the drug are hypertension and edema. These effects were easily managed by giving a drug to inhibit excess steroid production.

In clinical trials, abiraterone has been remarkably effective in patients with advanced prostate cancer that has progressed after ADT, causing marked declines in PSA levels and a decrease in the size of metastatic tumors. The overall response rate was greater than 50 percent. More patients responded when dexamethasone was added to the regimen to shut down the excess adrenal steroids thought to stimulate the promiscuous AR in these tumors.

NOTE: The level of response to new antiandrogens like MDV3100 and abiraterone offers clear proof that many prostate cancers are hormonally active even in the late stages of the disease and remain dependent on the function of the AR. The term "hormone-refractory" has been rendered obsolete, opening the way for many new approaches to controlling advanced prostate cancer.

RADIATION THERAPY

In addition to treating cancer within the prostate, radiation therapy is very useful in controlling metastatic sites in men with advanced prostate cancer. In fact, radiation has become an integral part of the therapeutic strategy for these patients, often in conjunction with first- and second-line hormonal manipulation. Radiation typically is administered to sites of cancer spread in bone, where it can lessen the risk of "pathological fracture" of a bone weakened by cancer and alleviate intractable bone pain. While treating the primary tumor in the prostate requires daily doses for seven to ten weeks, metastases can be controlled with 20 Gy given over two weeks. Even shorter regimens are widely used, with as few as three daily fractions, and even a single dose of 8 Gy is being explored at MSKCC for control of metastatic sites.[25] The key principle in treating prostate cancer metastases with radiation is to focus on the actual metastatic lesion and spare normal tissue, since radiation causes permanent destruction of the bone marrow. As bone is replaced by cancer, men tend to have decreased marrow reserves, leading to anemia and a decreased ability to fight infections or tolerate chemotherapy.

External beam therapy with IMRT is the best form of radiation when there are only a few metastatic sites in bones. If widespread metastases are present and causing pain, irradiating all these sites would obliterate the bone marrow.

Radioactive isotopes, developed from chemicals, with an affinity for bones, can alleviate bone pain more effectively. One of these isotopes, strontium 89, mimics calcium. Taken up by bone, it provides a high level of local radiation to the bony metastases. Pain relief is common, but strontium has not been shown to reduce fractures or to increase survival. Samarium 153, a newer agent, appears to be as effective as strontium with fewer side effects. The half-life of strontium 89 is fifty days. For samarium, the half-life is only two days, so it leaves the system faster and recovery from bone marrow suppression is quicker. Both agents cause a temporary increase in bone pain (flare) hours or days after they are administered. Typically, because of their toxicity, these agents can be used only once.[26]

CHEMOTHERAPY

For many other cancers, chemotherapy has long been a standard weapon in the treatment arsenal. For most serious breast cancers, a combination of chemotherapy drugs is given after surgery and/or radiation for six months to reduce the risk of later metastases. For prostate cancer, the use of chemotherapy is distinctly different. Only recently has chemotherapy been proven to prolong life in advanced prostate cancer. There is no role for routine, adjuvant chemotherapy after radiation or surgery. The first study that hinted at any benefit from chemotherapy was published in 2002. Patients treated with the anticancer drug mitoxantrone (Novantrone) plus steroids had substantially better pain relief and slightly longer survival than patients treated with steroids alone.[27] Still, the real breakthrough came in 2004, when two large studies proved that combination chemotherapy clearly prolonged life compared with a regimen of mitoxantrone and prednisone (a steroid). The chemotherapy combinations in both studies included the powerful taxol-related drug docetaxel (Taxotere). In one study, docetaxel was combined with the estrogen-like estramustine; in the other, with prednisone. In both trials, the combined chemotherapy "cocktails" prolonged life by three to four months compared with the previous standard that used pain-relieving mitoxantrone and prednisone.[28] While a few months do not constitute a huge improvement, it is an encouraging start. These patients were at the end of their rope. All other treatments had failed. Prolonging their lives proved that chemotherapy does work in prostate cancer and strongly suggests that if these drugs were used earlier in the course of the disease, the benefit might be much greater.

In other cancers, greater success has come from combining individual drugs, each of which has limited efficacy. Unfortunately, many combinations have been tried in prostate cancer and none has been sufficiently promising alone or in combination with docetaxel to justify routine use today.

Once a drug has been shown to be effective in advanced cancer, it is typically tested earlier in the disease, when its activity may be even greater. The value of chemotherapy early in the course of prostate cancer has rarely been tested and its use is controversial. Typically, physicians recommend trying all nonchemotherapeutic options before resorting to chemotherapy, even for metastatic cancer, because the toxicity is significant and the benefit is limited.

NOTE: An important clinical trial is available for a man with a rapidly rising PSA but no metastases after radical prostatectomy. These men at high risk for developing metastases are randomly assigned to either ADT alone for two years or ADT plus six months of docetaxel. The goal is to see which approach is more likely to reduce the PSA level to less than 0.05 and keep it there after all treatment has stopped.[29]

EXPERIMENTAL THERAPIES

Medical science is in the midst of a historic revolution. Research and practice are changing dramatically, ushering in the age of molecular medicine. In this new approach, medical treatment targets specific molecules that drive the growth of the cancer rather than all rapidly dividing cells in the body. Traditional chemotherapy damaged the gastrointestinal tract, causing nausea and vomiting, and depleted bone marrow with resultant low platelets, anemia, and reduced white cells. Modern targeted therapy tends to have far fewer side effects.

Biological profiling has been highly effective in identifying targets for therapy in breast, leukemia, lung, and other cancers. The classic example of targeted therapy is imatinib (Gleevec) for a form of leukemia that is driven by an aberrant oncogene called Bcr-Abl. Imatinib specifically blocks the growth-promoting action of this mutant gene and causes a dramatic remission, and an occasional cure, for patients with chronic lymphocytic leukemia. Breast cancer patients who test positive for the estrogen receptor gene benefit from antiestrogen drugs. Those who have excess Her2Neu receptor, which stimulates cancer cell growth, respond well to the monoclonal antibody trastuzumab (Herceptin). Lung cancers that harbor alterations in the EGFR gene respond to erlotimib (Tarceva) and gefitimib (Iressa).

Similarly, biological profiling may enable us to identify specific prostate cancer–promoting genes and develop agents that target them. Most men with prostate cancer that progresses after initial hormonal therapy test positive for the androgen receptor. Designer drugs such as the new antiandrogens and abiraterone have been developed to block the androgen receptor[30] or eliminate its stimulants[31] to reduce PSA and slow the growth of the cancer. New drugs such as the ansamycins and the tongue-twistingly named histone deacetylase inhibitors (H-DACs) might stem the growth of prostate cancers by destroying the androgen receptors that enable cells in the gland to absorb cancer-promoting hormones.[32]

Antisense refers to synthetic genetic agents that slow or stop the growth of cancer cells. Antisense drugs, targeting genes such as BCL-2 or clusterin, slow the growth of prostate cancers by making them more susceptible to cell death (apoptosis).[33]

If you have advanced prostate cancer, look for clinical trials of the latest agents near your home by searching www.cancer.gov for NCI-approved clinical trials. There are 50 to100 drugs in the development pipeline for prostate cancer.[34]

IMMUNOTHERAPY

A unique approach to treating cancer is to harness the power of the body's immune system to identify, attack, and destroy cancers. The power of the immune system is evident in the way the body will quickly destroy an alien organ or an infection. With cancer, we've long believed that the immune system serves as a powerful early sentry system, destroying aberrant cells well before they can muster their forces and become a viable tumor. Critics of this approach point out how common cancer is and how quickly it grows and develops even in people with healthy immune systems. We now recognize that cancer has the ability to fool the immune system by impersonating normal cells or by secreting substances such as TGF-beta or B7x that inhibit the immune system or induce it to shut down.

Harnessing the immune system to treat cancer has been a challenge, and several strategies have been attempted. One approach, which has recently proven effective in prolonging survival in clinical trials, has been a dendritic cell immune booster called sipuleucel-T (Provenge). A blood sample is drawn and dendritic cells (which process antigens) are extracted and exposed to a slurry of prostate-specific antigens. The cells are grown in tissue culture and given back to patients as an injection under the skin. These dendritic cells are thought to charge up the immune system to attack the cancer. A recent clinical trial found prolonged survival in men with a rising PSA after ADT whose cancer had not yet metastasized. Provenge is not yet approved by the FDA, but it promises to be the first immunotherapy for advanced prostate cancer. Nevertheless, the lack of clear effect on the cancer and the uncertain mechanism of action of

Provenge suggest it may be the first but will probably not be the most effective immunotherapy for prostate cancer.

Normally, when challenged by an infection, the immune system rallies rapidly to attack the invader and then quickly shuts down. If the immune system failed to accelerate in response to invading organisms, the infected person would soon die. On the other hand, if the braking mechanism failed to kick in once the threat had passed, the immune system would spiral out of control, eventually taking over the body with fatal consequences. Dr. James Allison at Memorial Sloan-Kettering Cancer Center discovered a way to target and disarm the immune braking system with antibodies, enabling the body's own immune defenses to continue to fight the cancer. This new drug, ipilumimab, or anti-CTLA-4, is being developed by Bristol-Myers Squibb. Easy to administer intravenously, ipilumimab has been powerfully effective against a number of cancers, but it has serious toxicity as well. The drug can provoke an autoimmune attack on the gastrointestinal tract, resulting in colitis and severe diarrhea, which can be fatal if not recognized and treated immediately. Some men with prostate cancer have developed an autoimmune reaction against their pituitary gland that may require lifelong replacement of pituitary hormones essential for life. While ipilumimab has been successful against several forms of cancer when used alone, Dr. Allison theorizes that it will work even better in combination with treatments that kill cancer cells, releasing their contents into the tissues, where the immune system can recognize cancer antigens and mount a broad response to them.[35] Radiation, hormone therapy, chemotherapy, and other anticancer regimens followed by anti-CTLA-4 are now being tested in clinical trials.

Another approach under development is to link monoclonal antibodies (laboratory-developed substances designed to seek out and bind to cancer cells) with toxic drugs or radiation emitters to deliver a lethal dose of drugs or radiation directly to the cancer cells with minimal damage to normal nearby tissues. Think of a ray gun targeting an enemy close up. This has proven effective in battling small lymphomas and some leukemias, and it is being studied in prostate cancer.[36]

Cancers are extraordinarily complex, but the essential features they require to grow and spread are steadily being identified. To survive in the body, cancer cells must be able to divide, to avoid apoptosis, to break through normal tissue barriers, to spread through the bloodstream or lymphatic system, and to induce the growth of the blood vessels (angiogenesis) they require for oxygen and nutrients. Each of these activities is controlled by a number of enzymes, signaling proteins, and growth regulators, all of which are potential targets for therapeutic assault. Major research efforts are currently in progress to develop drugs that will bring the cancer to its knees by arresting these conspirators and putting them out of commission for good. I have never witnessed a more exciting time in the field, when new technology holds such promise for men with advanced prostate cancer.

IS A CLINICAL TRIAL RIGHT FOR YOU?

Though many people initially balk at the idea of entering a clinical trial, experimental or investigational treatments actually offer several distinct advantages. Patients enrolled in a study are typically offered top-notch care and scrupulous monitoring. Experts in various disciplines review planned trials carefully to make sure they are well thought out and that the potential benefits outweigh the risks before investigators get the go-ahead to proceed.[37]

Since we have no approved medications as yet that cure advanced prostate cancer, a new drug or novel combination therapy may be the best way to improve your odds. A clinical trial gives you an early opportunity to try a novel therapy that might eventually prove to be more effective than treatments that are currently available. Remember, every drug treatment we have to battle diseases today was once experimental.

Through these trials, scientists using impeccable methodology may devise groundbreaking treatments. Most trials are rigorously designed and overseen by experts, but do be aware that a small percentage of research efforts is unquestionably misguided. Beware of trials you might find on the Internet that are not in the Physician Data Query (PDQ) database of the National Cancer Institute, conducted under the auspices of the NCI, or overseen by a major cancer center. To decide whether a given approach makes sense in your particular situation, it's important to understand how studies and clinical trials are constructed. (See the Resources section at the back of this book, and the NIH, NCI, PDQ websites.)

A medical study or clinical trial seeks to answer a question about the cause, treatment, or prevention of a medical condition or disease. The questions vary enormously. A trial may look at imaging techniques or pathology, or it may be designed to demonstrate the effectiveness of a new medication or medical device. To win approval by the Food and Drug Administration (FDA) or similar agencies in other countries, new drugs and devices are put through a series of increasingly challenging, rigorous, and expensive hoops.

Phase 1 clinical drug trials involve twenty to eighty subjects. These preliminary studies are intended to demonstrate that the drug under investigation can be safely administered to humans after their safety has been established in a laboratory setting. During a phase 1 trial, scientists observe the impact of the experimental drug and monitor its side effects at varying dose levels to establish the maximum safe dose.

Once a treatment appears safe in a phase 1 trial, a **phase 2 clinical drug trial** evaluates the drug's effectiveness on a larger group of patients who have the target condition or disease. Risks and side effects are carefully monitored, but the main goal of the trial is to see whether the drug works at the maximum safe dosage and confirm its safety in a larger number of patients.

During **phase 3 clinical trials**, a drug that has been proven safe and effective in smaller studies is administered to many hundreds or even thousands of patients to examine the overall risks and benefits. Usually, phase 3 trials compare new treatments with standard approaches to determine if the new treatment is as safe as and more effective than the best standard regimen. If an experimental regimen passes phase 2 and phase 3 trials, the sponsor applies for FDA approval to market the drug.

Once a drug is approved, **phase 4 scrutiny** is an effort to learn more about an approved drug's optimal dosage level, long-term effectiveness, and negative effects in the wider population as the drug is given in routine clinical practice. The main goal is to look for rare but serious side effects that may emerge when many people take the drug, and to detect long-term side effects or unexpected interactions with other medications. The trials that showed the unexpected increase in the risk of breast cancer, stroke, and blood clots in women taking hormone replacement after menopause are a good example of phase 4 trials.[38]

The value and validity of clinical trials hinge on how strictly they conform to the long-established principles of scientific investigation. Medical studies can range from the observation of a few people (which can yield highly misleading results) to scientifically rigorous assessments involving large groups that are carefully controlled to prevent extraneous factors from affecting the outcome. Prospective studies, where a question is asked and then the experimental groups are formed and followed over time, are considered more reliable than retrospective ones, though we have derived valuable information from retrospective studies as well, and sometimes retrospective information is all we have to go on.

While participants in clinical trials are fully informed about the nature of the study, to prevent bias that can affect results, they may be kept in the dark about which arm of a trial they are in. Experimental subjects get the drug under study, while control subjects get a standard medication or a placebo (see below). In single-blind studies, medical personnel know which therapy subjects are getting, but the patients remain unaware. Double-blind trials withhold this information from both patients and physicians, whose perceptions or practices might be influenced by the knowledge.

A placebo is an inactive substance that looks identical to and is administered in precisely the same way as an experimental drug. In clinical trials, placebos are often used to ensure that the observed effects are actually the result of the therapy being studied and not some extraneous factor such as a patient's expectation that he'll get better or experience fewer symptoms. Large, placebo-controlled, double-blind studies in which experimental subjects are carefully matched and randomly assigned to treatment and control groups are far more likely to yield reliable results than a study involving a small number of subjects and a less rigorous experimental design. The gold standard in medical investigation is the large, randomized, prospective, double-blind clinical trial.

The endpoint refers to the predefined event or outcome that completes the study. In medical investigations, total mortality or the overall survival rate is considered the easiest endpoint to define and the least subject to reporting bias (not to mention of crucial importance to patients). Did the experimental subjects live longer, and if so, how much longer? If there was a survival advantage, how long was it, and what percentage of subjects were alive five or ten years later?

Cause-specific survival refers to the numbers of deaths that resulted from the disease being studied. While this may say more about the effectiveness of the drug than overall survival, the measure is more subject to investigator bias. When a subject dies, the cause of death can be a judgment call. Pneumonia or the spread of prostate cancer to the lungs could reasonably be entered on the death certificate and in the researcher's databank.

Even when they do nothing to increase survival, therapies may confer other important benefits, such as symptom control. Treatments that improve quality of life are of critical importance to patients, and many studies focus on endpoints related to well-being in deciding whether a therapy should be included in medical practice. Did the treatment alleviate pain? Did the experimental subjects have fewer bowel problems than those in control groups? Were the experimental subjects able to have better erections and more satisfactory sexual function than those in the control groups?

Other endpoints focus on surrogate or secondary issues such as the amount of time subjects remain free of any signs of the disease (i.e. a measurable PSA after radical prostatectomy), the amount of time that elapses before their disease progresses (e.g., a new abnormality on bone scan), or how much tumors shrink as a result of the treatment. Since prostate cancer can take many years or even decades to become lethal, surrogate endpoints such as freedom from metastases or from a rapidly rising PSA can be highly useful in gauging the effectiveness of a new therapy.

NOTE: In clinical trials for men with metastatic prostate cancer, placebos would not be used. Men in both arms of the study would get potentially beneficial treatment, so valuable time would not be lost.

NOTE: Famed British statesman, orator, and novelist Benjamin Disraeli noted that "there are three kinds of lies: lies, damned lies and statistics." Study outcomes can be affected by subtle alterations in interpretation or experimental design. Clinical trials can cost many millions of dollars, and a company's fortunes, or even its very survival, might hinge on the outcome. It's wise to be aware of who sponsored a study and what, if anything, that sponsor had to gain. Where results are confusing or contradictory, experts should be able to help you sort things out and assess what is most significant and believable.

ALTERNATIVE AND COMPLEMENTARY MEDICINE

Alternative medicine utilizes substances such as vitamins and herbal or homeopathic remedies whose safety and effectiveness have not been established by proven scientific means. These "natural" agents are exempt from government oversight, and no agency guarantees their purity or consistency. In a particularly egregious example, shipments of PC-SPES that contained eight Chinese herbs and appeared to be effective in some men with hormone refractory prostate cancer were found to be contaminated with female hormones and hazardous blood thinners to counteract the blood clots those hormones cause. Obviously, the company that added these dangerous drugs did not believe in the efficacy of PC-SPES alone. Understandably, people are often drawn to such treatments by extravagant (though also unregulated and generally unproven) claims. In fact, if they were appropriately tested and scrupulously manufactured, some of these agents would be found to be harmless, while others might prove useful. The problem is separating the innocent suspects and positive players from those capable of doing serious harm.

If you decide to take alternative substances, be sure to discuss them with your doctor. Investigate any agent you plan to take—whether a supplement, an herb, or any other "natural" remedy—thoroughly before you start. Consider carefully the possible effects of the dose you plan to take. Beware of the foolhardy concept that if a little is good, a lot must be better. Some supplements and herbs can interact dangerously with prescribed medications. Others may drive your PSA down artificially without affecting the cancer, or change your testosterone level with the attendant side effects. If your physician is unaware that you're taking these drugs, the diagnostic significance of a change in these values could be misinterpreted, triggering a risky modification in your treatment.

Complementary medicine refers to therapies designed to improve well-being by reducing symptoms or making them more tolerable. Common approaches include prayer, meditation, exercise, acupuncture, guided imagery, and massage. Increasingly, complementary methods are gaining acceptance in conventional medical circles, and medical insurance may cover some of them, especially those that have been proven effective in randomized trials.

One group found that an intensive regimen of diet, supplements, exercise, and relaxation techniques decreased the rate of rise of PSA and slowed the progression of the prostate cancer in men with advanced disease.[39] Of course, the problem is in identifying which aspect of this regimen was responsible for the beneficial effect.

An estimated 70 percent of all cancer patients turn to alternative and complementary methods at some point in their treatment. If you decide to do so, be sure to seek referrals to reputable practitioners and substances that are considered safe. A reasonable doctor should be willing to explore these options with you and help you to take advantage of interventions that might ease the course of treatment and improve your quality of life.

PAIN MANAGEMENT AND PALLIATION

For patients with metastatic disease, pain is a central concern. Many of us remember losing relatives or friends to cancer, and those memories are often shadowed by the specter of suffering. Historically, pain control took a backseat to issues considered more medically relevant, such as prolonging life or alleviating dangerous symptoms. Today, in recognition of the enormous impact that pain and discomfort can have on quality of life, palliation and pain management receive far greater attention. In fact, pain management has spawned its own medical discipline. Most hospitals have pain-management teams dedicated to keeping patients comfortable throughout all stages of any given disease and reducing the pain and discomfort associated with treatments. Where no such team exists, attending physicians can and should see to the important business of keeping patients comfortable.

Nevertheless, an estimated 50 percent of cancer patients worldwide still receive inadequate analgesia. Sometimes this results from a discrepancy between the level of pain patients experience and how much discomfort doctors judge them to have. In some cases, physicians are reluctant to prescribe adequate pain relief, fearing that the patient may become addicted, develop a tolerance that would render the drugs ineffective, or experience unacceptable side effects. Patients may refuse to request sufficient pain medication for the same misguided reasons. Also, with serious illness, the primary focus still tends to be on medical issues such as prolonging life and relieving dangerous symptoms, rather than pain control. Nevertheless, adequate analgesic relief is critical to a patient's overall sense of well-being, central to how well he tolerates and complies with necessary treatments, and, quite possibly, crucial to how long he lives.

Recognizing this, the World Health Organization (WHO) recommends a sequential "ladder" approach to pain management and palliation for cancer patients. Following this approach, more than 80 percent of people with advanced cancer have their pain relieved.[40]

Under the WHO guidelines, a primary goal is to prevent the onset of pain by administering analgesics at regular intervals, rather than waiting for the pain to become severe and then try to relieve it with drugs. "By the clock" dosage is determined after a careful evaluation of how long an analgesic drug stays in the system (**half-life**) and the duration of its palliative effects. The best pain control is carefully tailored to meet each patient's needs, with constant adjustments as necessary to achieve the best pain control with the fewest possible side effects. Ideally, analgesics should be simple to administer so they can be taken by the patient or given by family members at home. For this reason, oral medications, patches, and nasal sprays are preferable to those that must be injected or administered intravenously.

Mild pain can often be managed with non-opioid drugs such as paracetamol (acetaminophen, Tylenol) or NSAIDs (aspirin, ibuprofen, Motrin, Advil). As a tumor grows, it can trigger the synthesis and release of substances called **prostaglandins**, which cause inflammation in adjacent tissues. NSAIDs work by blocking prostaglandin production, allowing the inflammation and the pain it causes to subside.

All drugs have effects and side effects. Taken persistently in high doses, NSAIDs can cause indigestion, nausea, and vomiting. Regular monitoring is necessary to ensure that serious problems such as ulcers or gastrointestinal bleeding do not develop. Extended use may compromise normal kidney function and lead to swelling in the extremities or cause easy bruising of the skin.

Non-opioids have limited analgesic effects. Above a certain recommended level, increasing the dose would only increase the risk of side effects while failing to alleviate the pain. At that point, it's necessary to add or switch to low-dose opioids, such as codeine or tramadol for mild to moderate pain, or stronger opioids, such as morphine, methadone, hydrocodone, buprenorphine, or fentanyl, if the pain is moderate to severe.

NOTE: It is important to speak with your family and your physician to plan your care during the late stages of prostate cancer, while you are still strong enough and your thinking is clear enough to give this the consideration it deserves. Modern hospice care is usually provided at home, but there are also very good hospice centers when home care is not feasible. Hospice workers are thoroughly trained in controlling pain and managing the other symptoms common to this stage of the disease. There does come a time when the focus should shift from ineffective treatment to maximizing the quality of your remaining life.

Morphine has long been the mainstay in pain management for advanced cancer. Though it has provided blessed relief for so many, patients (and some health professionals) continue to misunderstand and mistrust it. With this and all opioids, they worry about severe sedation, though, in reality, doses can be carefully regulated to minimize this risk. They believe that morphine will suppress breathing, but with proper dosing this is not the case. Addiction is not a concern in a patient with intractable pain from metastatic cancer.

Oral morphine comes in two forms. The short-release variety works in twenty to ninety minutes and effects last for four to six hours. The twelve-hour, slow-release variety requires only two doses per day. Morphine can also be administered by rectal suppository, by skin patch, or by injection.

Methadone, despite its unfortunate association with illegal narcotics, is a powerful, long-acting pain reliever that avoids some of the side effects of morphine. Hydromorphone is faster-acting (though not as long-lasting), and fentanyl is seventy-five times as potent as morphine. Several other powerful opioids are approved for the treatment of severe pain, and the best relief may require a trial of several of these alone or in combination.

Opioids can cause some sedation, constipation, and nausea, as well as many other unpleasant effects. Additional (adjuvant) drugs might be needed to counteract these problems and keep you comfortable. The treatment arsenal includes antidepressants, laxatives, amphetamines, corticosteroids, and anti-emetics (to counteract vomiting), to name a few. Some patients have severe anxiety or difficulty sleeping, requiring the use of tranquilizers. Anorexia or malnutrition may call for appetite stimulants. Anticonvulsants may be necessary if the disease causes damage to the nervous system.

Pain is a subjective sensation, and successful pain management depends on a careful assessment of and response to each patient's needs. A person's pain tolerance or pain threshold can be boosted by such simple measures as adequate rest, diverting activities, understanding, and empathy. On the other hand, psychological negatives like fear, anger, fatigue, isolation, or depression, all common in patients with advanced disease, can make pain seem worse and harder to tolerate. Cultural, spiritual, physical, and psychological issues also factor into our highly personal perception and tolerance of pain.

Try to think of your doctor as your quarterback, there to run interference, plan strategic moves, and ease your way past the problems and obstacles that arise. Be sure to discuss pain management before it becomes an issue and to seek help for issues like depression, fatigue, and anxiety that can make symptoms harder to tolerate. If you are not receiving adequate relief, or if the pain medication is causing unacceptable side effects, don't hesitate to request a more effective regime. Your medical team should work with you to alleviate symptoms and keep you feeling and functioning well for as long as possible.

In addition to pain medications, bone-seeking radiopharmaceuticals like Strontium 89, bisphosphonates, targeted external beam radiation, and chemotherapy are useful tools to alleviate the pain of bone metastases.

IN SUMMARY

Given steady advances in our understanding of prostate cancer and the emergence of novel, increasingly effective therapies, the outlook for men with advanced prostate cancer has improved considerably and continues to brighten all the time. For men with a rising PSA after surgery or radiation, standard hormone therapy is effective for nearly a decade. The average survival for men with bone metastases has risen from two to three years in the 1980s to five to six years today. As new drugs under investigation become part of the standard treatment arsenal, we will move ever nearer to the goal of eliminating suffering and death from this disease for all men. As we work toward that goal, we are also developing ever better means to palliate symptoms and prolong survival for men with metastatic disease.

NOTES

1. THE PROSTATE

1. Litwin, M. S., and C. S. Saigal, eds. *Urologic Diseases in America.* NIH Publication No. 07-5512. Washington, DC: U.S. Department of Health and Human Services, Public Health Service, National Institutes of Health, National Institute of Diabetes and Digestive and Kidney Diseases, U.S. Government Printing Office, 2007.
2. Pearson, J. D., H. H. Lei, T. H. Beaty, K. E. Wiley, S. D. Isaacs, W. B. Isaacs, E. Stoner, and P. C. Walsh. "Familial Aggregation of Bothersome Benign Prostatic Hyperplasia Symptoms." *Urology* 61, no. 4 (2003): 781–85.

3. CHANGES WITH AGING

1. Hijazi, R. A., and G. R. Cunningham. "Andropause: Is Androgen Replacement Therapy Indicated for the Aging Male?" *Ann Rev Med* 56 (2005): 117–37.
2. Araujo, A. B., G. R. Esche, V. Kupelian, A. B. O'Donnell, T. G. Travison, R. E. Williams, R. V. Clark, J. B. McKinlay. "Prevalence of Symptomatic Androgen Deficiency in Men." *J Clin Endocrinol Metab* 92, no. 11 (2007):4241–47.
3. Bhasin, S., G. R. Cunningham, F. J. Hayes, A. M. Matsumoto, P. J. Snyder, R. S. Swerdloff, and V. M. Montori. "Clinical Practice: Testosterone Therapy in Adult Men with Androgen Deficiency Syndromes: An Endocrine Society Clinical Practice Guideline." *J Clin Endocrinol Metab* 91, no. 6 (2006): 1995–2010.
4. Mulhall, J. P. Saving Your Sex Life: A Guide for Men with Prostate Cancer. Chicago: Hilton, 2008; and Rosen, R. C., and A. D. Seftel. "Validated Questionnaires for Assessing Sexual Dysfunction and Bph/Luts: Solidifying the Common Pathophysiologic Link." *Int J Impot Res* 20 Suppl 3 (2008): S27–32.

4. PROSTATITIS

1. Roberts, R. O., M. M. Lieber, T. Rhodes, C. J. Girman, D. G. Bostwick, and S. J. Jacobsen. "Prevalence of a Physician-Assigned Diagnosis of Prostatitis: The Olmsted County Study of Urinary Symptoms and Health Status Among Men." *Urology* 51, no. 4 (1998): 578–84; and Collins, M. M., R. S. Stafford, M. P. O'Leary, and M. J. Barry. "How Common Is Prostatitis? A National Survey of Physician Visits." *J Urol* 159, no. 4 (1998): 1224–28.
2. Stamey, T. A. "Prostatitis." *J R Soc Med* 74, no. 1 (1981): 22–40.
3. Schaeffer, A. J., J. R. Landis, J. S. Knauss, K. J. Propert, R. B. Alexander, M. S. Litwin, J. C. Nickel, M. P. O'Leary, R. B. Nadler, M. A. Pontari, D. A. Shoskes, S. I. Zeitlin, J. E. Fowler Jr., C. A. Mazurick, L. Kishel, J. W. Kusek, and L. M. Nyberg; Chronic Prostatitis Collaborative Research Network Group. "Demographics and Clinical Characteristics of Men with Chronic Prostatitis: the National Institutes of Health Chronic Prostatitis Cohort Study." *J Urol* 168, no. 2 (2002): 593–98.

4. McNaughton-Collins, M. M., and M.A. Pontari, "Prostatitis." In M. S. Litwin and C. S. Saigal, eds., *Urologic Diseases in America*, pp. 9–42. Washington, DC: U.S. Department of Health and Human Services, Public Health Service, National Institutes of Health, National Institute of Diabetes and Digestive and Kidney Diseases, U.S. Government Printing Office, 2007.

5. Krieger, J. N., L. Nyberg Jr., and J. C. Nickel. "NIH Consensus Definition and Classification of Prostatitis." *JAMA* 282, no. 3 (1999): 236–37.

6. Naber, K. G., F. M. E. Wagenlehner, and W. Weidner. "Acute Bacterial Prostatis." In D. A. Shoskes, ed., *Chronic Prostatitis/Chronic Pelvic Pain Syndrome*. Totowa, NJ: Humana Press, 2008, pp. 17–30.

7. Schaeffer, A. J. "Clinical Practice: Chronic Prostatitis and the Chronic Pelvic Pain Syndrome." *New Engl J Med* 355, no. 16 (2006): 1690–98.

8. Litwin, M. S., M. McNaughton-Collins, F. J. Fowler Jr., J. C. Nickel, E. A. Calhoun, M. A. Pontari, R. B. Alexander, J. T. Farrar, and M. P. O'Leary; Chronic Prostatitis Collaborative Research Network Group. "The National Institutes of Health Chronic Prostatitis Symptom Index: Development and Validation of a New Outcome Measure." *J Urol* 162, no. 2 (1999) 369–75.

9. Ponatri, M. A. "Chronic Prostatitis/Chronic Pelvic Pain Syndrome." *Urol Clin North Am* 35 (2008): 81–89.

10. Nickel, J. C., J. N. Krieger, M. McNaughton-Collins, et al. "Alfuzosin and Symptoms of Chronic Prostatitis-Chronic Pelvic Pain Syndrome. The Chronic Prostatitis Collaborative Research Network." *New Engl J Med* 359, no. 25 (2008): 2663–73.

11. Nickel, J. C., J. Downey, M. A. Pontari, D. A. Shoskes, and S. I. Zeitlin. "A Randomized Placebo-Controlled Multicenter Study to Evaluate the Safety and Efficacy of Finasteride for Male Chronic Pelvic Pain Syndrome (Category IIIA Chronic Nonbacterial Prostatitis)." *BJU Int* 93, no. 7 (2004): 991–95.

12. Nickel, J. C., J. B. Forrest, K. Tomera, et al. "Pentosan Polysulfate Sodium Therapy for Men with Chronic Pelvic Pain Syndrome: A Multicenter, Randomized, Placebo Controlled Study." *J Urol* 173, no. 4 (2005): 1252–55.

13. Cassileth, B. R. *The Alternative Medicine Handbook*. New York: W. W. Norton, 1998.

14. Miller, P., C. Kastner, H. Fletcher, et al. "Cooled Thermotherapy (TUMT) for Chronic Abacterial Prostatis (CP/CPPS): 2 Years After Treatment." *Urology* 66, no. 3 Suppl 1 (2005): 23.

15. Shoskes, D. A., J. C. Nickel, R. R. Rackley, et al. "Clinical Phenotyping in Chronic Prostatits/ Chronic Pelvic Pain Syndrome and Interstitial Cystitis: A Management Strategy for Urologic Chronic Pelvic Pain Syndromes." *Prostate Cancer Prostatic Dis* 12, no. 2 (2009): 177–83.

16. Potts, J. M. "Prospective Identification of National Institutes of Health Category IV Prostatitis in Men with Elevated Prostate Specific Antigen." *J Urol* 164, no. 5 (2000): 1550–53.

17. Nickel, J. C. "Inflammation and Benign Prostatic Hyperplasia." *Urol Clin North Am* 35, no. 1 (2008): 109–15.

18. Nelson, W. G., A. M. De Marzo, and W. B. Isaacs. "Prostate Cancer." *New Engl J Med* 349, no. 4 (2003): 366–81; and Hu, J. C., G. S. Palapattu, M. W. Kattan, P. T. Scardino, and T. M. Wheeler. "The Association of Selected Pathological Features with Prostate Cancer in a Single-Needle Biopsy Accession." *Hum Pathol* 29, no. 12 (1998): 1536–38.

19. Taylor, B. C., S. Noorbaloochi, M. McNaughton-Collins, et al. "Excessive Antibiotic Use in Men with Prostatitis." *Am J Med* 121 (2008): 444–49.

20 Eastham, J. A., E. Riedel, P. T. Scardino, M. Shike, M. Fleisher, A. Schatzkin, E. Lanza, L. Latkany, and C. B. Begg. "Variation of Serum Prostate-Specific Antigen Levels: An Evaluation of Year-to-Year Fluctuations." *JAMA* 289, no. 20 (2003): 2695–700.

21. Scardino, P. T. "The Responsible Use of Antibiotics for an Elevated PSA Level." *Nat Clin Pract Urol* 4, no. 1 (2007): 1.

5. BPH (BENIGN PROSTATIC ENLARGEMENT)

1. Isaacson, Walter. *Benjamin Franklin: An American Life*. New York: Simon & Schuster, 2003.

2. Murphy, L. J. T. *The History of Urology*. Springfield, IL: Charles C. Thomas, 1972.

3. Murphy, L. J. T. *The History of Urology*. Springfield, IL: Charles C. Thomas, 1972.

4. McNeal, J. E., E. A. Redwine, F. S. Freiha, and T. A. Stamey. "Zonal Distribution of Prostatic Adenocarcinoma. Correlation with Histologic Pattern and Direction of Spread." *Am J Surg Pathol* 12, no. 12 (1988): 897–906.

5. Jacobsen, S. J., C. J. Girman, and M. M. Lieber. "Natural History of Benign Prostatic Hyperplasia." *Urology* 58, no. 6 Suppl 1 (2001): 5–16; discussion 16.

6. Kristal, A. R., J. M. Schenk, Y. Song, K. B. Arnold, M. L. Neuhouser, P. J. Goodman, D. W. Lin, F. Z. Stanczyk, and I. M. Thompson. "Serum Steroid and Sex Hormone-Binding Globulin Concentrations and the Risk of Incident Benign Prostatic Hyperplasia: Results from the Prostate Cancer Prevention Trial." *Am J Epidemiol* 168, no. 12 (2008): 1416–24.

7. Imperato-McGinley, J., R. E. Peterson, T. Gautier, and E. Sturla. "Male Pseudohermaphroditism Secondary to 5 Alpha-Reductase Deficiency—A Model for the Role of Androgens in Both the Development of the Male Phenotype and the Evolution of a Male Gender Identity." *J Steroid Biochem* 11, no. 1B (1979): 637–45.

8. Gormley, G. J., E. Stoner, R. C. Bruskewitz, J. Imperato-McGinley, P. C. Walsh, J. D. McConnell, G. L. Andriole, J. Geller, B. R. Bracken, J. S. Tenover, et al. "The Effect of Finasteride in Men with Benign Prostatic Hyperplasia. The Finasteride Study Group." *N Engl J Med* 327, no. 17 (1992): 1185–91.

9. Rushton, D. H. "Androgenetic Alopecia in Men: The Scale of the Problem and Prospects for Treatment." *Int J Clin Pract* 53, no. 1 (1999): 50–53.

10. Jaffe, W. I., S. A. Kaplan, and J. D. McConnell. "Epidemiology and Pathophysiology of Benign Prostatic Hyperplasia." In P. T. Scardino and K. M. Slawin, eds., *Atlas of the Prostate*, 3rd ed. Philadelphia: Current Medicine, 2006.

11. Carter, H. B., and D. S. Coffey. "The Prostate—An Increasing Medical Problem." *Prostate* 16, no. 1 (1990): 39–48.

12. Wei, J. T. "Benign Prostatic Hyperplasia: Urologic Diseases in America." *J Urol* (2005).

13. McConnell, J. D., C. G. Roehrborn, O. M. Bautista, G. L. Andriole, Jr., C. M. Dixon, J. W. Kusek, H. Lepor, K. T. McVary, L. M. Nyberg, Jr., H. S. Clarke, E. D. Crawford, A. Diokno, J. P. Foley, H. E. Foster, S. C. Jacobs, S. A. Kaplan, K. J. Kreder, M. M. Lieber, M. S. Lucia, G. J. Miller, M. Menon, D. F. Milam, J. W. Ramsdell, N. S. Schenkman, K. M. Slawin, and J. A. Smith. "The Long-Term Effect of Doxazosin, Finasteride, and Combination Therapy on the Clinical Progression of Benign Prostatic Hyperplasia." *N Engl J Med* 349, no. 25 (2003): 2387–98.

14. Costabile, R. A., and W. D. Steers. "How Can We Best Characterize the Relationship Between Erectile Dysfunction and Benign Prostatic Hyperplasia?" *J Sex Med* 3, no. 4 (2006): 676–81.

15. Pearson, J. D., H. H. Lei, T. H. Beaty, K. E. Wiley, S. D. Isaacs, W. B. Isaacs, E. Stoner, and P. C. Walsh. "Familial Aggregation of Bothersome Benign Prostatic Hyperplasia Symptoms." *Urology* 61, no. 4 (2003): 781–85.

16. Moyad, M. A., and F. C. Lowe. "Educating Patients About Lifestyle Modifications for Prostate Health." *Am J Med* 121, no. 8 Suppl 2 (2008): S34–42.

17. Barry, M. J., F. J. Fowler, Jr., M. P. O'Leary, R. C. Bruskewitz, H. L. Holtgrewe, W. K. Mebust, A. T. K. Cockett, and the Measurement Committee of the American Urological Association. "The American Urological Association Symptom Index for Benign Prostatic Hyperplasia." *J Urol* 148, no. 5 (1992): 1549–57.

18. Makarov, D. V., S. Loeb, R. H. Getzenberg, and A. W. Partin. "Biomarkers for Prostate Cancer." *Ann Rev Med* 60 (2009): 139–51.

19. Thompson, I. M., C. Chi, D. P. Ankerst, P. J. Goodman, C. M. Tangen, S. M. Lippman, M. S. Lucia, H. L. Parnes, and C. A. Coltman, Jr. "Effect of Finasteride on the Sensitivity of PSA for Detecting Prostate Cancer." *J Natl Cancer Inst* 98, no. 16 (2006): 1128–33.

20. Emberton, M., G. L. Andriole, J. de la Rosette, B. Djavan, K. Hoefner, R. Vela Navarrete, J. Nordling, C. Roehrborn, C. Schulman, P. Teillac, A. Tubaro, and J. C. Nickel. "Benign Prostatic Hyperplasia: A Progressive Disease of Aging Men." *Urology* 61, no. 2 (2003): 267–73.

21. McConnell, J. D., C. G. Roehrborn, O. M. Bautista, G. L. Andriole, Jr., C. M. Dixon, J. W. Kusek, H. Lepor, K. T. McVary, L. M. Nyberg, Jr., H. S. Clarke, E. D. Crawford, A. Diokno, J. P. Foley, H. E. Foster, S. C. Jacobs, S. A. Kaplan, K. J. Kreder, M. M. Lieber, M. S. Lucia, G. J. Miller, M. Menon, D. F. Milam, J. W. Ramsdell, N. S. Schenkman, K. M. Slawin, and J. A. Smith. "The Long-Term Effect of Doxazosin, Finasteride, and Combination Therapy on the Clinical Progression of Benign Prostatic Hyperplasia." *N Engl J Med* 349, no. 25 (2003): 2387–98.

22. Slawin, K. M., and M. W. Kattan. "The Use of Nomograms for Selecting Bph Candidates for Dutasteride Therapy." *Rev Urol* 6 Suppl 9 (2004): S40–45.

23. Sutaria, P. M., and D. R. Staskin. "Hydronephrosis and Renal Deterioration in the Elderly Due to Abnormalities of the Lower Urinary Tract and Ureterovesical Junction." *Int Urol Nephrol* 32, no. 1 (2000): 119–26.

24. McConnell, J. D., C. G. Roehrborn, O. M. Bautista, G. L. Andriole, Jr., C. M. Dixon, J. W. Kusek, H. Lepor, K. T. McVary, L. M. Nyberg, Jr., H. S. Clarke, E. D. Crawford, A. Diokno, J. P. Foley, H. E. Foster, S. C. Jacobs, S. A. Kaplan, K. J. Kreder, M. M. Lieber, M. S. Lucia, G. J. Miller, M. Menon, D. F. Milam, J. W. Ramsdell, N. S. Schenkman, K. M. Slawin, and J. A. Smith. "The Long-Term Effect of Doxazosin, Finasteride, and Combination Therapy on the Clinical Progression of Benign Prostatic Hyperplasia." *N Engl J Med* 349, no. 25 (2003): 2387–98.

25. Issa, M. M., and T. S. Regan. "Medical Therapy for Benign Prostatic Hyperplasia—Present and Future Impact." *Am J Manag Care* 13 Suppl 1 (2007): S4–9; and Kaplan, S. A. "Update on the American Urological Association Guidelines for the Treatment of Benign Prostatic Hyperplasia." *Rev Urol* 8 Suppl 4 (2006): S10–17.

26. Lepor, H. "Alpha Blockers for the Treatment of Benign Prostatic Hyperplasia." *Rev Urol* 9, no. 4 (2007): 181–90.

27. McConnell, J. D., C. G. Roehrborn, O. M. Bautista, G. L. Andriole, Jr., C. M. Dixon, J. W. Kusek, H. Lepor, K. T. McVary, L. M. Nyberg, Jr., H. S. Clarke, E. D. Crawford, A. Diokno, J. P. Foley, H. E. Foster, S. C. Jacobs, S. A. Kaplan, K. J. Kreder, M. M. Lieber, M. S. Lucia, G. J. Miller, M. Menon, D. F. Milam, J. W. Ramsdell, N. S. Schenkman, K. M. Slawin, and J. A. Smith. "The Long-Term Effect of Doxazosin, Finasteride, and Combination Therapy on the Clinical Progression of Benign Prostatic Hyperplasia." *N Engl J Med* 349, no. 25 (2003): 2387–98; and Issa, M. M., and T. S. Regan. "Medical Therapy for Benign Prostatic Hyperplasia—Present and Future Impact." *Am J Manag Care* 13 Suppl 1 (2007): S4–9; and Kaplan, S. A. "Update on the American Urological Association Guidelines for the Treatment of Benign Prostatic Hyperplasia." *Rev Urol* 8 Suppl 4 (2006): S10–17.

28. McVary, K. T. "A Review of Combination Therapy in Patients with Benign Prostatic Hyperplasia." *Clin Ther* 29, no. 3 (2007): 387–98; and McConnell, J. D., C. G. Roehrborn, O. M. Bautista, G. L. Andriole, Jr., C. M. Dixon, J. W. Kusek, H. Lepor, K. T. McVary, L. M. Nyberg, Jr., H. S. Clarke, E. D. Crawford, A. Diokno, J. P. Foley, H. E. Foster, S. C. Jacobs, S. A. Kaplan, K. J. Kreder, M. M. Lieber, M. S. Lucia, G. J. Miller, M. Menon, D. F. Milam, J. W. Ramsdell, N. S. Schenkman, K. M. Slawin, and J. A. Smith. "The Long-Term Effect of Doxazosin, Finasteride, and Combination Therapy on the Clinical Progression of Benign Prostatic Hyperplasia." *N Engl J Med* 349, no. 25 (2003): 2387–98.

29. Thompson, I. M., P. J. Goodman, C. M. Tangen, M. S. Lucia, G. J. Miller, L. G. Ford, M. M. Lieber, R. D. Cespedes, J. N. Atkins, S. M. Lippman, S. M. Carlin, A. Ryan, C. M. Szczepanek, J. J.

Crowley, and C. A. Coltman, Jr. "The Influence of Finasteride on the Development of Prostate Cancer." *N Engl J Med* 349, no. 3 (2003): 215–24.

30. Lucia, M. S., A. K. Darke, P. J. Goodman, F. G. La Rosa, H. L. Parnes, L. G. Ford, C. A. Coltman, Jr., and I. M. Thompson. "Pathologic Characteristics of Cancers Detected in the Prostate Cancer Prevention Trial: Implications for Prostate Cancer Detection and Chemoprevention." *Cancer Prev Res* (Philadelphia) 1, no. 3 (2008): 167–73; Redman, M. W., C. M. Tangen, P. J. Goodman, M. S. Lucia, C. A. Coltman, Jr., and I. M. Thompson. "Finasteride Does Not Increase the Risk of High-Grade Prostate Cancer: A Bias-Adjusted Modeling Approach." *Cancer Prev Res* (Philadelphia) 1, no. 3 (2008): 174–81; and Thompson, I. M., C. M. Tangen, P. J. Goodman, M. S. Lucia, and E. A. Klein. "Chemoprevention of Prostate Cancer." *J Urol* 182, no. 2 (2009): 499–507; discussion 508.

31. McConnell, J. D., C. G. Roehrborn, O. M. Bautista, G. L. Andriole, Jr., C. M. Dixon, J. W. Kusek, H. Lepor, K. T. McVary, L. M. Nyberg, Jr., H. S. Clarke, E. D. Crawford, A. Diokno, J. P. Foley, H. E. Foster, S. C. Jacobs, S. A. Kaplan, K. J. Kreder, M. M. Lieber, M. S. Lucia, G. J. Miller, M. Menon, D. F. Milam, J. W. Ramsdell, N. S. Schenkman, K. M. Slawin, and J. A. Smith. "The Long-Term Effect of Doxazosin, Finasteride, and Combination Therapy on the Clinical Progression of Benign Prostatic Hyperplasia." *N Engl J Med* 349, no. 25 (2003): 2387–98; and McVary, K. T. "A Review of Combination Therapy in Patients with Benign Prostatic Hyperplasia." *Clin Ther* 29, no. 3 (2007): 387–98.

32. Slawin, K. M., and M. W. Kattan. "The Use of Nomograms for Selecting Bph Candidates for Dutasteride Therapy." *Rev Urol* 6 Suppl 9 (2004): S40–45.

33. DiPaola, R. S. & Morton, R. A. Proven and unproven therapy for benign prostatic hyperplasia. *N Engl J Med* 354, 632–34 (2006).

34. Moyad, M. A. & Lowe, F. C. Educating patients about lifestyle modifications for prostate health. *Am J Med* 121, S34–42 (2008).

35. Wasson, J. H., D. J. Reda, R. C. Bruskewitz, J. Elinson, A. M. Keller, and W. G. Henderson. "A Comparison of Transurethral Surgery with Watchful Waiting for Moderate Symptoms of Benign Prostatic Hyperplasia. The Veterans Affairs Cooperative Study Group on Transurethral Resection of the Prostate." *N Engl J Med* 332, no. 2 (1995): 75–79.

36. Schatzl, G., S. Madersbacher, B. Djavan, T. Lang, and M. Marberger. "Two-Year Results of Transurethral Resection of the Prostate Versus Four 'Less Invasive' Treatment Options." *Eur Urol* 37, no. 6 (2000): 695–701; and de la Rosette, J. J., S. Gravas, and J. M. Fitzpatrick. "Minimally Invasive Treatment of Male Lower Urinary Tract Symptoms." *Urol Clin North Am* 35, no. 3 (2008): 505–18, ix.

37. Lourenco, T., R. Pickard, L. Vale, A. Grant, C. Fraser, G. MacLennan, J. N'Dow; Benign Prostatic Enlargement Team. "Alternative Approaches to Endoscopic Ablation for Benign Enlargement of the Prostate: Systematic Review of Randomised Controlled Trials." *BMJ* 337 (2008): a449; and Te, A. E. "The Development of Laser Prostatectomy." *BJU Int* 93, no. 3 (2004): 262–65.

38. Humphreys, M. R., N. L. Miller, S. E. Handa, C. Terry, L. C. Munch, and J. E. Lingeman. "Holmium Laser Enucleation of the Prostate—Outcomes Independent of Prostate Size?" *J Urol* 180, no. 6 (2008): 2431–35; discussion 2435.

39. Schatzl, G., S. Madersbacher, B. Djavan, T. Lang, and M. Marberger. "Two-Year Results of Transurethral Resection of the Prostate Versus Four 'Less Invasive' Treatment Options." *Eur Urol* 37, no. 6 (2000): 695–701; and de la Rosette, J. J., S. Gravas, and J. M. Fitzpatrick. "Minimally Invasive Treatment of Male Lower Urinary Tract Symptoms." *Urol Clin North Am* 35, no. 3 (2008): 505–18, ix.

40. Schatzl, G., S. Madersbacher, B. Djavan, T. Lang, and M. Marberger. "Two-Year Results of Transurethral Resection of the Prostate Versus Four 'Less Invasive' Treatment Options." *Eur Urol* 37, no. 6 (2000): 695–701; and de la Rosette, J. J., S. Gravas, and J. M. Fitzpatrick. "Minimally

Invasive Treatment of Male Lower Urinary Tract Symptoms." *Urol Clin North Am* 35, no. 3 (2008): 505–18, ix.

41. Schatzl, G., S. Madersbacher, B. Djavan, T. Lang, and M. Marberger. "Two-Year Results of Transurethral Resection of the Prostate Versus Four 'Less Invasive' Treatment Options." *Eur Urol* 37, no. 6 (2000): 695–701; and de la Rosette, J. J., S. Gravas, and J. M. Fitzpatrick. "Minimally Invasive Treatment of Male Lower Urinary Tract Symptoms." *Urol Clin North Am* 35, no. 3 (2008): 505–18, ix.

42. Schatzl, G., S. Madersbacher, B. Djavan, T. Lang, and M. Marberger. "Two-Year Results of Transurethral Resection of the Prostate Versus Four 'Less Invasive' Treatment Options." *Eur Urol* 37, no. 6 (2000): 695–701; and de la Rosette, J. J., S. Gravas, and J. M. Fitzpatrick. "Minimally Invasive Treatment of Male Lower Urinary Tract Symptoms." *Urol Clin North Am* 35, no. 3 (2008): 505–18, ix.

6. PROSTATE CANCER FACTS

1. American Cancer Society. "Cancer Facts and Figures 2009." American Cancer Society. http://www.cancer.org/downloads/STT/500809web.pdf (accessed May 5, 2009).

2. Moyad, M. A., and P. R. Carroll. "Lifestyle Recommendations to Prevent Prostate Cancer, Part I: Time to Redirect Our Attention?" *Urol Clin North Am* 31, no. 2 2004): 289–300.

3. American Cancer Society. "Cancer Facts and Figures 2009." American Cancer Society. http://www.cancer.org/downloads/STT/500809web.pdf (accessed May 5, 2009).

4. Tomlins, S. A., D. R. Rhodes, S. Perner, S. M. Dhanasekaran, R. Mehra, X. W. Sun, S. Varambally, X. Cao, J. Tchinda, R. Kuefer, C. Lee, J. E. Montie, R. B. Shah, K. J. Pienta, M. A. Rubin, and A. M. Chinnaiyan. "Recurrent Fusion of Tmprss2 and Ets Transcription Factor Genes in Prostate Cancer." *Science* 310, no. 5748 (2005): 644–48.

5. Folkman, J. "What Is the Evidence That Tumors Are Angiogenesis Dependent?" *J Natl Cancer Inst* 82, no. 1 (1990): 4–6.

6. Chen, C. D., D. S. Welsbie, C. Tran, S. H. Baek, R. Chen, R. Vessella, M. G. Rosenfeld, and C. L. Sawyers. "Molecular Determinants of Resistance to Antiandrogen Therapy." *Nat Med* 10, no. 1 (2004): 33–39.

7. Scher, H. I., and C. L. Sawyers. "Biology of Progressive, Castration-Resistant Prostate Cancer: Directed Therapies Targeting the Androgen-Receptor Signaling Axis." *J Clin Oncol* 23, no. 32 (2005): 8253–61.

8. Attard, G., A. H. Reid, T. A. Yap, F. Raynaud, M. Dowsett, S. Settatree, M. Barrett, C. Parker, V. Martins, E. Folkerd, J. Clark, C. S. Cooper, S. B. Kaye, D. Dearnaley, G. Lee, and J. S. de Bono. "Phase I Clinical Trial of a Selective Inhibitor of CYP17, Abiraterone Acetate, Confirms That Castration-Resistant Prostate Cancer Commonly Remains Hormone Driven." *J Clin Oncol* 26, no. 28 (2008): 4563–71.

9. Tran, C., S. Ouk, N. J. Clegg, Y. Chen, P. A. Watson, V. Arora, J. Wongvipat, P. M. Smith-Jones, D. Yoo, A. Kwon, T. Wasielewska, D. Welsbie, C. D. Chen, C. S. Higano, T. M. Beer, D. T. Hung, H. I. Scher, M. E. Jung, and C. L. Sawyers. "Development of a Second-Generation Antiandrogen for Treatment of Advanced Prostate Cancer." *Science* 324, no. 5928 (2009): 787–90.

10. Scardino, P. T., R. Weaver, and M. A. Hudson. "Early Detection of Prostate Cancer." *Hum Pathol* 23, no. 3 (1992): 211–22.

11. Ohori, M., T. M. Wheeler, J. K. Dunn, T. A. Stamey, and P. T. Scardino. "The Pathological Features and Prognosis of Prostate Cancer Detectable with Current Diagnostic Tests." *J Urol* 152, no. 5, pt. 2 (1994): 1714–20.

12. Eggener, S. E., A. Mueller, R. K. Berglund, R. Ayyathurai, C. Soloway, M. S. Soloway, R. Abouassaly, E. A. Klein, S. J. Jones, C. Zappavigna, L. Goldenberg, P. T. Scardino, J. A. Eastham, and

B. Guillonneau. "A Multi-Institutional Evaluation of Active Surveillance for Low Risk Prostate Cancer." *J Urol* 181, no. 4 (2009): 1635–41; discussion 1641.

13. Cuzick, J., G. Fisher, M. W. Kattan, D. Berney, T. Oliver, C. S. Foster, H. Moller, V. Reuter, P. Fearn, J. Eastham, and P. Scardino. "Long-Term Outcome Among Men with Conservatively Treated Localised Prostate Cancer." *Br J Cancer* 95, no. 9 (2006): 1186–94.

14. McNeal, J. E., E. A. Redwine, F. S. Freiha, and T. A. Stamey. "Zonal Distribution of Prostatic Adenocarcinoma. Correlation with Histologic Pattern and Direction of Spread." *Am J Surg Pathol* 12, no. 12 (1988): 897–906.

15. Scardino, P. T., and L. L. Abenhaim. "Focal Therapy for Prostate Cancer: Analysis by an International Panel." *Urology* 72, no. 6 Suppl (2008); and Ahmed, H. U. "The Index Lesion and the Origin of Prostate Cancer." *N Engl J Med* 361, no. 17 (2009): 1704–6.

16. Al-Ahmadie, H. A., S. K. Tickoo, S. Olgac, A. Gopalan, P. T. Scardino, V. E. Reuter, and S. W. Fine. "Anterior-Predominant Prostatic Tumors: Zone of Origin and Pathologic Outcomes at Radical Prostatectomy." *Am J Surg Pathol* 32, no. 2 (2008): 229–35.

17. Mattei, A., F. G. Fuechsel, N. Bhatta Dhar, S. H. Warncke, G. N. Thalmann, T. Krause, and U. E. Studer. "The Template of the Primary Lymphatic Landing Sites of the Prostate Should Be Revisited: Results of a Multimodality Mapping Study." *Eur Urol* 53, no. 1 (2008): 118–25.

18. Masterson, T. A., F. J. Bianco, Jr., A. J. Vickers, C. J. DiBlasio, P. A. Fearn, F. Rabbani, J. A. Eastham, and P. T. Scardino. "The Association Between Total and Positive Lymph Node Counts, and Disease Progression in Clinically Localized Prostate Cancer." *J Urol* 175, no. 4 (2006): 1320–24; discussion 1324–25.

19. Yossepowitch, O., S. E. Eggener, A. M. Serio, B. S. Carver, F. J. Bianco, Jr., P. T. Scardino, and J. A. Eastham. "Secondary Therapy, Metastatic Progression, and Cancer-Specific Mortality in Men with Clinically High-Risk Prostate Cancer Treated with Radical Prostatectomy." *Eur Urol* 53, no. 5 (2008): 950–59.

20. Cuzick, J., G. Fisher, M. W. Kattan, D. Berney, T. Oliver, C. S. Foster, H. Moller, V. Reuter, P. Fearn, J. Eastham, and P. Scardino. "Long-Term Outcome Among Men with Conservatively Treated Localised Prostate Cancer." *Br J Cancer* 95, no. 9 (2006): 1186–94; and Albertsen, P. C., J. A. Hanley, and J. Fine. "20-Year Outcomes Following Conservative Management of Clinically Localized Prostate Cancer." *JAMA* 293, no. 17 (2005): 2095–101.

7. RISK FACTORS AND PREVENTION

1. National Safety Council. "Odds of Dying." National Safety Council. http://www.nsc.org/news_resources/injury_and_death_statistics/Documents/Odds%20of%20Dying%201510.pdf (accessed June 20, 2009).

2. Reddy, S., M. Shapiro, R. Morton, Jr., and O. W. Brawley. "Prostate Cancer in Black and White Americans." *Cancer Metastasis Rev* 22, no. 1 (2003): 83–86.

3. Carter, H. B., and D. S. Coffey. "The Prostate—An Increasing Medical Problem." *Prostate* 16, no. 1 (1990): 39–48.

4. Dockser Marcus, A. "At 32, a Decision: Is Cancer Small Enough to Ignore?" *Wall Street Journal*, 2004.

5. Tominaga, S. "Cancer Incidence in Japanese in Japan, Hawaii, and Western United States." National Cancer Institute Monographs 69 (1985): 83–92.

6. Hsing, A. W., and A. P. Chokkalingam. "Prostate Cancer Epidemiology." *Front Biosci* 11 (2006): 1388–413.

7. Calle, E. E., C. Rodriguez, K. Walker-Thurmond, and M. J. Thun. "Overweight, Obesity, and Mortality from Cancer in a Prospectively Studied Cohort of U.S. Adults." *N Engl J Med* 348, no. 17 (2003): 1625–38.

8. Freedland, S. J., and E. A. Platz. "Obesity and Prostate Cancer: Making Sense Out of Apparently Conflicting Data." *Epidemiol Rev* 29 (2007): 88–97.

9. Stanford, J. L., E. A. Noonan, L. Iwasaki, S. Kolb, R. B. Chadwick, Z. Feng, and E. A. Ostrander. "A Polymorphism in the CYP17 Gene and Risk of Prostate Cancer." *Cancer Epidemiol Biomarkers Prev* 11, no. 3 (2002): 243–47.

10. Zeegers, M. P., A. Jellema, and H. Ostrer. "Empiric Risk of Prostate Carcinoma for Relatives of Patients with Prostate Carcinoma: A Meta-Analysis." *Cancer* 97, no. 8 (2003): 1894–903.

11. Lichtenstein, P., N. V. Holm, P. K. Verkasalo, A. Iliadou, J. Kaprio, M. Koskenvuo, E. Pukkala, A. Skytthe, and K. Hemminki. "Environmental and Heritable Factors in the Causation of Cancer—Analyses of Cohorts of Twins from Sweden, Denmark, and Finland." *N Engl J Med* 343, no. 2 (2000): 78–85.

12. Witte, J. S. "Prostate Cancer Genomics: Towards a New Understanding." *Nat Rev Genet* 10, no. 2 (2009): 77–82.

13. Hsing, A. W., and A. P. Chokkalingam. "Prostate Cancer Epidemiology." *Front Biosci* 11 (2006): 1388–413.

14. Hsing, A. W., and A. P. Chokkalingam. "Prostate Cancer Epidemiology." *Front Biosci* 11 (2006): 1388–413.

15. Nelson, W. G., A. M. De Marzo, and W. B. Isaacs. "Prostate Cancer." *N Engl J Med* 349, no. 4 (2003): 366–81.

16. Verougstraete, V., D. Lison, and P. Hotz. "Cadmium, Lung and Prostate Cancer: A Systematic Review of Recent Epidemiological Data." *J Toxicol Environ Health B Crit Rev* 6, no. 3 (2003): 227–55.

17. *Veterans and Agent Orange: Health Effects of Herbicides Used in Vietnam: Update 1998.* Institute of Medicine. Washington, DC: National Academy Press, 1998.

18. Maravelias, C., A. Dona, M. Stefanidou, and C. Spiliopoulou. "Adverse Effects of Anabolic Steroids in Athletes. A Constant Threat." *Toxicol Lett* 158, no. 3 (2005): 167–75.

19. Thompson, I. M., P. J. Goodman, C. M. Tangen, M. S. Lucia, G. J. Miller, L. G. Ford, M. M. Lieber, R. D. Cespedes, J. N. Atkins, S. M. Lippman, S. M. Carlin, A. Ryan, C. M. Szczepanek, J. J. Crowley, and C. A. Coltman, Jr. "The Influence of Finasteride on the Development of Prostate Cancer." *N Engl J Med* 349, no. 3 (2003): 215–24.

20. Scardino, P. T. "The Prevention of Prostate Cancer—The Dilemma Continues." *N Engl J Med* 349, no. 3 (2003): 297–99.

21. Redman, M. W., C. M. Tangen, P. J. Goodman, M. S. Lucia, C. A. Coltman, Jr., and I. M. Thompson. "Finasteride Does Not Increase the Risk of High-Grade Prostate Cancer: A Bias-Adjusted Modeling Approach." *Cancer Prev Res* (Philadelphia) 1, no. 3 (2008): 174–81.

22. Cohen, Y. C., K. S. Liu, N. L. Heyden, A. D. Carides, K. M. Anderson, A. G. Daifotis, and P. H. Gann. "Detection Bias Due to the Effect of Finasteride on Prostate Volume: A Modeling Approach for Analysis of the Prostate Cancer Prevention Trial." *J Natl Cancer Inst* 99, no. 18 (2007): 1366–74; and Pinsky, P., H. Parnes, and L. Ford. "Estimating Rates of True High-Grade Disease in the Prostate Cancer Prevention Trial." *Cancer Prev Res* (Philadelphia) 1, no. 3 (2008): 182–86.

23. Andriole, G., D. Bostwick, O. Brawley, L. Gomella, M. Marberger, D. Tindall, S. Breed, M. Somerville, and R. Rittmaster. "Chemoprevention of Prostate Cancer in Men at High Risk: Rationale and Design of the Reduction by Dutasteride of Prostate Cancer Events (Reduce) Trial." *J Urol* 172, no. 4, pt. 1 (2004): 1314–17; and Andriole, G., D. Bostwick, O. Brawley, L. Gomella, M. Marberger, F. Montorsi, C. Pettaway, T. Tammela, C. Teloken, D. Tindall, M. Somerville, I. Fowler, and R. Rittmaster. "Further Analysis from the REDUCE Prostate Cancer Risk Reduction Trial." Annual Meeting of the American Urological Association 2009. http://www.aua2009.org/abstracts/2009/LBA1.pdf (accessed June 20, 2009).

24. Moyad, M. A., and F. C. Lowe. "Educating Patients About Lifestyle Modifications for Prostate Health." *Am J Med* 121, no. 8 Suppl 2 (2008): S34–42.

25. Ornish, D., J. Lin, J. Daubenmier, G. Weidner, E. Epel, C. Kemp, M. J. Magbanua, R. Marlin, L. Yglecias, P. R. Carroll, and E. H. Blackburn. "Increased Telomerase Activity and Comprehensive Lifestyle Changes: A Pilot Study." *Lancet Oncol* 9, no. 11 (2008): 1048–57.

26. Ornish, D., G. Weidner, W. R. Fair, R. Marlin, E. B. Pettengill, C. J. Raisin, S. Dunn-Emke, L. Crutchfield, F. N. Jacobs, R. J. Barnard, W. J. Aronson, P. McCormac, D. J. McKnight, J. D. Fein, A. M. Dnistrian, J. Weinstein, T. H. Ngo, N. R. Mendell, and P. R. Carroll. "Intensive Lifestyle Changes May Affect the Progression of Prostate Cancer." *J Urol* 174, no. 3 (2005): 1065–70.

27. Cassileth, B. R. *The Alternative Medicine Handbook.* New York: W. W. Norton, 1998; and Sloan-Kettering, "About Herbs, Botanicals & Other Products." Memorial Sloan-Kettering Cancer Center. http://www.mskcc.org/aboutherbs (accessed June 20, 2009).

28. Lippman, S. M., E. A. Klein, P. J. Goodman, M. S. Lucia, I. M. Thompson, L. G. Ford, H. L. Parnes, L. M. Minasian, J. M. Gaziano, J. A. Hartline, J. K. Parsons, J. D. Bearden, 3rd, E. D. Crawford, G. E. Goodman, J. Claudio, E. Winquist, E. D. Cook, D. D. Karp, P. Walther, M. M. Lieber, A. R. Kristal, A. K. Darke, K. B. Arnold, P. A. Ganz, R. M. Santella, D. Albanes, P. R. Taylor, J. L. Probstfield, T. J. Jagpal, J. J. Crowley, F. L. Meyskens, Jr., L. H. Baker, and C. A. Coltman, Jr. "Effect of Selenium and Vitamin E on Risk of Prostate Cancer and Other Cancers: The Selenium and Vitamin E Cancer Prevention Trial (Select)." *JAMA* 301, no. 1.

29. Sloan-Kettering, "About Herbs, Botanicals & Other Products." Memorial Sloan-Kettering Cancer Center. http://www.mskcc.org/aboutherbs (accessed June 20, 2009).

8. DETECTING PROSTATE CANCER WITH PSA AND OTHER TESTS

1. Makarov, D. V., S. Loeb, R. H. Getzenberg, and A. W. Partin. "Biomarkers for Prostate Cancer." *Ann Rev Med* 60 (2009): 139–51.

2. Schroder, F. H., J. Hugosson, M. J. Roobol, T. L. Tammela, S. Ciatto, V. Nelen, M. Kwiatkowski, M. Lujan, H. Lilja, M. Zappa, L. J. Denis, F. Recker, A. Berenguer, L. Maattanen, C. H. Bangma, G. Aus, A. Villers, X. Rebillard, T. van der Kwast, B. G. Blijenberg, S. M. Moss, H. J. de Koning, and A. Auvinen. "Screening and Prostate-Cancer Mortality in a Randomized European Study." *N Engl J Med* 360, no. 13 (2009): 1320–28.

3. Draisma, G., R. Etzioni, A. Tsodikov, A. Mariotto, E. Wever, R. Gulati, E. Feuer, and H. de Koning. "Lead Time and Overdiagnosis in Prostate-Specific Antigen Screening: Importance of Methods and Context." *J Natl Cancer Inst* 101, no. 6 (2009): 374–83.

4. Andriole, G. L., E. D. Crawford, R. L. Grubb, 3rd, S. S. Buys, D. Chia, T. R. Church, M. N. Fouad, E. P. Gelmann, P. A. Kvale, D. J. Reding, J. L. Weissfeld, L. A. Yokochi, B. O'Brien, J. D. Clapp, J. M. Rathmell, T. L. Riley, R. B. Hayes, B. S. Kramer, G. Izmirlian, A. B. Miller, P. F. Pinsky, P. C. Prorok, J. K. Gohagan, and C. D. Berg. "Mortality Results from a Randomized Prostate-Cancer Screening Trial." *N Engl J Med* 360, no. 13 (2009): 1310–19.

5. Barry, M. J. "Screening for Prostate Cancer—The Controversy That Refuses to Die." *N Engl J Med* 360, no. 13 (2009): 1351–54.

6. U.S. Preventive Services Task Force. "Screening for Prostate Cancer." U.S. Department of Health and Human Services. http://www.ahrq.gov/CLINIC/uspstf08/prostate/prostaters .htm (accessed June 22, 2009).

7. U.S. Preventive Services Task Force. "Screening for Prostate Cancer." U.S. Department of Health and Human Services. http://www.ahrq.gov/CLINIC/uspstf08/prostate/prostaters .htm (accessed June 22, 2009).

8. American Cancer Society. "Guidelines for the Early Detection of Cancer." American Cancer Society. http://www.cancer.org/docroot/ped/content/ped_2_3x_acs_cancer_detection _guidelines_36.asp (accessed June 10, 2009).

9. Urology Health. "American Urological Society. What You Should Know About Prostate Cancer Screening." AUA Foundation. http://www.urologyhealth.org/6578_BrochureR1.pdf (accessed June 19, 2009).

10. Lilja, H. "Biology of Prostate-Specific Antigen." *Urology* 62, no. 5 Suppl 1 (2003): 27–33.

11. Thompson, I. M., D. P. Ankerst, C. Chi, P. J. Goodman, C. M. Tangen, M. S. Lucia, Z. Feng, H. L. Parnes, and C. A. Coltman, Jr. "Assessing Prostate Cancer Risk: Results from the Prostate Cancer Prevention Trial." *J Natl Cancer Inst* 98, no. 8 (2006): 529–34; and Thompson, I. M., D. K. Pauler, P. J. Goodman, C. M. Tangen, M. S. Lucia, H. L. Parnes, L. M. Minasian, L. G. Ford, S. M. Lippman, E. D. Crawford, J. J. Crowley, and C. A. Coltman, Jr. "Prevalence of Prostate Cancer Among Men with a Prostate-Specific Antigen Level < or =4.0 Ng Per Milliliter." *N Engl J Med* 350, no. 22 (2004): 2239–46; and University of Texas Health Science Center. "Risk of Biopsy-Detectable Prostate Cancer." UT Health Science Center San Antonio. http://deb.uthscsa.edu/URORiskCalc/Pages/uroriskcalc.jsp (accessed June 23, 2009).

12. Crawford, E. D., S. Leewansangtong, S. Goktas, K. Holthaus, and M. Baier. "Efficiency of Prostate-Specific Antigen and Digital Rectal Examination in Screening, Using 4.0 Ng/Ml and Age-Specific Reference Range as a Cutoff for Abnormal Values." *Prostate* 38, no. 4 (1999): 296–302.

13. Catalona, W. J., J. P. Richie, F. R. Ahmann, M. A. Hudson, P. T. Scardino, R. C. Flanigan, J. B. deKernion, T. L. Ratliff, L. R. Kavoussi, B. L. Dalkin, et al. "Comparison of Digital Rectal Examination and Serum Prostate Specific Antigen in the Early Detection of Prostate Cancer: Results of a Multicenter Clinical Trial of 6,630 Men." *J Urol* 151, no. 5 (1994): 1283–90.

14. Thompson, I. M., D. K. Pauler, P. J. Goodman, C. M. Tangen, M. S. Lucia, H. L. Parnes, L. M. Minasian, L. G. Ford, S. M. Lippman, E. D. Crawford, J. J. Crowley, and C. A. Coltman, Jr. "Prevalence of Prostate Cancer Among Men with a Prostate-Specific Antigen Level < or =4.0 Ng Per Milliliter." *N Engl J Med* 350, no. 22 (2004): 2239–46.

15. Makarov, D. V., S. Loeb, R. H. Getzenberg, and A. W. Partin. "Biomarkers for Prostate Cancer." *Ann Rev Med* 60 (2009): 139–51.

16. Scardino, P. T. "The Responsible Use of Antibiotics for an Elevated PSA Level." *Natl Clin Pract Urol* 4, no. 1 (2007): 1.

17. Crawford, E. D., M. J. Schutz, S. Clejan, J. Drago, M. I. Resnick, G. W. Chodak, L. G. Gomella, M. Austenfeld, N. N. Stone, and B. J. Miles. "The Effect of Digital Rectal Examination on Prostate-Specific Antigen Levels." *JAMA* 267, no. 16 (1992): 2227–28; and Stenner, J., K. Holthaus, S. H. Mackenzie, and E. D. Crawford. "The Effect of Ejaculation on Prostate-Specific Antigen in a Prostate Cancer-Screening Population." *Urology* 51, no. 3 (1998): 455–59.

18. Catalona, W. J., J. P. Richie, F. R. Ahmann, M. A. Hudson, P. T. Scardino, R. C. Flanigan, J. B. deKernion, T. L. Ratliff, L. R. Kavoussi, B. L. Dalkin, et al. "Comparison of Digital Rectal Examination and Serum Prostate Specific Antigen in the Early Detection of Prostate Cancer: Results of a Multicenter Clinical Trial of 6,630 Men." *J Urol* 151, no. 5 (1994): 1283–90.

19. Thompson, I. M., D. K. Pauler, P. J. Goodman, C. M. Tangen, M. S. Lucia, H. L. Parnes, L. M. Minasian, L. G. Ford, S. M. Lippman, E. D. Crawford, J. J. Crowley, and C. A. Coltman, Jr. "Prevalence of Prostate Cancer Among Men with a Prostate-Specific Antigen Level < or =4.0 Ng Per Milliliter." *N Engl J Med* 350, no. 22 (2004): 2239–46; and University of Texas Health Science Center. "Risk of Biopsy-Detectable Prostate Cancer." UT Health Science Center San Antonio. http://deb.uthscsa.edu/URORiskCalc/Pages/uroriskcalc.jsp (accessed June 23, 2009).

20. Eastham, J. A., E. Riedel, P. T. Scardino, M. Shike, M. Fleisher, A. Schatzkin, E. Lanza, L. Latkany, and C. B. Begg. "Variation of Serum Prostate-Specific Antigen Levels: An Evaluation of Year-to-Year Fluctuations." *JAMA* 289, no. 20 (2003): 2695–700.

21. Lilja, H., D. Ulmert, and A. J. Vickers. "Prostate-Specific Antigen and Prostate Cancer: Prediction, Detection and Monitoring." *Natl Rev Cancer* 8, no. 4 (2008): 268–78.
22. Gann, P. H., C. H. Hennekens, and M. J. Stampfer. "A Prospective Evaluation of Plasma Prostate-Specific Antigen for Detection of Prostatic Cancer." *JAMA* 273, no. 4 (1995): 289–94.
23. Lilja, H., D. Ulmert, and A. J. Vickers. "Prostate-Specific Antigen and Prostate Cancer: Prediction, Detection and Monitoring." *Natl Rev Cancer* 8, no. 4 (2008): 268–78.
24. Catalona, W. J., A. W. Partin, K. M. Slawin, M. K. Brawer, R. C. Flanigan, A. Patel, J. P. Richie, J. B. deKernion, P. C. Walsh, P. T. Scardino, P. H. Lange, E. N. Subong, R. E. Parson, G. H. Gasior, K. G. Loveland, and P. C. Southwick. "Use of the Percentage of Free Prostate-Specific Antigen to Enhance Differentiation of Prostate Cancer from Benign Prostatic Disease: A Prospective Multicenter Clinical Trial." *JAMA* 279, no. 19 (1998): 1542–47.
25. Benson, M. C., I. S. Whang, A. Pantuck, K. Ring, S. A. Kaplan, C. A. Olsson, and W. H. Cooner. "Prostate Specific Antigen Density: A Means of Distinguishing Benign Prostatic Hypertrophy and Prostate Cancer." *J Urol* 147, no. 3, pt. 2 (1992): 815–16.
26. Carter, H. B., J. D. Pearson, E. J. Metter, L. J. Brant, D. W. Chan, R. Andres, J. L. Fozard, and P. C. Walsh. "Longitudinal Evaluation of Prostate-Specific Antigen Levels in Men with and Without Prostate Disease." *JAMA* 267, no. 16 (1992): 2215–20.
27. O'Brien, M. F., A. M. Cronin, P. A. Fearn, B. Smith, J. Stasi, B. Guillonneau, P. T. Scardino, J. A. Eastham, A. J. Vickers, and H. Lilja. "Pretreatment Prostate-Specific Antigen (PSA) Velocity and Doubling Time Are Associated with Outcome but Neither Improves Prediction of Outcome Beyond Pretreatment PSA Alone in Patients Treated with Radical Prostatectomy." *J Clin Oncol* 27, no. 3 (2009): 3591–97.
28. Vickers, A. J., C. Savage, M. F. O'Brien, and H. Lilja. "Systematic Review of Pretreatment Prostate-Specific Antigen Velocity and Doubling Time as Predictors for Prostate Cancer." *J Clin Oncol* 27, no. 3 (2009): 398–403.
29. Fradet, Y. "Biomarkers in Prostate Cancer Diagnosis and Prognosis: Beyond Prostate-Specific Antigen." *Curr Opin Urol* 19, no. 3 (2009): 243–46.
30. Zheng, S. L., J. Sun, F. Wiklund, S. Smith, P. Stattin, G. Li, H. O. Adami, F. C. Hsu, Y. Zhu, K. Balter, A. K. Kader, A. R. Turner, W. Liu, E. R. Bleecker, D. A. Meyers, D. Duggan, J. D. Carpten, B. L. Chang, W. B. Isaacs, J. Xu, and H. Gronberg. "Cumulative Association of Five Genetic Variants with Prostate Cancer." *N Engl J Med* 358, no. 9 (2008): 910–19.

9. BIOPSY

1. Eastham, J. A., E. Riedel, P. T. Scardino, M. Shike, M. Fleisher, A. Schatzkin, E. Lanza, L. Latkany, and C. B. Begg. "Variation of Serum Prostate-Specific Antigen Levels: An Evaluation of Year-to-Year Fluctuations." *JAMA* 289, no. 20 (2003): 2695–700.
2. Makarov, D. V., S. Loeb, R. H. Getzenberg, and A. W. Partin. "Biomarkers for Prostate Cancer." *Ann Rev Med* 60 (2009): 139–51; and Lilja, H., D. Ulmert, and A. J. Vickers. "Prostate-Specific Antigen and Prostate Cancer: Prediction, Detection and Monitoring." *Natl Rev Cancer* 8, no. 4 (2008): 268–78.
3. Catalona, W. J., J. P. Richie, F. R. Ahmann, M. A. Hudson, P. T. Scardino, R. C. Flanigan, J. B. deKernion, T. L. Ratliff, L. R. Kavoussi, B. L. Dalkin, et al. "Comparison of Digital Rectal Examination and Serum Prostate Specific Antigen in the Early Detection of Prostate Cancer: Results of a Multicenter Clinical Trial of 6,630 Men." *J Urol* 151, no. 5 (1994): 1283–90.
4. Watanabe, H. "History of Ultrasound in Nephrourology." *Ultrasound Med Biol* 27, no. 4 (2001): 447–53.
5. Ragde, H., H. C. Aldape, and C. M. Bagley, Jr. "Ultrasound-Guided Prostate Biopsy. Biopsy Gun Superior to Aspiration." *Urology* 32, no. 6 (1988): 503–6.

6. Scattoni, V., A. Zlotta, R. Montironi, C. Schulman, P. Rigatti, and F. Montorsi. "Extended and Saturation Prostatic Biopsy in the Diagnosis and Characterisation of Prostate Cancer: A Critical Analysis of the Literature." *Eur Urol* 52, no. 5 (2007): 1309–22.

7. Barzell, W. E., and M. R. Melamed. "Appropriate Patient Selection in the Focal Treatment of Prostate Cancer: The Role of Transperineal 3-Dimensional Pathologic Mapping of the Prostate—a 4-Year Experience." *Urology* 70, no. 6 Suppl (2007): 27–35.

8. Carey, J. M., and H. J. Korman. "Transrectal Ultrasound Guided Biopsy of the Prostate. Do Enemas Decrease Clinically Significant Complications?" *J Urol* 166, no. 1 (2001): 82–85.

9. Rodriguez, L.V., and M. K. Terris. "Risks and Complications of Transrectal Ultrasound Guided Prostate Needle Biopsy: A Prospective Study and Review of the Literature." *J Urol* 160, no. 6, pt. 1 (1998): 2115–20.

10. American Urological Association Education and Research. "Antibiotic Prophylaxis Pocket Tables." American Urological Association. http://www.auanet.org/content/guidelines-and-quality-care/clinical-guidelines/appockettables.pdf (accessed June 24, 2009).

11. Obek, C., B. Ozkan, B. Tunc, G. Can, V. Yalcin, and V. Solok. "Comparison of 3 Different Methods of Anesthesia Before Transrectal Prostate Biopsy: A Prospective Randomized Trial." *J Urol* 172, no. 2 (2004): 502–5.

12. Roehl, K. A., J. A. Antenor, and W. J. Catalona. "Serial Biopsy Results in Prostate Cancer Screening Study." *J Urol* 167, no. 6 (2002): 2435–39.

13. Hricak, H., P. L. Choyke, S. C. Eberhardt, S. A. Leibel, and P. T. Scardino. "Imaging Prostate Cancer: A Multidisciplinary Perspective." *Radiology* 243, no. 1 (2007): 28–53.

14. Bastacky, S. S., P. C. Walsh, and J. I. Epstein. "Needle Biopsy Associated Tumor Tracking of Adenocarcinoma of the Prostate." *J Urol* 145, no. 5 (1991): 1003–7.

15. Bostwick, D. G., and J. Qian. "High-Grade Prostatic Intraepithelial Neoplasia." *Mod Pathol* 17, no. 3 (2004): 360–79.

16. National Cancer Institute. "Cancer Facts: Tumor Grade: Questions and Answers." U.S. National Institutes of Health. http://www.cancer.gov/cancertopics/factsheet/detection/tumor-grade (accessed June 24, 2009).

17. Humphrey, P. A. "Gleason Grading and Prognostic Factors in Carcinoma of the Prostate." *Mod Pathol* 17, no. 3 (2004): 292–306.

18. Stamey, T. A., C. M. Yemoto, J. E. McNeal, B. M. Sigal, and I. M. Johnstone. "Prostate Cancer Is Highly Predictable: A Prognostic Equation Based on All Morphological Variables in Radical Prostatectomy Specimens." *J Urol* 163, no. 4 (2000): 1155–60.

19. Tarkan, L. "Value of Second Opinion Is Underscored in a Study of Biopsies." Published April 4, 2000. *New York Times*. http://www.nytimes.com/2000/04/04/health/value-of-second-opinions-is-underscored-in-study-of-biopsies.html?pagewanted=all (accessed June 24, 2009).

20. Albertsen, P. C., J. A. Hanley, G. H. Barrows, D. F. Penson, P. D. Kowalczyk, M. M. Sanders, and J. Fine. "Prostate Cancer and the Will Rogers Phenomenon." *J Natl Cancer Inst* 97, no. 17 (2005): 1248–53.

21. Yossepowitch, O., S. E. Eggener, F. J. Bianco, Jr., B. S. Carver, A. Serio, P. T. Scardino, and J. A. Eastham. "Radical Prostatectomy for Clinically Localized, High Risk Prostate Cancer: Critical Analysis of Risk Assessment Methods." *J Urol* 178, no. 2 (2007): 493–99.

22. King, C. R., J. E. McNeal, H. Gill, and J. C. Presti, Jr. "Extended Prostate Biopsy Scheme Improves Reliability of Gleason Grading: Implications for Radiotherapy Patients." *Int J Radiat Oncol Biol Phys* 59, no. 2 (2004): 386–91.

23. Berglund, R. K., T. A. Masterson, K. C. Vora, S. E. Eggener, J. A. Eastham, and B. D. Guillonneau. "Pathological Upgrading and Up Staging with Immediate Repeat Biopsy in Patients Eligible for Active Surveillance." *J Urol* 180, no. 5 (2008): 1964–67; discussion 1967–68.

24. Nelson, E. C., A. J. Cambio, J. C. Yang, J. H. Ok, P. N. Lara, Jr., and C. P. Evans. "Clinical Implications of Neuroendocrine Differentiation in Prostate Cancer." *Prostate Cancer Prostatic Dis* 10, no. 1 (2007): 6–14.

25. Bock, B. J., and D. G. Bostwick. "Does Prostatic Ductal Adenocarcinoma Exist?" *Am J Surg Pathol* 23, no. 7 (1999): 781–85.

26. Habermacher, G. M., J. T. Chason, and A. J. Schaeffer. "Prostatitis/Chronic Pelvic Pain Syndrome." *Ann Rev Med* 57 (2006): 195–206.

27. Bostwick, D. G., and J. Qian. "High-Grade Prostatic Intraepithelial Neoplasia." *Mod Pathol* 17, no. 3 (2004): 360–79.

28. Epstein, J. I., and S. R. Potter. "The Pathological Interpretation and Significance of Prostate Needle Biopsy Findings: Implications and Current Controversies." *J Urol* 166, no. 2 (2001): 402–10.

29. Lopez-Corona, E., M. Ohori, P. T. Scardino, V. E. Reuter, M. Gonen, and M. W. Kattan. "A Nomogram for Predicting a Positive Repeat Prostate Biopsy in Patients with a Previous Negative Biopsy Session." *J Urol* 170, no. 4, pt. 1 (2003): 1184–88; discussion 1188.

10. UNDERSTANDING YOUR CANCER

1. American Cancer Society. "Cancer Facts and Figures 2009." American Cancer Society. http://www.cancer.org/downloads/STT/500809web.pdf (accessed July 1, 2009); and American Cancer Society, "How Many Men Get Prostate Cancer." American Cancer Society. http://www.cancer.org/docroot/CRI/content/CRI_2_2_1X_How_many_men_get_prostate_cancer_36.asp (accessed July 1, 2009).

2. Makarov, D.V., S. Loeb, R. H. Getzenberg, and A. W. Partin. "Biomarkers for Prostate Cancer." *Ann Rev Med* 60 (2009): 139–51.

3. Kikuchi, E., P. T. Scardino, T. M. Wheeler, K. M. Slawin, and M. Ohori. "Is Tumor Volume an Independent Prognostic Factor in Clinically Localized Prostate Cancer?" *J Urol* 172, no. 2 (2004): 508–11.

4. Kundu, S. D., K. A. Roehl, X. Yu, J. A. Antenor, B. K. Suarez, and W. J. Catalona. "Prostate Specific Antigen Density Correlates with Features of Prostate Cancer Aggressiveness." *J Urol* 177, no. 2 (2007): 505–9.

5. Singh, H., E. I. Canto, S. F. Shariat, D. Kadmon, B. J. Miles, T. M. Wheeler, and K. M. Slawin. "Six Additional Systematic Lateral Cores Enhance Sextant Biopsy Prediction of Pathological Features at Radical Prostatectomy." *J Urol* 171, no. 1 (2004): 204–9.

6. Shinohara, K., T. M. Wheeler, and P. T. Scardino. "The Appearance of Prostate Cancer on Transrectal Ultrasonography: Correlation of Imaging and Pathological Examinations." *J Urol* 142, no. 1 (1989): 76–82.

7. Halpern, E. J., F. Frauscher, S. E. Strup, L. N. Nazarian, P. O'Kane, and L. G. Gomella. "Prostate: High-Frequency Doppler US Imaging for Cancer Detection." *Radiology* 225, no. 1 (2002): 71–77.

8. Hricak, H., P. L. Choyke, S. C. Eberhardt, S. A. Leibel, and P. T. Scardino. "Imaging Prostate Cancer: A Multidisciplinary Perspective." *Radiology* 243, no. 1 (2007): 28–53.

9. Hricak, H., and P. T. Scardino, eds. *Contemporary Issues in Cancer Imaging: Prostate Cancer.* New York: Cambridge University Press, 2009.

10. Edge, S. B., D. R. Byrd, M. Carducci, C. C. Compton, A. G. Fritz, F. L. Greene, and A. Trotti, eds. *AJCC Cancer Staging Manual*, 7th ed. New York: Springer-Verlag, 2009.

11. Makarov, D.V., B.J. Trock, E.B. Humphreys, L.A. Mangold, P.C. Walsh, J.I. Epstein, and A.W. Partin. "Prostate Cancer: The Partin Tables." Johns-Hopkins University. http://urology.jhu.edu/prostate/partintables.php (accessed July 2, 2009).

12. Ohori, M., M. W. Kattan, H. Koh, N. Maru, K. M. Slawin, S. Shariat, M. Muramoto, V. E. Reuter, T. M. Wheeler, and P. T. Scardino. "Predicting the Presence and Side of Extracapsular Extension: A Nomogram for Staging Prostate Cancer." *J Urol* 171, no. 5 (2004): 1844–49.

13. D'Amico, A. V., M. H. Chen, K. A. Roehl, and W. J. Catalona. "Preoperative PSA Velocity and the Risk of Death from Prostate Cancer After Radical Prostatectomy." *N Engl J Med* 351, no. 2 (2004): 125–35.

14. Vickers, A. J., C. Savage, M. F. O'Brien, and H. Lilja. "Systematic Review of Pretreatment Prostate-Specific Antigen Velocity and Doubling Time as Predictors for Prostate Cancer." *J Clin Oncol* 27, no. 3 (2009): 398–403.

15. Eastham, J. A., E. Riedel, P. T. Scardino, M. Shike, M. Fleisher, A. Schatzkin, E. Lanza, L. Latkany, and C. B. Begg. "Variation of Serum Prostate-Specific Antigen Levels: An Evaluation of Year-to-Year Fluctuations." *JAMA* 289, no. 20 (2003): 2695–700.

16. Lilja, H., D. Ulmert, and A. J. Vickers. "Prostate-Specific Antigen and Prostate Cancer: Prediction, Detection and Monitoring." *Nat Rev Cancer* 8, no. 4 (2008): 268–78; and Ulmert, D., A. M. Cronin, T. Bjork, M. F. O'Brien, P. T. Scardino, J. A. Eastham, C. Becker, G. Berglund, A. J. Vickers, and H. Lilja. "Prostate-Specific Antigen at or before Age 50 as a Predictor of Advanced Prostate Cancer Diagnosed up to 25 Years Later: A Case-Control Study." *BMC Med* 6 (2008): 6.

17. D'Amico, A. V., M. H. Chen, K. A. Roehl, and W. J. Catalona. "Preoperative PSA Velocity and the Risk of Death from Prostate Cancer After Radical Prostatectomy." *N Engl J Med* 351, no. 2 (2004): 125–35.

18. Bianco, F. J., Jr., M. W. Kattan, and P. T. Scardino. "PSA Velocity and Prostate Cancer." *N Engl J Med* 351, no. 17 (2004): 1800–802; author reply 1800–802; and O'Brien, M. F., A. M. Cronin, P. A. Fearn, B. Smith, J. Stasi, B. Guillonneau, P. T. Scardino, J. A. Eastham, A. J. Vickers, and H. Lilja. "Pretreatment Prostate-Specific Antigen (PSA) Velocity and Doubling Time Are Associated with Outcome but Neither Improves Prediction of Outcome Beyond Pretreatment PSA Alone in Patients Treated with Radical Prostatectomy." *J Clin Oncol* 27, no. 22 (2009): 3591–97.

19. NCCN Subscriptions. "Practice Guidelines in Oncology—v. 2, 2009. Prostate Cancer." National Comprehensive Cancer Network. http://www.nccn.org/professionals/physician _gls/PDF/prostate.pdf (accessed July 1, 2009).

20. Shariat, S. F., P. I. Karakiewicz, N. Suardi, and M. W. Kattan. "Comparison of Nomograms with Other Methods for Predicting Outcomes in Prostate Cancer: A Critical Analysis of the Literature." *Clin Cancer Res* 14, no. 14 (2008): 4400–407; and Stephenson, A. J., and M. W. Kattan. "Nomograms for Prostate Cancer." *BJU Int* 98, no. 1 (2006): 39–46.

21. Dotan, Z. A., F. J. Bianco, Jr., F. Rabbani, J. A. Eastham, P. Fearn, H. I. Scher, K. W. Kelly, H. N. Chen, H. Schoder, H. Hricak, P. T. Scardino, and M. W. Kattan. "Pattern of Prostate-Specific Antigen (PSA) Failure Dictates the Probability of a Positive Bone Scan in Patients with an Increasing PSA After Radical Prostatectomy." *J Clin Oncol* 23, no. 9 (2005): 1962–68.

22. Hricak, H., and P. T. Scardino, eds. *Contemporary Issues in Cancer Imaging: Prostate Cancer*. New York: Cambridge University Press, 2009.

23. Cooperberg, M. R., D. P. Lubeck, G. D. Grossfeld, S. S. Mehta, and P. R. Carroll. "Contemporary Trends in Imaging Test Utilization for Prostate Cancer Staging: Data from the Cancer of the Prostate Strategic Urologic Research Endeavor." *J Urol* 168, no. 2 (2002): 491–95; and American Urological Association Education and Research Inc. "Guideline for the Management of Clinically Localized Prostate Cancer: 2007 Update." American Urological Association. http://www.auanet.org/content/guidelines-and-quality-care/clinical-guidelines/main-reports/proscan07/content.pdf (accessed July 2, 2009).

24. D'Amico, A. V., R. Whittington, S. B. Malkowicz, D. Schultz, K. Blank, G. A. Broderick, J. E. Tomaszewski, A. A. Renshaw, I. Kaplan, C. J. Beard, and A. Wein. "Biochemical Outcome After Radical Prostatectomy, External Beam Radiation Therapy, or Interstitial Radiation Therapy for Clinically Localized Prostate Cancer." *JAMA* 280, no. 11 (1998): 969–74.

25. Yossepowitch, O., S. E. Eggener, F. J. Bianco, Jr., B. S. Carver, A. Serio, P. T. Scardino, and J. A. Eastham. "Radical Prostatectomy for Clinically Localized, High Risk Prostate Cancer: Critical Analysis of Risk Assessment Methods." *J Urol* 178, no. 2 (2007): 493–99; discussion 499.

26. Stephenson, A. J., and M. W. Kattan. "Nomograms for Prostate Cancer." *BJU Int* 98, no. 1 (2006): 39–46.

27. Makarov, D. V., B. J. Trock, E. B. Humphreys, L. A. Mangold, P. C. Walsh, J. I. Epstein, and A. W. Partin. "Updated Nomogram to Predict Pathologic Stage of Prostate Cancer Given Prostate-Specific Antigen Level, Clinical Stage, and Biopsy Gleason Score (Partin Tables) Based on Cases from 2000 to 2005." *Urology* 69, no. 6 (2007): 1095–101.

28. Stephenson, A. J., P. T. Scardino, J. A. Eastham, F. J. Bianco, Jr., Z. A. Dotan, P. A. Fearn, and M. W. Kattan. "Preoperative Nomogram Predicting the 10-Year Probability of Prostate Cancer Recurrence After Radical Prostatectomy." *J Natl Cancer Inst* 98, no. 10 (2006): 715–17.

29. Yossepowitch, O., S. E. Eggener, A. M. Serio, B. S. Carver, F. J. Bianco, Jr., P. T. Scardino, and J. A. Eastham. "Secondary Therapy, Metastatic Progression, and Cancer-Specific Mortality in Men with Clinically High-Risk Prostate Cancer Treated with Radical Prostatectomy." *Eur Urol* 53, no. 5 (2008): 950–59.

11. UNDERSTANDING YOURSELF

1. Roth, A. J., B. Rosenfeld, A. B. Kornblith, C. Gibson, H. I. Scher, T. Curley-Smart, J. C. Holland, and W. Breitbart. "The Memorial Anxiety Scale for Prostate Cancer: Validation of a New Scale to Measure Anxiety in Men with Prostate Cancer." *Cancer* 97, no. 11 (2003): 2910–18.

2. NCCN. "NCCN Practice Guidelines for the Management of Psychosocial Distress. National Comprehensive Cancer Network." *Oncology* (Huntington) 13, no. 5A (1999): 113–47.

3. Us TOO "Us TOO International Prostate Cancer Education and Support Network." Us TOO International. http://www.ustoo.com/ (accessed July 2, 2009).

4. Ross, P. L., B. Littenberg, P. Fearn, P. T. Scardino, P. I. Karakiewicz, and M. W. Kattan. "Paper Standard Gamble: A Paper-Based Measure of Standard Gamble Utility for Current Health." *Int J Technol Assess Health Care* 19, no. 1 (2003): 135–47.

12. DECIDING HOW TO TREAT LOCALIZED PROSTATE CANCER

1. Howard, K. "Quality Adjusted Life Years (QALYs)." In M. W. Kattan, ed., *Encyclopedia of Medical Decision Making*. Thousand Oaks, CA: SAGE, 2009.

2. Bill-Axelson, A., L. Holmberg, F. Filen, M. Ruutu, H. Garmo, C. Busch, S. Nordling, M. Haggman, S. O. Andersson, S. Bratell, A. Spangberg, J. Palmgren, H. O. Adami, and J. E. Johansson. "Radical Prostatectomy Versus Watchful Waiting in Localized Prostate Cancer: The Scandinavian Prostate Cancer Group-4 Randomized Trial." *J Natl Cancer Inst* 100, no. 16 (2008): 1144–54.

3. D'Amico, A. V., R. Whittington, S. B. Malkowicz, D. Schultz, K. Blank, G. A. Broderick, J. E. Tomaszewski, A. A. Renshaw, I. Kaplan, C. J. Beard, and A. Wein. "Biochemical Outcome After Radical Prostatectomy, External Beam Radiation Therapy, or Interstitial Radiation Therapy for Clinically Localized Prostate Cancer." *JAMA* 280, no. 11 (1998): 969–74.

4. CDC Home. "CDC. FASTSTATS: Life Expectancy." Centers for Disease Control and Prevention. http://www.cdc.gov/nchs/fastats/lifexpec.htm (accessed July 2, 2009).

5. de Groot, V., H. Beckerman, G. J. Lankhorst, and L. M. Bouter. "How to Measure Comorbidity. A Critical Review of Available Methods." *J Clin Epidemiol* 56, no. 3 (2003): 221–29.

6. Berglund, R. K., T. A. Masterson, K. C. Vora, S. E. Eggener, J. A. Eastham, and B. D. Guillonneau. "Pathological Upgrading and Up Staging with Immediate Repeat Biopsy in Patients Eligible for Active Surveillance." *J Urol* 180, no. 5 (2008): 1964–67; discussion 1967–68.

7. Zelefsky M, et al. "A Comparison of Surgery and Radiation for the Treatment of Localized Prostate Cancer: A Case Control Analysis." *J Clin Oncol.* In press (2010).

8. Shipley, W. U., P. T. Scardino, D. S. Kaufman, and M. W. Kattan. "Advising Patients with Early Prostatic Cancer on Their Treatment Decision." In N. J. Vogelzang, P. T. Scardino, W. U. Shipley, and C. S. Coffey, eds., *The Comprehensive Textbook of Genitourinary Oncology*. Philadelphia: Lippincott Williams & Wilkins, 2005.

9. Sloan-Kettering. "Prediction Tools." Memorial Sloan-Kettering Cancer Center. http://www.mskcc. org/mskcc/html/5794.cfm (accessed July 2, 2009).

10. Stephenson, A. J., and M. W. Kattan. "Nomograms for Prostate Cancer." *BJU Int* 98, no. 1 (2006): 39–46.

11. Shariat, S. F., P. I. Karakiewicz, N. Suardi, and M. W. Kattan. "Comparison of Nomograms with Other Methods for Predicting Outcomes in Prostate Cancer: A Critical Analysis of the Literature." Clin Cancer Res 14, no. 14 (2008): 4400–407.

12. Bill-Axelson, A., L. Holmberg, F. Filen, M. Ruutu, H. Garmo, C. Busch, S. Nordling, M. Haggman, S. O. Andersson, A. Bratell, A. Spangberg, J. Palmgren, H. O. Adami, and J. E. Johansson. "Radical Prostatectomy Versus Watchful Waiting in Localized Prostate Cancer: The Scandinavian Prostate Cancer Group-4 Randomized Trial." *J Natl Cancer Inst* 100, no. 16 (2008): 1144–54.

13. Wilt, T. J., R. MacDonald, I. Rutks, T. A. Shamliyan, B. C. Taylor, and R. L. Kane. "Systematic Review: Comparative Effectiveness and Harms of Treatments for Clinically Localized Prostate Cancer." *Ann Intern Med* 148, no. 6 (2008): 435–48.

14. Hu, J. C., X. Gu, S. R. Lipsitz, M. J. Barry, A. V. D'Amico, A. C. Weinberg, and N. L. Keating. "Comparative Effectiveness of Minimally Invasive Vs Open Radical Prostatectomy." *JAMA* 302, no. 14 (2009): 1557–64.

15. Begg, C. B., E. R. Riedel, P. B. Bach, M. W. Kattan, D. Schrag, J. L. Warren, and P. T. Scardino. "Variations in Morbidity After Radical Prostatectomy." *N Engl J Med* 346, no. 15 (2002): 1138–44; Bianco, F. J., Jr., E. R. Riedel, C. B. Begg, M. W. Kattan, and P. T. Scardino. "Variations Among High Volume Surgeons in the Rate of Complications After Radical Prostatectomy: Further Evidence That Technique Matters." *J Urol* 173, no. 6 (2005): 2099–103; and Vickers, A. J., F. J. Bianco, A. M. Serio, J. A. Eastham, D. Schrag, E. A. Klein, A. M. Reuther, M. W. Kattan, J. E. Pontes, and P. T. Scardino. "The Surgical Learning Curve for Prostate Cancer Control After Radical Prostatectomy." *J Natl Cancer Inst* 99, no. 15 (2007): 1171–77.

16. Schroeck, F. R., T. L. Krupski, L. Sun, D. M. Albala, M. M. Price, T. J. Polascik, C. N. Robertson, A. K. Tewari, and J. W. Moul. "Satisfaction and Regret After Open Retropubic or Robot-Assisted Laparoscopic Radical Prostatectomy." *Eur Urol* 54, no. 4 (2008): 785–93.

17. Sanda, M. G., R. L. Dunn, J. Michalski, H. M. Sandler, L. Northouse, L. Hembroff, X. Lin, T. K. Greenfield, M. S. Litwin, C. S. Saigal, A. Mahadevan, E. Klein, A. Kibel, L. L. Pisters, D. Kuban, I. Kaplan, D. Wood, J. Ciezki, N. Shah, and J. T. Wei. "Quality of Life and Satisfaction with Outcome Among Prostate-Cancer Survivors." *N Engl J Med* 358, no. 12 (2008): 1250–61.

13. WATCHFUL WAITING

1. Scardino, P. T., R. Weaver, and M. A. Hudson. "Early Detection of Prostate Cancer." *Human Pathology* 23, no. 3 (1992): 211–22.

2. Berglund, R. K., T. A. Masterson, K. C. Vora, S. E. Eggener, J. A. Eastham, and B. D. Guillonneau. "Pathological Upgrading and Up Staging with Immediate Repeat Biopsy in Patients Eligible for Active Surveillance." *J Urol* 180, no. 5 (2008): 1964–67; discussion 1967–68; and Shukla-Dave, A., H. Hricak, M. W. Kattan, D. Pucar, K. Kuroiwa, H. N. Chen, J. Spector, J. A. Koutcher, K. L. Zakian, and P. T. Scardino. "The Utility of Magnetic Resonance Imaging and Spectroscopy for Predicting Insignificant Prostate Cancer: An Initial Analysis." *BJU Int* 99, no. 4 (2007): 786–93.

3. Johansson, J. E., L. Holmberg, S. Johansson, R. Bergstrom, and H. O. Adami. "Fifteen-Year Survival in Prostate Cancer. A Prospective, Population-Based Study in Sweden [see comments] [published erratum appears in *JAMA* 278, no. 3 (July 16,1997): 206." *JAMA* 277, no. 6 (1997): 467–71.

4. Holmberg, L., A. Bill-Axelson, F. Helgesen, J. O. Salo, P. Folmerz, M. Haggman, S. O. Andersson, A. Spangberg, C. Busch, S. Nordling, J. Palmgren, H. O. Adami, J. E. Johansson, and B. J. Norlen. "A Randomized Trial Comparing Radical Prostatectomy with Watchful Waiting in Early Prostate Cancer." *N Engl J Med* 347, no. 11 (2002): 781–89.

5. Bill-Axelson, A., L. Holmberg, F. Filen, M. Ruutu, H. Garmo, C. Busch, S. Nordling, M. Haggman, S. O. Andersson, S. Bratell, A. Spangberg, J. Palmgren, H. O. Adami, and J. E. Johansson. "Radical Prostatectomy Versus Watchful Waiting in Localized Prostate Cancer: The Scandinavian Prostate Cancer Group-4 Randomized Trial." *J Natl Cancer Inst* 100, no. 16 (2008): 1144–54.

6. Draisma, G., R. Etzioni, A. Tsodikov, A. Mariotto, E. Wever, R. Gulati, E. Feuer, and H. de Koning. "Lead Time and Overdiagnosis in Prostate-Specific Antigen Screening: Importance of Methods and Context." *J Natl Cancer Inst* 101, no. 6 (2009): 374–83.

7. Klotz, L. "Active Surveillance for Favorable Risk Prostate Cancer: Rationale, Risks, and Results." *Urol Oncol* 25, no. 6 (2007): 505–9.

8. Ohori, M., T. M. Wheeler, N. Maru, A. Erbersdobler, M. Graefen, H. Huland, H. Koh, S. F. Shariat, K. M. Slawin, J. A. Eastham, P. T. Scardino, and M. W. Kattan. "Counseling Men with Prostate Cancer (PCA): A Nomogram for Predicting the Presence of Indolent (Small, Well-Moderately Differentiated, Confined) Tumors." *J Urol* 169, no. 4 (2003): 425–26.

9. Ohori, M., T. M. Wheeler, N. Maru, A. Erbersdobler, M. Graefen, H. Huland, H. Koh, S. F. Shariat, K. M. Slawin, J. A. Eastham, P. T. Scardino, and M. W. Kattan. "Counseling Men with Prostate Cancer (PCA): A Nomogram for Predicting the Presence of Indolent (Small, Well-Moderately Differentiated, Confined) Tumors." *J Urol* 169, no. 4 (2003): 425–26.

10. Eggener, S. E., A. Mueller, R. K. Berglund, R. Ayyathurai, C. Soloway, M. S. Soloway, R. Abouassaly, E. A. Klein, S. J. Jones, C. Zappavigna, L. Goldenberg, P. T. Scardino, J. A. Eastham, and B. Guillonneau. "A Multi-Institutional Evaluation of Active Surveillance for Low Risk Prostate Cancer." *J Urol* 181, no. 4 (2009): 1635–41; discussion 1641.

11. Patel, M. I., D. T. DeConcini, E. Lopez-Corona, M. Ohori, T. Wheeler, and P. T. Scardino. "An Analysis of Men with Clinically Localized Prostate Cancer Who Deferred Definitive Therapy." *J Urol* 171, no. 4 (2004): 1520–24.

12. Shukla-Dave, A., H. Hricak, M. W. Kattan, D. Pucar, K. Kuroiwa, H. N. Chen, J. Spector, J. A. Koutcher, K. L. Zakian, and P. T. Scardino. "The Utility of Magnetic Resonance Imaging and Spectroscopy for Predicting Insignificant Prostate Cancer: An Initial Analysis." *BJU Int* 99, no. 4 (2007): 786–93.

13. CDC Home. "CDC. FASTSTATS: Life Expectancy." Centers for Disease Control and Prevention. http://www.cdc.gov/nchs/fastats/lifexpec.htm (accessed July 2, 2009).

14. Patel, M. I., D. T. DeConcini, E. Lopez-Corona, M. Ohori, T. Wheeler, and P. T. Scardino. "An Analysis of Men with Clinically Localized Prostate Cancer Who Deferred Definitive Therapy." *J Urol* 171, no. 4 (2004): 1520–24; and Klotz, L. "Active Surveillance for Favorable Risk Prostate Cancer: Rationale, Risks, and Results." *Urol Oncol* 25, no. 6 (2007): 505–9; and Eggener, S. E., A. Mueller, R. K. Berglund, R. Ayyathurai, C. Soloway, M. S. Soloway, R. Abouassaly, E. A. Klein, S. J. Jones, C. Zappavigna, L. Goldenberg, P. T. Scardino, J. A. Eastham, and B. Guillonneau. "A Multi-Institutional Evaluation of Active Surveillance for Low Risk Prostate Cancer." *J Urol* 181, no. 4 (2009): 1635–41; discussion 1641.

15. Eastham, J. A., E. Riedel, P. T. Scardino, M. Shike, M. Fleisher, A. Schatzkin, E. Lanza, L. Latkany, and C. B. Begg. "Variation of Serum Prostate-Specific Antigen Levels: An Evaluation of Year-to-Year Fluctuations." *JAMA* 289, no. 20 (2003): 2695–700.

16. Makarov, D.V., S. Loeb, R. H. Getzenberg, and A.W. Partin. "Biomarkers for Prostate Cancer." *Ann Rev Med* 60 (2009): 139–51.

17. Vickers, A. J., C. Savage, M. F. O'Brien, and H. Lilja. "Systematic Review of Pretreatment Prostate-Specific Antigen Velocity and Doubling Time as Predictors for Prostate Cancer." *J Clin Oncol* 27, no. 3 (2009): 398–403.

18. Berglund, R. K., T. A. Masterson, K. C.Vora, S. E. Eggener, J. A. Eastham, and B. D. Guillonneau. "Pathological Upgrading and Up Staging with Immediate Repeat Biopsy in Patients Eligible for Active Surveillance." *J Urol* 180, no. 5 (2008): 1964–67; discussion 1967–68.

19. Patel, M. I., D. T. DeConcini, E. Lopez-Corona, M. Ohori, T. Wheeler, and P. T. Scardino. "An Analysis of Men with Clinically Localized Prostate Cancer Who Deferred Definitive Therapy." *J Urol* 171, no. 4 (2004): 1520–24; and Klotz, L. "Active Surveillance for Favorable Risk Prostate Cancer: Rationale, Risks, and Results." *Urol Oncol* 25, no. 6 (2007): 505–9; and Eggener, S. E., A. Mueller, R. K. Berglund, R. Ayyathurai, C. Soloway, M. S. Soloway, R. Abouassaly, E. A. Klein, S. J. Jones, C. Zappavigna, L. Goldenberg, P. T. Scardino, J. A. Eastham, and B. Guillonneau. "A Multi-Institutional Evaluation of Active Surveillance for Low Risk Prostate Cancer." *J Urol* 181, no. 4 (2009): 1635–41; discussion 1641.

20. Klotz, L. "Active Surveillance for Favorable Risk Prostate Cancer: Rationale, Risks, and Results." *Urol Oncol* 25, no. 6 (2007): 505–9; and Eggener, S. E., A. Mueller, R. K. Berglund, R. Ayyathurai, C. Soloway, M. S. Soloway, R. Abouassaly, E. A. Klein, S. J. Jones, C. Zappavigna, L. Goldenberg, P. T. Scardino, J. A. Eastham, and B. Guillonneau. "A Multi-Institutional Evaluation of Active Surveillance for Low Risk Prostate Cancer." *J Urol* 181, no. 4 (2009): 1635–41; discussion 1641.

21. Schatzkin, A., E. Lanza, D. Corle, P. Lance, F. Iber, B. Caan, M. Shike, J. Weissfeld, R. Burt, M. R. Cooper, J. W. Kikendall, J. Cahill, L. Freedman, J. Marshall, R. E. Schoen, and M. Slattery. "Lack of Effect of a Low-Fat, High-Fiber Diet on the Recurrence of Colorectal Adenomas." *N Engl J Med* 342, no. 16 (2000): 1149–55; and Shike, M., L. Latkany, E. Riedel, M. Fleisher, A. Schatzkin, E. Lanza, D. Corle, and C. B. Begg. "Lack of Effect of a Low-Fat, High-Fruit, -Vegetable, and -Fiber Diet on Serum Prostate-Specific Antigen of Men Without Prostate Cancer: Results from a Randomized Trial." *J Clin Oncol* 20, no. 17 (2002): 3592–98.

22. Lippman, S. M., E. A. Klein, P. J. Goodman, M. S. Lucia, I. M. Thompson, L. G. Ford, H. L. Parnes, L. M. Minasian, J. M. Gaziano, J. A. Hartline, J. K. Parsons, J. D. Bearden, 3rd, E. D. Crawford, G. E. Goodman, J. Claudio, E. Winquist, E. D. Cook, D. D. Karp, P. Walther, M. M. Lieber, A. R. Kristal, A. K. Darke, K. B. Arnold, P. A. Ganz, R. M. Santella, D. Albanes, P. R. Taylor, J. L. Probstfield, T. J. Jagpal, J. J. Crowley, F. L. Meyskens, Jr., L. H. Baker, and C. A. Coltman, Jr. "Effect of Selenium and Vitamin E on Risk of Prostate Cancer and Other Cancers: The Selenium and Vitamin E Cancer Prevention Trial (Select)." *JAMA* 301, no. 1 (2009): 39–51.

23. Fleshner, N., L. G. Gomella, M. S. Cookson, A. Finelli, A. Evans, S. S. Taneja, M. S. Lucia, E. Wolford, M. C. Somerville, and R. Rittmaster. "Delay in the Progression of Low-Risk Prostate Cancer: Rationale and Design of the Reduction by Dutasteride of Clinical Progression Events in Expectant Management (Redeem) Trial." *Contemp Clin Trials* 28, no. 6 (2007): 763–69.

14. SURGERY

1. Murphy, L. J. T. *The History of Urology*. Springfield, IL: Charles C. Thomas, 1972; and Skrepetis, K., and N. Antoniou. "History of Radical Perineal Prostatectomy." *J Pelvic Med Surg* 9, no. 2 (2003): 49–57.

2. Young, H. H. "The Early Diagnosis and Cure of Carcinoma of the Prostate: Being a Study of 40 Cases and Presentation of a Radical Operation Which Was Carried Out in Four Cases." *Johns Hopkins Hosp Bull* 16 (1905): 315.

3. Walsh, P. C., and P. J. Donker. "Impotence Following Radical Prostatectomy: Insight into Etiology and Prevention." *J Urol* 128, no. 3 (1982): 492–97.

4. Kim, E. D., R. Nath, K. M. Slawin, D. Kadmon, B. J. Miles, and P. T. Scardino. "Bilateral Nerve Grafting During Radical Retropubic Prostatectomy: Extended Follow-Up." *J Urol* 168, no. 1 (2002): 376–77.

5. Satkunasivam, R., S. Appu, R. Al-Azab, K. Hersey, G. Lockwood, J. Lipa, and N. E. Fleshner. "Recovery of Erectile Function After Unilateral and Bilateral Cavernous Nerve Interposition Grafting During Radical Pelvic Surgery." *J Urol* 181, no. 3 (2009): 1258–63.

6. Rabbani, F., A. M. Stapleton, M. W. Kattan, T. M. Wheeler, and P. T. Scardino. "Factors Predicting Recovery of Erections After Radical Prostatectomy." *J Urol* 164, no. 6 (2000): 1929–34.

7. Secin, F. P., T. M. Koppie, P. T. Scardino, J. A. Eastham, M. Patel, F. J. Bianco, R. Tal, J. Mulhall, J. J. Disa, P. G. Cordeiro, and F. Rabbani. "Bilateral Cavernous Nerve Interposition Grafting During Radical Retropubic Prostatectomy: Memorial Sloan-Kettering Cancer Center Experience." *J Urol* 177, no. 2 (2007): 664–68.

8. Davis, J. W., D. W. Chang, P. Chevray, R. Wang, Y. Shen, S. Wen, C. A. Pettaway, L. L. Pisters, D. A. Swanson, L. T. Madsen, N. Huber, P. Troncoso, R. J. Babaian, and C. G. Wood. "Randomized Phase II Trial Evaluation of Erectile Function After Attempted Unilateral Cavernous Nerve-Sparing Retropubic Radical Prostatectomy with Versus Without Unilateral Sural Nerve Grafting for Clinically Localized Prostate Cancer." *Eur Urol* 55, no. 5 (2009): 1135–43.

9. Eastham, J. A., and P. T. Scardino. "Radical Prostatectomy for Clinical Stage T1 and T2 Prostate Cancer." In N. J. Vogelzang, P. T. Scardino, W. U. Shipley, F. M. J. Debruyne, W. M. Linehan, eds., *The Comprehensive Textbook of Genitourinary Oncology*, pp. 166–89. Philadelphia: Lippincott Williams & Wilkins, 2005.

10. Walz, J., A. L. Burnett, A. J. Costello, J. A. Eastham, M. Graefen, B. Guillonneau, M. Menon, F. Montorsi, R. P. Myers, B. Rocco, and A. Villers. "A Critical Analysis of the Current Knowledge of Surgical Anatomy Related to Optimization of Cancer Control and Preservation of Continence and Erection in Candidates for Radical Prostatectomy." *Eur Urol* 57, no. 2 (2010): 179–92.

11. Saranchuk, J. W., M. W. Kattan, E. Elkin, A. K. Touijer, P. T. Scardino, and J. A. Eastham. "Achieving Optimal Outcomes After Radical Prostatectomy." *J Clin Oncol* 23, no. 18 (2005): 4146–51.

12. Eastham, J. A., P. T. Scardino, and M. W. Kattan. "Predicting an Optimal Outcome After Radical Prostatectomy: The Trifecta Nomogram." *J Urol* 179, no. 6 (2008): 2207–10; discussion 2210–11.

13. Sanda, M. G., R. L. Dunn, J. Michalski, H. M. Sandler, L. Northouse, L. Hembroff, X. Lin, T. K. Greenfield, M. S. Litwin, C. S. Saigal, A. Mahadevan, E. Klein, A. Kibel, L. L. Pisters, D. Kuban, I. Kaplan, D. Wood, J. Ciezki, N. Shah, and J. T. Wei. "Quality of Life and Satisfaction with Outcome Among Prostate-Cancer Survivors." *N Engl J Med* 358, no. 12 (2008): 1250–61.

14. Begg, C. B., E. R. Riedel, P. B. Bach, M. W. Kattan, D. Schrag, J. L. Warren, and P. T. Scardino. "Variations in Morbidity After Radical Prostatectomy." *N Engl J Med* 346, no. 15 (2002): 1138–44; and Vickers, A. J., F. J. Bianco, A. M. Serio, J. A. Eastham, D. Schrag, E. A. Klein, A. M. Reuther, M. W. Kattan, J. E. Pontes, and P. T. Scardino. "The Surgical Learning Curve for Prostate Cancer Control After Radical Prostatectomy." *J Natl Cancer Inst* 99, no. 15 (2007): 1171–77.

15. Guillonneau, B., I. S. Gill, G. Janetschek, and I. Tuerk. *Laparoscopic Techniques in Uro-Oncology*. London: Springer Verlag, 2009.

16. Tewari, A., J. Peabody, R. Sarle, G. Balakrishnan, A. Hemal, A. Shrivastava, and M. Menon. "Technique of da Vinci Robot–Assisted Anatomic Radical Prostatectomy." *Urology* 60, no. 4 (2002): 569–72.

17. Hu, J. C., X. Gu, S. R. Lipsitz, M. J. Barry, A. V. D'Amico, A. C. Weinberg, and N. L. Keating. "Comparative Effectiveness of Minimally Invasive Vs Open Radical Prostatectomy." *JAMA* 302, no. 14 (2009): 1557–64; and Caryn Rabin, R. "Study Finds Pros and Cons to Prostate Surgeries." October 13 2009. *New York Times.* http://www.nytimes.com/2009/10/14/health/research/14prostate.html (accessed November 2, 2009).

18. Touijer, K., J. A. Eastham, F. P. Secin, J. Romero Otero, A. Serio, J. Stasi, R. Sanchez-Salas, A. Vickers, V. E. Reuter, P. T. Scardino, and B. Guillonneau. "Comprehensive Prospective Comparative Analysis of Outcomes Between Open and Laparoscopic Radical Prostatectomy Conducted in 2003 to 2005." *J Urol* 179, no. 5 (2008): 1811–17; discussion 1817.

19. Vickers, A. J., C. J. Savage, M. Hruza, I. Tuerk, P. Koenig, L. Martinez-Pineiro, G. Janetschek, and B. Guillonneau. "The Surgical Learning Curve for Laparoscopic Radical Prostatectomy: A Retrospective Cohort Study." *Lancet Oncol* 10, no. 5 (2009): 475–80.

20. Hu, J. C., X. Gu, S. R. Lipsitz, M. J. Barry, A. V. D'Amico, A. C. Weinberg, and N. L. Keating. "Comparative Effectiveness of Minimally Invasive Vs Open Radical Prostatectomy." *JAMA* 302, no. 14 (2009): 1557–64; and Lowrance, J., et al. "Comparative Effectiveness of Surgical Treatments for Prostate Cancer: A Population-Based Analysis of Postoperative Outcomes." *J Urol.* In press (2010).

21. Bianco, F. J., Jr., A. J. Vickers, A. M. Cronin, E. A. Klein, J. A. Eastham, J. E. Pontes, and P. T. Scardino. "Variations Among Experienced Surgeons in Cancer Control After Open Radical Prostatectomy." *J Urol* (2010); epub.

22. Vickers, A. J., C. J. Savage, M. Hruza, I. Tuerk, P. Koenig, L. Martinez-Pineiro, G. Janetschek, and B. Guillonneau. "The Surgical Learning Curve for Laparoscopic Radical Prostatectomy: A Retrospective Cohort Study." *Lancet Oncol* 10, no. 5 (2009): 475–80.

23. Stephenson, A. J., M. W. Kattan, J. A. Eastham, F. J. Bianco, O. Yossepowitch, A. Vickers, E. A. Klein, D. P. Wood, and P. T. Scardino. "Prostate Cancer–Specific Mortality After Radical Prostatectomy for Patients Treated in the Prostate-Specific Antigen Era." *J Clin Oncol* 27, no. 26 (2009): 4300–305.

24. Eastham, J. A., J. R. Goad, E. Rogers, M. Ohori, M. W. Kattan, T. B. Boone, and P. T. Scardino. "Risk Factors for Urinary Incontinence After Radical Prostatectomy." *J Urol* 156, no. 5 (1996): 1707–13.

25. Rabbani, F., A. M. Stapleton, M. W. Kattan, T. M. Wheeler, and P. T. Scardino. "Factors Predicting Recovery of Erections After Radical Prostatectomy." *J Urol* 164, no. 6 (2000): 1929–34.

26. Eastham, J. A., and P. T. Scardino. "Radical Prostatectomy for Clinical Stage T1 and T2 Prostate Cancer." In N. J. Vogelzang, N. J., P. T. Scardino, W. U. Shipley, F. M. J. Debruyne, W. M. Linehan, eds., *The Comprehensive Textbook of Genitourinary Oncology*, pp. 166–89. Philadelphia: Lippincott Williams & Wilkins, 2005.

27. Catalona, W. J., and D. S. Smith. "Cancer Recurrence and Survival Rates After Anatomic Radical Retropubic Prostatectomy for Prostate Cancer: Intermediate-Term Results." *J Urol* 160, no. 6, pt. 2 (1998): 2428–34; and Dillioglugil, O., B. D. Leibman, N. S. Leibman, M. W. Kattan, A. L. Rosas, and P. T. Scardino. "Risk Factors for Complications and Morbidity After Radical Retropubic Prostatectomy." *J Urol* 157, no. 5 (1997): 1760–67.

28. Begg, C. B., E. R. Riedel, P. B. Bach, M. W. Kattan, D. Schrag, J. L. Warren, and P. T. Scardino. "Variations in Morbidity After Radical Prostatectomy." *N Engl J Med* 346, no. 15 (2002): 1138–44.

29. Bianco, F. J., Jr., A. J. Vickers, A. M. Cronin, E. A. Klein, J. A. Eastham, J. E. Pontes, and P. T. Scardino. "Variations Among Experienced Surgeons in Cancer Control After Open Radical Prostatectomy." *J Urol* (2010); epub.

30. Eastham, J. A., J. R. Goad, E. Rogers, M. Ohori, M. W. Kattan, T. B. Boone, and P. T. Scardino. "Risk Factors for Urinary Incontinence After Radical Prostatectomy." *J Urol* 156, no. 5 (1996): 1707–13.

31. Wille, S., A. Sobottka, A. Heidenreich, and R. Hofmann. "Pelvic Floor Exercises, Electrical Stimulation and Biofeedback After Radical Prostatectomy: Results of a Prospective Randomized Trial." *J Urol* 170, no. 2, pt. 1 (2003): 490–93.

32. Rabbani, F., A. M. Stapleton, M. W. Kattan, T. M. Wheeler, and P. T. Scardino. "Factors Predicting Recovery of Erections After Radical Prostatectomy." *J Urol* 164, no. 6 (2000): 1929–34.

33. Eastham, J. A., M. W. Kattan, E. Riedel, C. B. Begg, T. M. Wheeler, C. Gerigk, M. Gonen, V. Reuter, and P. T. Scardino. "Variations Among Individual Surgeons in the Rate of Positive Surgical Margins in Radical Prostatectomy Specimens." *J Urol* 170, no. 6, pt. 1 (2003): 2292–95.

34. Swindle, P., J. A. Eastham, M. Ohori, M. W. Kattan, T. Wheeler, N. Maru, K. Slawin, and P. T. Scardino. "Do Margins Matter? The Prognostic Significance of Positive Surgical Margins in Radical Prostatectomy Specimens." *J Urol* 174, no. 3 (2005): 903–7.

35. Castle Connolly Top Doctors. "Finding Castle Connolly Top Doctor Listings." Castle Connolly Medical Ltd. http://www.castleconnolly.com/doctors/index.cfm (accessed July 7, 2009).

36. Savage, C. J., and A. J. Vickers. "Low Annual Caseloads of United States Surgeons Conducting Radical Prostatectomy." *J Urol* 182, no. 6 (2009): 2677–79.

37. Feifer, A. H., E. B. Elkin, W. T. Lowrance, L. Jacks, D. S. Yee, J. A. Coleman, V. P. Laudone, P. T. Scardino, and J. A. Eastham. "Temporal Trends and Predictors of Lymphadenectomy in Open or Minimally Invasive Radical Prostatectomy." *J Urol*. In press (2010).

38. Hu, J. C., X. Gu, S. R. Lipsitz, M. J. Barry, A. V. D'Amico, A. C. Weinberg, and N. L. Keating. "Comparative Effectiveness of Minimally Invasive Vs. Open Radical Prostatectomy." *JAMA* 302, no. 14 (2009): 1557–64; Lowrance, J., et al. "Comparative Effectiveness of Surgical Treatments for Prostate Cancer: A Population-Based Analysis of Postoperative Outcomes." *J Urol*. In press (2010); and Mulhall, J. P., C. Rojaz-Cruz, and A. Muller. "An Analysis of Sexual Health Information on Radical Prostatectomy Websites." *BJU Int* (2009).

39. Touijer, K., J. A. Eastham, F. P. Secin, J. Romero Otero, A. Serio, J. Stasi, R. Sanchez-Salas, A. Vickers, V. E. Reuter, P. T. Scardino, and B. Guillonneau. "Comprehensive Prospective Comparative Analysis of Outcomes Between Open and Laparoscopic Radical Prostatectomy Conducted in 2003 to 2005." *J Urol* 179, no. 5 (2008): 1811–17; discussion 1817.

40. Ang-Lee, M. K., J. Moss, and C. S. Yuan. "Herbal Medicines and Perioperative Care." *JAMA* 286, no. 2 (2001): 208–16; and Sloan-Kettering. "About Herbs, Botanicals & Other Products." Memorial Sloan-Kettering Cancer Center. http://www.mskcc.org/aboutherbs (accessed June 20, 2009).

41. Guillonneau, B., I. S. Gill, G. Janetschek, and I. Tuerk. *Laparoscopic Techniques in Uro-Oncology*. London: Springer Verlag, 2009.

42. Thompson, I. M., C. M. Tangen, J. Paradelo, M. S. Lucia, G. Miller, D. Troyer, E. Messing, J. Forman, J. Chin, G. Swanson, E. Canby-Hagino, and E. D. Crawford. "Adjuvant Radiotherapy for Pathological T3n0m0 Prostate Cancer Significantly Reduces Risk of Metastases and Improves Survival: Long-Term Followup of a Randomized Clinical Trial." *J Urol* 181, no. 3 (2009): 956–62; and Bolla, M., H. van Poppel, L. Collette, P. van Cangh, K. Vekemans, L. Da Pozzo, T. M. de Reijke, A. Verbaeys, J. F. Bosset, R. van Velthoven, J. M. Marechal, P. Scalliet, K. Haustermans, and M. Pierart. "Postoperative Radiotherapy After Radical Prostatectomy: A Randomised Controlled Trial (Eortc Trial 22911)." *Lancet* 366, no. 9485 (2005): 572–78.

43. Stephenson, A. J., P. T. Scardino, M. W. Kattan, T. M. Pisansky, K. M. Slawin, E. A. Klein, M. S. Anscher, J. M. Michalski, H. M. Sandler, D. W. Lin, J. D. Forman, M. J. Zelefsky, L. L. Kestin,

C. G. Roehrborn, C. N. Catton, T. L. DeWeese, S. L. Liauw, R. K. Valicenti, D. A. Kuban, and A. Pollack. "Predicting the Outcome of Salvage Radiation Therapy for Recurrent Prostate Cancer After Radical Prostatectomy." *J Clin Oncol* 25, no. 15 (2007): 2035–41.

15. RADIATION THERAPY

1. Fuks, Z., and R. Kolesnick. "Engaging the Vascular Component of the Tumor Response." *Cancer Cell* 8, no. 2 (2005): 89–91; and Garcia-Barros, M., F. Paris, C. Cordon-Cardo, D. Lyden, S. Rafii, A. Haimovitz-Friedman, Z. Fuks, and R. Kolesnick. "Tumor Response to Radiotherapy Regulated by Endothelial Cell Apoptosis." *Science* 300, no. 5622 (2003): 1155–59.

2. Zelefsky, M. J., V. E. Reuter, Z. Fuks, P. Scardino, and A. Shippy. "Influence of Local Tumor Control on Distant Metastases and Cancer Related Mortality After External Beam Radiotherapy for Prostate Cancer." *J Urol* 179, no. 4 (2008): 1368–73; discussion 1373.

3. Barringer, B. "Radium in the Treatment of Carcinoma of the Bladder and Prostate." *JAMA* 68 (1917): 1227–30.

4. Aronowitz, J. N. "The 'Golden Age' of Prostate Brachytherapy: A Cautionary Tale." *Brachytherapy* 7, no. 1 (2008): 55–59.

5. Bagshaw, M. A. "Definitive Radiotherapy in Carcinoma of the Prostate." *JAMA* 210, no. 2 (1969): 326–27.

6. Fuks, Z., S. A. Leibel, K. E. Wallner, C. B. Begg, W. R. Fair, L. L. Anderson, B. S. Hilaris, and W. F. Whitmore. "The Effect of Local Control on Metastatic Dissemination in Carcinoma of the Prostate: Long-Term Results in Patients Treated with 125i Implantation." *Int J Radiat Oncol Biol Phys* 21, no. 3 (1991): 537–47.

7. Bogdanich, W. "Radiation Offers New Cures, Ways to Do Harm." January 23, 2010. *New York Times*. http://www.nytimes.com/2010/01/24/health/24radiation.html (accessed February 2, 2010).

8. Hanks, G. E., A. L. Hanlon, B. Epstein, and E. M. Horwitz. "Dose Response in Prostate Cancer with 8–12 Years' Follow-Up." *Int J Radiat Oncol Biol Phys* 54, no. 2 (2002): 427–35.

9. Zelefsky, M. J., Z. Fuks, M. Hunt, H. J. Lee, D. Lombardi, C. C. Ling, V. E. Reuter, E. S. Venkatraman, and S. A. Leibel. "High Dose Radiation Delivered by Intensity Modulated Conformal Radiotherapy Improves the Outcome of Localized Prostate Cancer." *J Urol* 166, no. 3 (2001): 876–81.

10. Zelefsky, M. J., Z. Fuks, M. Hunt, H. J. Lee, D. Lombardi, C. C. Ling, V. E. Reuter, E. S. Venkatraman, and S. A. Leibel. "High Dose Radiation Delivered by Intensity Modulated Conformal Radiotherapy Improves the Outcome of Localized Prostate Cancer." *J Urol* 166, no. 3 (2001): 876–81.

11. Zelefsky, M. J., Z. Fuks, M. Hunt, H. J. Lee, D. Lombardi, C. C. Ling, V. E. Reuter, E. S. Venkatraman, and S. A. Leibel. "High Dose Radiation Delivered by Intensity Modulated Conformal Radiotherapy Improves the Outcome of Localized Prostate Cancer." *J Urol* 166, no. 3 (2001): 876–81.

12. Zietman, A. L., M. L. DeSilvio, J. D. Slater, C. J. Rossi, Jr., D. W. Miller, J. A. Adams, and W. U. Shipley. "Comparison of Conventional-Dose Vs. High-Dose Conformal Radiation Therapy in Clinically Localized Adenocarcinoma of the Prostate: A Randomized Controlled Trial." *JAMA* 294, no. 10 (2005): 1233–39.

13. Bogdanich, W. "As Technology Surges, Radiation Safeguards Lag." January 26, 2010. *New York Times*. http://www.nytimes.com/2010/01/27/us/27radiation.html (accessed February 2, 2010).

14. Caloglu, M., and J. Ciezki. "Prostate-Specific Antigen Bounce After Prostate Brachytherapy: Review of a Confusing Phenomenon." *Urology* (2009).

15. Cahlon, O., M. J. Zelefsky, A. Shippy, H. Chan, Z. Fuks, Y. Yamada, M. Hunt, S. Greenstein, and H. Amols. "Ultra-High Dose (86.4 Gy) Imrt for Localized Prostate Cancer: Toxicity and Biochemical Outcomes." *Int J Radiat Oncol Biol Phys* 71, no. 2 (2008): 330–37.

16. Zelefsky, M. J., D. Cowen, Z. Fuks, M. Shike, C. Burman, A. Jackson, E. S. Venkatraman, and S. A. Leibel. "Long Term Tolerance of High Dose Three-Dimensions Conformal Radiotherapy in Patients with Localized Prostate Carcinoma." *Cancer* 85, no. 11 (1999): 2460–68.

17. Ellis, R. J., and E. Kim. "Brachytherapy: Update and Results." *Curr Urol Rep* 4, no. 3 (2003): 233–9.

18. Zelefsky, M. J., Y. Yamada, G. N. Cohen, N. Sharma, A. M. Shippy, D. Fridman, and M. Zaider. "Intraoperative Real-Time Planned Conformal Prostate Brachytherapy: Post-Implantation Dosimetric Outcome and Clinical Implications." *Radiother Oncol* 84, no. 2 (2007): 185–89.

19. Zelefsky, M. J. "PSA Bounce Versus Biochemical Failure Following Prostate Brachytherapy." *Nat Clin Pract Urol* 3, no. 11 (2006): 578–79.

20. Roach, M., 3rd, G. Hanks, H. Thames, Jr., P. Schellhammer, W. U. Shipley, G. H. Sokol, and H. Sandler. "Defining Biochemical Failure Following Radiotherapy with or Without Hormonal Therapy in Men with Clinically Localized Prostate Cancer: Recommendations of the RTOG-ASTRO Phoenix Consensus Conference." *Int J Radiat Oncol Biol Phys* 65, no. 4 (2006): 965–74.

21. Sanda, M. G., R. L. Dunn, J. Michalski, H. M. Sandler, L. Northouse, L. Hembroff, X. Lin, T. K. Greenfield, M. S. Litwin, C. S. Saigal, A. Mahadevan, E. Klein, A. Kibel, L. L. Pisters, D. Kuban, I. Kaplan, D. Wood, J. Ciezki, N. Shah, and J. T. Wei. "Quality of Life and Satisfaction with Outcome Among Prostate-Cancer Survivors." *N Engl J Med* 358, no. 12 (2008): 1250–61.

22. Sanda, M. G., R. L. Dunn, J. Michalski, H. M. Sandler, L. Northouse, L. Hembroff, X. Lin, T. K. Greenfield, M. S. Litwin, C. S. Saigal, A. Mahadevan, E. Klein, A. Kibel, L. L. Pisters, D. Kuban, I. Kaplan, D. Wood, J. Ciezki, N. Shah, and J. T. Wei. "Quality of Life and Satisfaction with Outcome Among Prostate-Cancer Survivors." *N Engl J Med* 358, no. 12 (2008): 1250–61.

23. Zelefsky, M. J., Y. Yamada, G. N. Cohen, N. Sharma, A. M. Shippy, D. Fridman, and M. Zaider. "Intraoperative Real-Time Planned Conformal Prostate Brachytherapy: Post-Implantation Dosimetric Outcome and Clinical Implications." *Radiother Oncol* 84, no. 2 (2007): 185–89.

24. Zelefsky, M. J., M. A. Nedelka, Z. L. Arican, Y. Yamada, G. N. Cohen, A. M. Shippy, J. J. Park, and M. Zaider. "Combined Brachytherapy with External Beam Radiotherapy for Localized Prostate Cancer: Reduced Morbidity with an Intraoperative Brachytherapy Planning Technique and Supplemental Intensity-Modulated Radiation Therapy." *Brachytherapy* 7, no. 1 (2008): 1–6.

25. Bolla, M., T. M. de Reijke, G. Van Tienhoven, A. C. Van den Bergh, J. Oddens, P. M. Poortmans, E. Gez, P. Kil, A. Akdas, G. Soete, O. Kariakine, E. M. van der Steen-Banasik, E. Musat, M. Pierart, M. E. Mauer, and L. Collette. "Duration of Androgen Suppression in the Treatment of Prostate Cancer." *N Engl J Med* 360, no. 24 (2009): 2516–27.

26. Widmark, A., O. Klepp, A. Solberg, J. E. Damber, A. Angelsen, P. Fransson, J. A. Lund, I. Tasdemir, M. Hoyer, F. Wiklund, and S. D. Fossa. "Endocrine Treatment, with or Without Radiotherapy, in Locally Advanced Prostate Cancer (Spcg-7/Sfuo-3): An Open Randomised Phase III Trial." *Lancet* 373, no. 9660 (2009): 301–8.

27. Bolla, M., L. Collette, L. Blank, P. Warde, J. B. Dubois, R. O. Mirimanoff, G. Storme, J. Bernier, A. Kuten, C. Sternberg, J. Mattelaer, J. Lopez Torecilla, J. R. Pfeffer, C. Lino Cutajar, A. Zurlo, and M. Pierart. "Long-Term Results with Immediate Androgen Suppression and External Irradiation in Patients with Locally Advanced Prostate Cancer (an Eortc Study): A Phase III Randomised Trial." *Lancet* 360, no. 9327 (2002): 103–6; and Pilepich, M.V., K. Winter, C. A. Lawton, R. E. Krisch, H. B. Wolkov, B. Movsas, E. B. Hug, S. O. Asbell, and D. Grignon. "Androgen

Suppression Adjuvant to Definitive Radiotherapy in Prostate Carcinoma—Long-Term Results of Phase III RTOG 85-31." *Int J Radiat Oncol Biol Phys* 61, no. 5 (2005): 1285–90.

28. Pucar, D., H. Hricak, A. Shukla-Dave, K. Kuroiwa, M. Drobnjak, J. Eastham, P. T. Scardino, and M. J. Zelefsky. "Clinically Significant Prostate Cancer Local Recurrence After Radiation Therapy Occurs at the Site of Primary Tumor: Magnetic Resonance Imaging and Step-Section Pathology Evidence." *Int J Radiat Oncol Biol Phys* 69, no. 1 (2007): 62–69.

16. FOCAL AND OTHER "LOCAL" THERAPIES

1. Marberger, M., P. R. Carroll, M. J. Zelefsky, J. A. Coleman, H. Hricak, P. T. Scardino, and L. L. Abenhaim. "New Treatments for Localized Prostate Cancer." *Urology* 72, no. 6 Suppl (2008): S36–43.

2. Shelley, M., T. J. Wilt, B. Coles, and M. D. Mason. "Cryotherapy for Localised Prostate Cancer." *Cochrane Database Syst Rev*, no. 3 (2007): CD005010.

3. American Urological Association Education and Research Inc. "Best Practice Policy Statement on Cryosurgery for the Treatment of Localized Prostate Cancer." American Urological Association. http://www.auanet.org/content/guidelines-and-quality-care/clinical-guidelines/main-reports/cryosurgery08.pdf (accessed August 4, 2009); and Heidenreich, A., M. Bolla, S. Joniau, T. H. van der Kwast, V. Mateev, M. D. Mason, N. Mottet, H.-P. Schmid, T. Wiegel, and F. Zattoni. "Guidelines on Prostate Cancer 2009." European Association of Urology. http://www.uroweb.org/fileadmin/tx_eauguidelines/2009/Full/Prostate_Cancer.pdf (accessed August 4, 2009).

4. Wilt, T. J., R. MacDonald, I. Rutks, T. A. Shamliyan, B. C. Taylor, and R. L. Kane. "Systematic Review: Comparative Effectiveness and Harms of Treatments for Clinically Localized Prostate Cancer." *Ann Intern Med* 148, no. 6 (2008): 435–48.

5. Huang, W. C., K. Kuroiwa, A. M. Serio, F. J. Bianco, Jr., S. W. Fine, B. Shayegan, P. T. Scardino, and J. A. Eastham. "The Anatomical and Pathological Characteristics of Irradiated Prostate Cancers May Influence the Oncological Efficacy of Salvage Ablative Therapies." *J Urol* 177, no. 4 (2007): 1324–29; quiz 591.

6. Shelley, M., T. J. Wilt, B. Coles, and M. D. Mason. "Cryotherapy for Localised Prostate Cancer." *Cochrane Database Syst Rev*, no. 3 (2007): CD005010.

7. Heidenreich, A., M. Bolla, S. Joniau, T. H. van der Kwast, V. Mateev, M. D. Mason, N. Mottet, H.-P. Schmid, T. Wiegel, and F. Zattoni. "Guidelines on Prostate Cancer 2009." European Association of Urology: p. 72–73. http://www.uroweb.org/fileadmin/tx_eauguidelines/2009/Full/Prostate_Cancer.pdf (accessed August 4, 2009).

8. Pisters, L. L., J. C. Rewcastle, B. J. Donnelly, F. M. Lugnani, A. E. Katz, and J. S. Jones. "Salvage Prostate Cryoablation: Initial Results from the Cryo on-Line Data Registry." *J Urol* 180, no. 2 (2008): 559–63; discussion 63–64.

9. Pisters, L. L., D. Leibovici, M. Blute, H. Zincke, T. J. Sebo, J. M. Slezak, J. Izawa, J. F. Ward, S. M. Scott, L. Madsen, P. E. Spiess, and B. C. Leibovich. "Locally Recurrent Prostate Cancer After Initial Radiation Therapy: A Comparison of Salvage Radical Prostatectomy Versus Cryotherapy." *J Urol* 182, no. 2 (2009): 517–25; discussion 525–27.

10. Blana, A., F. J. Murat, B. Walter, S. Thuroff, W. F. Wieland, C. Chaussy, and A. Gelet. "First Analysis of the Long-Term Results with Transrectal HIFU in Patients with Localised Prostate Cancer." *Eur Urol* 53, no. 6 (2008): 1194–201.

11. Aus, G. "Current Status of HIFU and Cryotherapy in Prostate Cancer—A Review." *Eur Urol* 50, no. 5 (2006): 927–34; discussion 934.

12. Blana, A., F. J. Murat, B. Walter, S. Thuroff, W. F. Wieland, C. Chaussy, and A. Gelet. "First Analysis of the Long-Term Results with Transrectal HIFU in Patients with Localised Prostate Cancer." *Eur Urol* 53, no. 6 (2008): 1194–201.

13. Marberger, M., P. R. Carroll, M. J. Zelefsky, J. A. Coleman, H. Hricak, P. T. Scardino, and L. L. Abenhaim. "New Treatments for Localized Prostate Cancer." *Urology* 72, no. 6 Suppl (2008): S36–43.

14. Boukaram, C., and J. M. Hannoun-Levi. "Management of Prostate Cancer Recurrence After Definitive Radiation Therapy." *Cancer Treat Rev* (2010).

15. Moore, C. M., D. Pendse, and M. Emberton. "Photodynamic Therapy for Prostate Cancer—A Review of Current Status and Future Promise." *Nat Clin Pract Urol* 6, no. 1 (2009): 18–30.

16. Eggener, S. E., P. T. Scardino, P. R. Carroll, M. J. Zelefsky, O. Sartor, H. Hricak, T. M. Wheeler, S. W. Fine, J. Trachtenberg, M. A. Rubin, M. Ohori, K. Kuroiwa, M. Rossignol, and L. Abenhaim. "Focal Therapy for Localized Prostate Cancer: A Critical Appraisal of Rationale and Modalities." *J Urol* 178, no. 6 (2007): 2260–67.

17. Barzell, W. E., and M. R. Melamed. "Appropriate Patient Selection in the Focal Treatment of Prostate Cancer: The Role of Transperineal 3-Dimensional Pathologic Mapping of the Prostate—A 4-Year Experience." *Urology* 70, no. 6 Suppl (2007): 27–35.

18. Scardino, P. T., ed. "Focal Therapy for Prostate Cancer: Analysis by an International Panel." *Urology* 72, no. 6 Suppl (2008).

19. Onik, G., D. Vaughan, R. Lotenfoe, M. Dineen, and J. Brady. "'Male Lumpectomy': Focal Therapy for Prostate Cancer Using Cryoablation." *Urology* 70, no. 6 Suppl (2007): 16–21.

20. Hou, A. H., K. F. Sullivan, and E. D. Crawford. "Targeted Focal Therapy for Prostate Cancer: A Review." *Curr Opin Urol* 19, no. 3 (2009): 283–89.

21. Jolesz, F. A. "Mri-Guided Focused Ultrasound Surgery." *Ann Rev Med* 60 (2009): 417–30.

22. Ahmed, H. U., C. Moore, and M. Emberton. "Minimally-Invasive Technologies in Uro-Oncology: The Role of Cryotherapy, HIFU and Photodynamic Therapy in Whole Gland and Focal Therapy of Localised Prostate Cancer." *Surg Oncol* 18, no. 3 (2009): 219–32.

23. Schenk, E., M. Essand, and C. Bangma. "Clinical Adenoviral Gene Therapy for Prostate Cancer." *Hum Gene Ther* (2009); epub.

24. Salvador-Morales, C., W. Gao, P. Ghatalia, F. Murshed, W. Aizu, R. Langer, and O. C. Farokhzad. "Multifunctional Nanoparticles for Prostate Cancer Therapy." *Expert Rev Anticancer Ther* 9, no. 2 (2009): 211–21.

17. URINARY SIDE EFFECTS

1. Sanda, M. G., R. L. Dunn, J. Michalski, H. M. Sandler, L. Northouse, L. Hembroff, X. Lin, T. K. Greenfield, M. S. Litwin, C. S. Saigal, A. Mahadevan, E. Klein, A. Kibel, L. L. Pisters, D. Kuban, I. Kaplan, D. Wood, J. Ciezki, N. Shah, and J. T. Wei. "Quality of Life and Satisfaction with Outcome Among Prostate-Cancer Survivors." *N Engl J Med* 358, no. 12 (2008): 1250–61.

2. Lepor, H., L. Kaci, and X. Xue. "Continence Following Radical Retropubic Prostatectomy Using Self-Reporting Instruments." *J Urol* 171, no. 3 (2004): 1212–15.

3. Kundu, S. D., K. A. Roehl, S. E. Eggener, J. A. Antenor, M. Han, and W. J. Catalona. "Potency, Continence and Complications in 3,477 Consecutive Radical Retropubic Prostatectomies." *J Urol* 172, no. 6, pt. 1 (2004): 2227–31; and Eastham, J. A., J. R. Goad, E. Rogers, M. Ohori, M. W. Kattan, T. B. Boone, and P. T. Scardino. "Risk Factors for Urinary Incontinence After Radical Prostatectomy." *J Urol* 156, no. 5 (1996): 1707–13.

4. Begg, C. B., E. R. Riedel, P. B. Bach, M. W. Kattan, D. Schrag, J. L. Warren, and P. T. Scardino. "Variations in Morbidity After Radical Prostatectomy." *N Engl J Med* 346, no. 15 (2002): 1138–44.

5. Touijer, K., J. A. Eastham, F. P. Secin, J. Romero Otero, A. Serio, J. Stasi, R. Sanchez-Salas, A. Vickers, V. E. Reuter, P. T. Scardino, and B. Guillonneau. "Comprehensive Prospective Comparative Analysis of Outcomes Between Open and Laparoscopic Radical Prostatectomy Conducted in 2003 to 2005." *J Urol* 179, no. 5 (2008): 1811–17; discussion 1817.

6. Stanford, J. L., Z. Feng, A. S. Hamilton, F. D. Gilliland, R. A. Stephenson, J. W. Eley, P. C. Albertsen, L. C. Harlan, and A. L. Potosky. "Urinary and Sexual Function After Radical Prostatectomy for

Clinically Localized Prostate Cancer: The Prostate Cancer Outcomes Study." *JAMA* 283, no. 3 (2000): 354–60.

7. Cooperberg, M. R., V. A. Master, and P. R. Carroll. "Health Related Quality of Life Significance of Single Pad Urinary Incontinence Following Radical Prostatectomy." *J Urol* 170, no. 2, pt. 1 (2003): 512–15.

8. Paparel, P., O. Akin, J. S. Sandhu, J. R. Otero, A. M. Serio, P. T. Scardino, H. Hricak, and B. Guillonneau. "Recovery of Urinary Continence After Radical Prostatectomy: Association with Urethral Length and Urethral Fibrosis Measured by Preoperative and Postoperative Endorectal Magnetic Resonance Imaging." *Eur Urol* 55, no. 3 (2009): 629–37.

9. Choi, J. M., C. J. Nelson, J. Stasi, and J. P. Mulhall. "Orgasm Associated Incontinence (Climacturia) Following Radical Pelvic Surgery: Rates of Occurrence and Predictors." *J Urol* 177, no. 6 (2007): 2223–26.

10. Erickson, B. A., J. J. Meeks, K. A. Roehl, C. M. Gonzalez, and W. J. Catalona. "Bladder Neck Contracture After Retropubic Radical Prostatectomy: Incidence and Risk Factors from a Large Single-Surgeon Experience." *BJU Int* 104, no. 11 (2009): 1615–19.

11. Bianco, F. J., Jr., E. R. Riedel, C. B. Begg, M. W. Kattan, and P. T. Scardino. "Variations Among High Volume Surgeons in the Rate of Complications After Radical Prostatectomy: Further Evidence That Technique Matters." *J Urol* 173, no. 6 (2005): 2099–103.

12. Sanda, M. G., R. L. Dunn, J. Michalski, H. M. Sandler, L. Northouse, L. Hembroff, X. Lin, T. K. Greenfield, M. S. Litwin, C. S. Saigal, A. Mahadevan, E. Klein, A. Kibel, L. L. Pisters, D. Kuban, I. Kaplan, D. Wood, J. Ciezki, N. Shah, and J. T. Wei. "Quality of Life and Satisfaction with Outcome Among Prostate-Cancer Survivors." *N Engl J Med* 358, no. 12 (2008): 1250–61.

13. Terk, M. D., R. G. Stock, and N. N. Stone. "Identification of Patients at Increased Risk for Prolonged Urinary Retention Following Radioactive Seed Implantation of the Prostate." *J Urol* 160, no. 4 (1998): 1379–82.

14. Sanda, M. G., R. L. Dunn, J. Michalski, H. M. Sandler, L. Northouse, L. Hembroff, X. Lin, T. K. Greenfield, M. S. Litwin, C. S. Saigal, A. Mahadevan, E. Klein, A. Kibel, L. L. Pisters, D. Kuban, I. Kaplan, D. Wood, J. Ciezki, N. Shah, and J. T. Wei. "Quality of Life and Satisfaction with Outcome Among Prostate-Cancer Survivors." *N Engl J Med* 358, no. 12 (2008): 1250–61.

15. Zelefsky, M. J., Y. Yamada, G. N. Cohen, N. Sharma, A. M. Shippy, D. Fridman, and M. Zaider. "Intraoperative Real-Time Planned Conformal Prostate Brachytherapy: Post-Implantation Dosimetric Outcome and Clinical Implications." *Radiother Oncol* 84, no. 2 (2007): 185–89.

16. Zelefsky, M. J., M. A. Nedelka, Z. L. Arican, Y. Yamada, G. N. Cohen, A. M. Shippy, J. J. Park, and M. Zaider. "Combined Brachytherapy with External Beam Radiotherapy for Localized Prostate Cancer: Reduced Morbidity with an Intraoperative Brachytherapy Planning Technique and Supplemental Intensity-Modulated Radiation Therapy." *Brachytherapy* 7, no. 1 (2008): 1–6.

17. Shelley, M., T. J. Wilt, B. Coles, and M. D. Mason. "Cryotherapy for Localised Prostate Cancer." Cochrane Database Syst Rev, no. 3 (2007): CD005010.

18. Wilt, T. J., R. MacDonald, I. Rutks, T. A. Shamliyan, B. C. Taylor, and R. L. Kane. "Systematic Review: Comparative Effectiveness and Harms of Treatments for Clinically Localized Prostate Cancer." *Ann Intern Med* 148, no. 6 (2008): 435–48.

19. Paparel, P., O. Akin, J. S. Sandhu, J. R. Otero, A. M. Serio, P. T. Scardino, H. Hricak, and B. Guillonneau. "Recovery of Urinary Continence After Radical Prostatectomy: Association with Urethral Length and Urethral Fibrosis Measured by Preoperative and Postoperative Endorectal Magnetic Resonance Imaging." *Eur Rol* 55, no. 3 (2009): 629–37; and Nguyen, L., J. Jhaveri, and A. Tewari. "Surgical Technique to Overcome Anatomical Shortcoming: Balancing Post-Prostatectomy Continence Outcomes of Urethral Sphincter Lengths on Preoperative Magnetic Resonance Imaging." *J Urol* 179, no. 5 (2008): 1907–11.

20. Kegel, A. H. "Progressive Resistance Exercise in the Functional Restoration of the Perineal Muscles." *Am J Obstet Gynecol* 56, no. 2 (1948): 238–48.

21. Van Kampen, M., W. De Weerdt, H. Van Poppel, D. De Ridder, H. Feys, and L. Baert. "Effect of Pelvic-Floor Re-Education on Duration and Degree of Incontinence After Radical Prostatectomy: A Randomised Controlled Trial." *Lancet* 355, no. 9198 (2000): 98–102.

22. Kerr, L. A. "Bulking Agents in the Treatment of Stress Urinary Incontinence: History, Outcomes, Patient Populations, and Reimbursement Profile." *Rev Urol* 7 Suppl 1 (2005): S3–S11.

23. Triaca, V., C. O. Twiss, and S. Raz. "Urethral Compression for the Treatment of Postprostatectomy Urinary Incontinence: Is History Repeating Itself?" *Eur Rol* 51, no. 2 (2007): 304–5.

24. Dalkin, B. L., H. Wessells, and H. Cui. "A National Survey of Urinary and Health Related Quality of Life Outcomes in Men with an Artificial Urinary Sphincter for Post-Radical Prostatectomy Incontinence." *J Urol* 169, no. 1 (2003): 237–39.

18. SEXUAL SIDE EFFECTS

1. Mulhall, John P. *Sexual Function in the Prostate Cancer Patient.* New York: Springer-Verlag, 2009.

2. Ong, A. M., L. M. Su, I. Varkarakis, T. Inagaki, R. E. Link, S. B. Bhayani, A. Patriciu, B. Crain, and P. C. Walsh. "Nerve Sparing Radical Prostatectomy: Effects of Hemostatic Energy Sources on the Recovery of Cavernous Nerve Function in a Canine Model." *J Urol* 172, no. 4, pt. 1 (2004): 1318–22.

3. Munarriz, R., J. Hwang, I. Goldstein, A. M. Traish, and N. N. Kim. "Cocaine and Ephedrine-Induced Priapism: Case Reports and Investigation of Potential Adrenergic Mechanisms." *Urology* 62, no. 1 (2003): 187–92.

4. Mulhall, John P. *Sexual Function in the Prostate Cancer Patient.* New York: Springer-Verlag, 2009.

5. Mulhall, John P. *Sexual Function in the Prostate Cancer Patient.* New York: Springer-Verlag, 2009.

6. Potosky, A. L., W. W. Davis, R. M. Hoffman, J. L. Stanford, R. A. Stephenson, D. F. Penson, and L. C. Harlan. "Five-Year Outcomes After Prostatectomy or Radiotherapy for Prostate Cancer: The Prostate Cancer Outcomes Study." *J Natl Cancer Inst* 96, no. 18 (2004): 1358–67.

7. Sanda, M. G., R. L. Dunn, J. Michalski, H. M. Sandler, L. Northouse, L. Hembroff, X. Lin, T. K. Greenfield, M. S. Litwin, C. S. Saigal, A. Mahadevan, E. Klein, A. Kibel, L. L. Pisters, D. Kuban, I. Kaplan, D. Wood, J. Ciezki, N. Shah, and J. T. Wei. "Quality of Life and Satisfaction with Outcome Among Prostate-Cancer Survivors." *N Engl J Med* 358, no. 12 (2008): 1250–61.

8. Rabbani, F., A. M. Stapleton, M. W. Kattan, T. M. Wheeler, and P. T. Scardino. "Factors Predicting Recovery of Erections After Radical Prostatectomy." *J Urol* 164, no. 6 (2000): 1929–34.

9. Schlosshauer, B., L. Dreesmann, H. E. Schaller, and N. Sinis. "Synthetic Nerve Guide Implants in Humans: A Comprehensive Survey." *Neurosurgery* 59, no. 4 (2006): 740–47; discussion 747–48.

10. Rabbani, F., R. Ramasamy, M. I. Patel, P. Cozzi, J. J. Disa, P. G. Cordeiro, B. J. Mehrara, J. A. Eastham, P. T. Scardino, and J. P. Mulhall. "Predictors of Recovery of Erectile Function After Unilateral Cavernous Nerve Graft Reconstruction at Radical Retropubic Prostatectomy." *J Sex Med* 7, 1, pt. 1 (2010): 166–81.

11. Rogers, C. G., B. P. Trock, and P. C. Walsh. "Preservation of Accessory Pudendal Arteries During Radical Retropubic Prostatectomy: Surgical Technique and Results." *Urology* 64, no. 1 (2004): 148–51.

12. Mulhall, John P. *Sexual Function in the Prostate Cancer Patient.* New York: Springer-Verlag, 2009.

13. Savoie, M., S. S. Kim, and M. S. Soloway. "A Prospective Study Measuring Penile Length in Men Treated with Radical Prostatectomy for Prostate Cancer." *J Urol* 169, no. 4 (2003): 1462–64.

14. Briganti, A., and Montorsi, F. "Rebuttal from Authors re: John Mulhall. Can Penile Size Be Preserved After Radical Prostatectomy?" *Eur Rol* 52, no. 3: 626–28.

15. Mulhall, John P. *Sexual Function in the Prostate Cancer Patient.* New York: Springer-Verlag, 2009.

16. Mulhall, John P. *Sexual Function in the Prostate Cancer Patient.* New York: Springer-Verlag, 2009.

17. Montorsi, F., G. Brock, J. Lee, J. Shapiro, H. Van Poppel, M. Graefen, and C. Stief. "Effect of Nightly Versus on-Demand Vardenafil on Recovery of Erectile Function in Men Following Bilateral Nerve-Sparing Radical Prostatectomy." *Eur Urol* 54, no. 4 (2008): 924–31.

18. Montorsi, F., G. Brock, J. Lee, J. Shapiro, H. Van Poppel, M. Graefen, and C. Stief. "Effect of Nightly Versus on-Demand Vardenafil on Recovery of Erectile Function in Men Following Bilateral Nerve-Sparing Radical Prostatectomy." *Eur Urol* 54, no. 4 (2008): 924–31.

19. Mulhall, John P. *Sexual Function in the Prostate Cancer Patient*. New York: Springer-Verlag, 2009.

20. Sanda, M. G., R. L. Dunn, J. Michalski, H. M. Sandler, L. Northouse, L. Hembroff, X. Lin, T. K. Greenfield, M. S. Litwin, C. S. Saigal, A. Mahadevan, E. Klein, A. Kibel, L. L. Pisters, D. Kuban, I. Kaplan, D. Wood, J. Ciezki, N. Shah, and J. T. Wei. "Quality of Life and Satisfaction with Outcome Among Prostate-Cancer Survivors." *N Engl J Med* 358, no. 12 (2008): 1250–61.

21. Miller, D. C., M. G. Sanda, R. L. Dunn, J. E. Montie, H. Pimentel, H. M. Sandler, W. P. McLaughlin, and J. T. Wei. "Long-Term Outcomes Among Localized Prostate Cancer Survivors: Health-Related Quality-of-Life Changes After Radical Prostatectomy, External Radiation, and Brachytherapy." *J Clin Oncol* 23, no. 12 (2005): 2772–80.

22. Wei, J. T., R. L. Dunn, H. M. Sandler, P. W. McLaughlin, J. E. Montie, M. S. Litwin, L. Nyquist, and M. G. Sanda. "Comprehensive Comparison of Health-Related Quality of Life After Contemporary Therapies for Localized Prostate Cancer." *J Clin Oncol* 20, no. 2 (2002): 557–66.

23. Sanda, M. G., R. L. Dunn, J. Michalski, H. M. Sandler, L. Northouse, L. Hembroff, X. Lin, T. K. Greenfield, M. S. Litwin, C. S. Saigal, A. Mahadevan, E. Klein, A. Kibel, L. L. Pisters, D. Kuban, I. Kaplan, D. Wood, J. Ciezki, N. Shah, and J. T. Wei. "Quality of Life and Satisfaction with Outcome Among Prostate-Cancer Survivors." *N Engl J Med* 358, no. 12 (2008): 1250–61.

24. Higano, C. S. "Side Effects of Androgen Deprivation Therapy: Monitoring and Minimizing Toxicity." *Urology* 61, no. 2, Suppl 1 (2003): 32–38.

25. Mulhall, John P. *Sexual Function in the Prostate Cancer Patient*. New York: Springer-Verlag, 2009.

26. Hatzimouratidis, K., A. L. Burnett, D. Hatzichristou, A. R. McCullough, F. Montorsi, and J. P. Mulhall. "Phosphodiesterase Type 5 Inhibitors in Postprostatectomy Erectile Dysfunction: A Critical Analysis of the Basic Science Rationale and Clinical Application." *Eur Rol* 55, no. 2 (2009): 334–47.

27. Brock, G., L. M. Tu, and O. I. Linet. "Return of Spontaneous Erection During Long-Term Intracavernosal Alprostadil (Caverject) Treatment." *Urology* 57, no. 3 (2001): 536–41.

28. Raina, R., A. Agarwal, C. E. Zaramo, S. Ausmundson, D. Mansour, and C. D. Zippe. "Long-Term Efficacy and Compliance of Muse for Erectile Dysfunction Following Radical Prostatectomy: Shim (Iief-5) Analysis." *Int J Impot Res* 17, no. 1 (2005): 86–90.

29. Mulhall, J. P., A. Ahmed, J. Branch, and M. Parker. "Serial Assessment of Efficacy and Satisfaction Profiles Following Penile Prosthesis Surgery." *J Urol* 169, no. 4 (2003): 1429–33.

19. BOWEL SIDE EFFECTS

1. Van Appledorn, S., and A. J. Costello. "Complications of Robotic Surgery and How to Prevent Them." In V. Patel, ed., *Robotic Urology Surgery*, pp. 169–70. London: Springer, 2007.

2. Michaelson, M. D., S. E. Cotter, P. C. Gargollo, A. L. Zietman, D. M. Dahl, and M.R. Smith. "Management of Complications of Prostate Cancer Treatment." *CA Cancer J Clin* 58, no. 4 (2008): 196–213; and Thomas, C., J. Jones, W. Jager, C. Hampel, J. W. Thuroff, and R. Gillitzer. "Incidence, Clinical Symptoms and Management of Rectourethral Fistulas After Radical Prostatectomy." *J Urol* 183, no. 2 (2010): 608–12.

3. Zelefsky, M. J., H. Chan, M. Hunt, Y. Yamada, A. M. Shippy, and H. Amols. "Long-Term Outcome of High Dose Intensity Modulated Radiation Therapy for Patients with Clinically Localized Prostate Cancer." *J Urol* 176, no. 4, pt. 1 (2006): 1415–19.

4. Yeoh, E. E., R. H. Holloway, R. J. Fraser, R. J. Botten, A. C. Di Matteo, J. W. Moore, M. N. Schoeman, and F. D. Bartholomeusz. "Anorectal Dysfunction Increases with Time Following Radiation Therapy for Carcinoma of the Prostate." *Am J Gastroenterol* 99, no. 2 (2004): 361–69.

5. Miller, D. C., M. G. Sanda, R. L. Dunn, J. E. Montie, H. Pimentel, H. M. Sandler, W. P. McLaughlin, and J. T. Wei. "Long-Term Outcomes Among Localized Prostate Cancer Survivors: Health-Related Quality-of-Life Changes After Radical Prostatectomy, External Radiation, and Brachytherapy." *J Clin Oncol* 23, no. 12 (2005): 2772–80.

6. Sanda, M. G., R. L. Dunn, J. Michalski, H. M. Sandler, L. Northouse, L. Hembroff, X. Lin, T. K. Greenfield, M. S. Litwin, C. S. Saigal, A. Mahadevan, E. Klein, A. Kibel, L. L. Pisters, D. Kuban, I. Kaplan, D. Wood, J. Ciezki, N. Shah, and J. T. Wei. "Quality of Life and Satisfaction with Outcome Among Prostate-Cancer Survivors." *N Engl J Med* 358, no. 12 (2008): 1250–61.

7. Zelefsky, M. J., H. Chan, M. Hunt, Y. Yamada, A. M. Shippy, and H. Amols. "Long-Term Outcome of High Dose Intensity Modulated Radiation Therapy for Patients with Clinically Localized Prostate Cancer." *J Urol* 176, no. 4, pt. 1 (2006): 1415–19.

8. Shelley, M., T. J. Wilt, B. Coles, and M. D. Mason. "Cryotherapy for Localised Prostate Cancer." Cochrane Database Syst Rev, no. 3 (2007): CD005010 American Urological Association Education and Research Inc. "Best Practice Policy Statement on Cryosurgery for the Treatment of Localized Prostate Cancer." American Urological Association. http://www.auanet .org/content/guidelines-and-quality-care/clinical-guidelines/main-reports/cryosurgery08 .pdf (accessed August 4, 2009); and Heidenreich, A., M. Bolla, S. Joniau, T. H. van der Kwast, V. Mateev, M. D. Mason, N. Mottet, H.-P. Schmid, T. Wiegel, and F. Zattoni. "Guidelines on Prostate Cancer 2009." European Association of Urology. http://www.uroweb.org/fileadmin/ tx_eauguidelines/2009/Full/Prostate_Cancer.pdf (accessed August 4, 2009).

9. Anastasiadis, A. G., R. Sachdev, L. Salomon, M. A. Ghafar, B. C. Stisser, R. Shabsigh, and A. E. Katz. "Comparison of Health-Related Quality of Life and Prostate-Associated Symptoms After Primary and Salvage Cryotherapy for Prostate Cancer." *J Cancer Res Clin Oncol* 129, no. 12 (2003): 676–82.

20. RISING PSA AFTER SURGERY, RADIATION, OR OTHER THERAPY

1. Trock, B. J., M. Han, S. J. Freedland, E. B. Humphreys, T. L. DeWeese, A. W. Partin, and P. C. Walsh. "Prostate Cancer-Specific Survival Following Salvage Radiotherapy Vs Observation in Men with Biochemical Recurrence After Radical Prostatectomy." *JAMA* 299, no. 23 (2008): 2760–69; and Thompson, I. M., C. M. Tangen, J. Paradelo, M. S. Lucia, G. Miller, D. Troyer, E. Messing, J. Forman, J. Chin, G. Swanson, E. Canby-Hagino, and E. D. Crawford. "Adjuvant Radiotherapy for Pathological T3n0m0 Prostate Cancer Significantly Reduces Risk of Metastases and Improves Survival: Long-Term Followup of a Randomized Clinical Trial." *J Urol* 181, no. 3 (2009): 956–62.

2. Amling, C. L., E. J. Bergstralh, M. L. Blute, J. M. Slezak, and H. Zincke. "Defining Prostate Specific Antigen Progression After Radical Prostatectomy: What Is the Most Appropriate Cut Point?" *J Urol* 165, no. 4 (2001): 1146–51.

3. Thaxton, C. S., R. Elghanian, A. D. Thomas, S. I. Stoeva, J. S. Lee, N. D. Smith, A. J. Schaeffer, H. Klocker, W. Horninger, G. Bartsch, and C. A. Mirkin. "Nanoparticle-Based Bio-Barcode Assay Redefines "Undetectable" Psa and Biochemical Recurrence After Radical Prostatectomy." *Proc Natl Acad Sci USA* 106, no. 44 (2009): 18437–42.

4. Roach, M., 3rd, G. Hanks, H. Thames, Jr., P. Schellhammer, W. U. Shipley, G. H. Sokol, and H. Sandler. "Defining Biochemical Failure Following Radiotherapy with or Without Hormonal Therapy in Men with Clinically Localized Prostate Cancer: Recommendations of the RTOG-ASTRO Phoenix Consensus Conference." *Int J Radiat Oncol Biol Phys* 65, no. 4 (2006): 965–74.

5. Fowler, J. E., Jr., J. Brooks, P. Pandey, and L. E. Seaver. "Variable Histology of Anastomotic Biopsies with Detectable Prostate Specific Antigen After Radical Prostatectomy." *J Urol* 153, no. 3, pt. 2 (1995): 1011–14.

6. Stephenson, A. J., P. T. Scardino, M. W. Kattan, T. M. Pisansky, K. M. Slawin, E. A. Klein, M. S. Anscher, J. M. Michalski, H. M. Sandler, D. W. Lin, J. D. Forman, M. J. Zelefsky, L. L. Kestin, C. G. Roehrborn, C. N. Catton, T. L. DeWeese, S. L. Liauw, R. K. Valicenti, D. A. Kuban, and A. Pollack. "Predicting the Outcome of Salvage Radiation Therapy for Recurrent Prostate Cancer After Radical Prostatectomy." *J Clin Oncol* 25, no. 15 (2007): 2035–41.

7. Bill-Axelson, A., L. Holmberg, F. Filen, M. Ruutu, H. Garmo, C. Busch, S. Nordling, M. Haggman, S. O. Andersson, S. Bratell, A. Spangberg, J. Palmgren, H. O. Adami, and J. E. Johansson. "Radical Prostatectomy Versus Watchful Waiting in Localized Prostate Cancer: The Scandinavian Prostate Cancer Group-4 Randomized Trial." *J Natl Cancer Inst* 100, no. 16 (2008): 1144–54.

8. Thompson, I. M., C. M. Tangen, J. Paradelo, M. S. Lucia, G. Miller, D. Troyer, E. Messing, J. Forman, J. Chin, G. Swanson, E. Canby-Hagino, and E. D. Crawford. "Adjuvant Radiotherapy for Pathological T3n0m0 Prostate Cancer Significantly Reduces Risk of Metastases and Improves Survival: Long-Term Followup of a Randomized Clinical Trial." *J Urol* 181, no. 3 (2009): 956–62.

9. Stephenson, A. J., S. F. Shariat, M. J. Zelefsky, M. W. Kattan, E. B. Butler, B. S. Teh, E. A. Klein, P. A. Kupelian, C. G. Roehrborn, D. A. Pistenmaa, H. D. Pacholke, S. L. Liauw, M. S. Katz, S. A. Leibel, P. T. Scardino, and K. M. Slawin. "Salvage Radiotherapy for Recurrent Prostate Cancer After Radical Prostatectomy." *JAMA* 291, no. 11 (2004): 1325–32; and Trock, B. J., M. Han, S. J. Freedland, E. B. Humphreys, T. L. DeWeese, A. W. Partin, and P. C. Walsh. "Prostate Cancer-Specific Survival Following Salvage Radiotherapy Vs Observation in Men with Biochemical Recurrence After Radical Prostatectomy." *JAMA* 299, no. 23 (2008): 2760–69.

10. Pucar, D., H. Hricak, A. Shukla-Dave, K. Kuroiwa, M. Drobnjak, J. Eastham, P. T. Scardino, and M. J. Zelefsky. "Clinically Significant Prostate Cancer Local Recurrence After Radiation Therapy Occurs at the Site of Primary Tumor: Magnetic Resonance Imaging and Step-Section Pathology Evidence." *Int J Radiat Oncol Biol Phys* 69, no. 1 (2007): 62–69.

11. Paparel, P., A. M. Cronin, C. Savage, P. T. Scardino, and J. A. Eastham. "Oncologic Outcome and Patterns of Recurrence After Salvage Radical Prostatectomy." *Eur Rol* 55, no. 2 (2009): 404–10.

12. D'Amico, A. V., J. W. Moul, P. R. Carroll, L. Sun, D. Lubeck, and M. H. Chen. "Surrogate End Point for Prostate Cancer-Specific Mortality After Radical Prostatectomy or Radiation Therapy." *J Natl Cancer Inst* 95, no. 18 (2003): 1376–83.

13. Stephenson, A. J., P. T. Scardino, M. W. Kattan, T. M. Pisansky, K. M. Slawin, E. A. Klein, M. S. Anscher, J. M. Michalski, H. M. Sandler, D. W. Lin, J. D. Forman, M. J. Zelefsky, L. L. Kestin, C. G. Roehrborn, C. N. Catton, T. L. DeWeese, S. L. Liauw, R. K. Valicenti, D. A. Kuban, and A. Pollack. "Predicting the Outcome of Salvage Radiation Therapy for Recurrent Prostate Cancer After Radical Prostatectomy." *J Clin Oncol* 25, no. 15 (2007): 2035–41.

14. Sella, T., L. H. Schwartz, P. W. Swindle, C. N. Onyebuchi, P. T. Scardino, H. I. Scher, and H. Hricak. "Suspected Local Recurrence After Radical Prostatectomy: Endorectal Coil Mr Imaging." *Radiology* 231, no. 2 (2004): 379–85.

15. Dotan, Z. A., F. J. Bianco, Jr., F. Rabbani, J. A. Eastham, P. Fearn, H. I. Scher, K. W. Kelly, H. N. Chen, H. Schoder, H. Hricak, P. T. Scardino, and M. W. Kattan. "Pattern of Prostate-Specific Antigen (PSA) Failure Dictates the Probability of a Positive Bone Scan in Patients with an Increasing PSA After Radical Prostatectomy." *J Clin Oncol* 23, no. 9 (2005): 1962–68.

16. Bander, N. H., M. I. Milowsky, D. M. Nanus, L. Kostakoglu, S. Vallabhajosula, and S. J. Goldsmith. "Phase I Trial of 177lutetium-Labeled J591, a Monoclonal Antibody to Prostate-Specific

Membrane Antigen, in Patients with Androgen-Independent Prostate Cancer." *J Clin Oncol* 23, no. 21 (2005): 4591–601.

17. Ornish, D., G. Weidner, W. R. Fair, R. Marlin, E. B. Pettengill, C. J. Raisin, S. Dunn-Emke, L. Crutchfield, F. N. Jacobs, R. J. Barnard, W. J. Aronson, P. McCormac, D. J. McKnight, J.D. Fein, A. M. Dnistrian, J. Weinstein, T. H. Ngo, N. R. Mendell, and P. R. Carroll. "Intensive Lifestyle Changes May Affect the Progression of Prostate Cancer." *J Urol* 174, no. 3 (2005): 1065–70.

18. Stephenson, A. J., S. F. Shariat, M. J. Zelefsky, M. W. Kattan, E. B. Butler, B. S. Teh, E. A. Klein, P. A. Kupelian, C. G. Roehrborn, D. A. Pistenmaa, H. D. Pacholke, S. L. Liauw, M. S. Katz, S. A. Leibel, P. T. Scardino, and K. M. Slawin. "Salvage Radiotherapy for Recurrent Prostate Cancer After Radical Prostatectomy." *JAMA* 291, no. 11 (2004): 1325–32.

19. Thompson, I. M., Jr., C. M. Tangen, J. Paradelo, M. S. Lucia, G. Miller, D. Troyer, E. Messing, J. Forman, J. Chin, G. Swanson, E. Canby-Hagino, and E. D. Crawford. "Adjuvant Radiotherapy for Pathologically Advanced Prostate Cancer: A Randomized Clinical Trial." *JAMA* 296, no. 19 (2006): 2329–35.

20. Stephenson, A. J., and J. A. Eastham. "Role of Salvage Radical Prostatectomy for Recurrent Prostate Cancer After Radiation Therapy." *J Clin Oncol* 23, no. 32 (2005): 8198–203; and Stephenson, A. J., P. T. Scardino, F. J. Bianco, Jr., C. J. DiBlasio, P. A. Fearn, and J. A. Eastham. "Morbidity and Functional Outcomes of Salvage Radical Prostatectomy for Locally Recurrent Prostate Cancer After Radiation Therapy." *J Urol* 172, no. 6, pt. 1 (2004): 2239–43.

21. Shelley, M., T. J. Wilt, B. Coles, and M. D. Mason. "Cryotherapy for Localised Prostate Cancer." Cochrane Database Syst Rev, no. 3 (2007): CD005010.

21. TREATING ADVANCED PROSTATE CANCER

1. Chen, C. D., D. S. Welsbie, C. Tran, S. H. Baek, R. Chen, R. Vessella, M. G. Rosenfeld, and C. L. Sawyers. "Molecular Determinants of Resistance to Antiandrogen Therapy." *Nat Med* 10, no. 1 (2004): 33–39.

2. Chen, Y., C. L. Sawyers, and H. I. Scher. "Targeting the Androgen Receptor Pathway in Prostate Cancer." *Curr Opin Pharmacol* 8, no. 4 (2008): 440–48.

3. Holzbeierlein, J., P. Lal, E. LaTulippe, A. Smith, J. Satagopan, L. Zhang, C. Ryan, S. Smith, H. Scher, P. Scardino, V. Reuter, and W. L. Gerald. "Gene Expression Analysis of Human Prostate Carcinoma During Hormonal Therapy Identifies Androgen-Responsive Genes and Mechanisms of Therapy Resistance." *Am J Pathol* 164, no. 1 (2004): 217–27; and Montgomery, R. B., E. A. Mostaghel, R. Vessella, D. L. Hess, T. F. Kalhorn, C. S. Higano, L. D. True, and P. S. Nelson. "Maintenance of Intratumoral Androgens in Metastatic Prostate Cancer: A Mechanism for Castration-Resistant Tumor Growth." *Cancer Res* 68, no. 11 (2008): 4447–54.

4. Knudsen, K. E., and H. I. Scher. "Starving the Addiction: New Opportunities for Durable Suppression of Ar Signaling in Prostate Cancer." *Clin Cancer Res* 15, no. 15 (2009): 4792–98.

5. Scher, H. I., and W. K. Kelly. "Flutamide Withdrawal Syndrome: Its Impact on Clinical Trials in Hormone-Refractory Prostate Cancer." *J Clin Oncol* 11, no. 8 (1993): 1566–72; and Kelly, W. K., S. Slovin, and H. I. Scher. "Steroid Hormone Withdrawal Syndromes: Pathophysiology and Clinical Significance." *Urol Clin North Am* 24, no. 2 (1997): 421–31.

6. Zhou, P., M. H. Chen, D. McLeod, P. R. Carroll, J. W. Moul, and A. V. D'Amico. "Predictors of Prostate Cancer-Specific Mortality After Radical Prostatectomy or Radiation Therapy." *J Clin Oncol* 23, no. 28 (2005): 6992–98.

7. Shahinian, V. B., Y. F. Kuo, J. L. Freeman, and J. S. Goodwin. "Risk of Fracture After Androgen Deprivation for Prostate Cancer." *N Engl J Med* 352, no. 2 (2005): 154–64.

8. Keating, N. L., A. J. O'Malley, S. J. Freedland, and M. R. Smith. "Diabetes and Cardiovascular Disease During Androgen Deprivation Therapy: Observational Study of Veterans with Prostate Cancer." *J Natl Cancer Inst* 102, no. 1 (2010): 39–46.

9. Bianco, F. J., Z. A. Dotan, M. W. Kattan, P. Fearn, H. Scher, J. A. Eastham, and P. T. Scardino. "Duration of Response to Androgen Deprivation Therapy and Survival After Subsequent Biochemical Relapse in Men Initially Treated with Radical Prostatectomy." *J Clin Oncol* 22, no. 14S (2004): 4552.

10. D'Amico, A. V., J. W. Moul, P. R. Carroll, L. Sun, D. Lubeck, and M. H. Chen. "Surrogate End Point for Prostate Cancer-Specific Mortality After Radical Prostatectomy or Radiation Therapy." *J Natl Cancer Inst* 95, no. 18 (2003): 1376–83.

11. Dotan, Z. A., F. J. Bianco, Jr., F. Rabbani, J. A. Eastham, P. Fearn, H. I. Scher, K. W. Kelly, H. N. Chen, H. Schoder, H. Hricak, P. T. Scardino, and M. W. Kattan. "Pattern of Prostate-Specific Antigen (PSA) Failure Dictates the Probability of a Positive Bone Scan in Patients with an Increasing PSA After Radical Prostatectomy." *J Clin Oncol* 23, no. 9 (2005): 1962–68.

12. Conti, P. D., A. N. Atallah, H. Arruda, B. G. Soares, R. P. El Dib, and T. J. Wilt. "Intermittent Versus Continuous Androgen Suppression for Prostatic Cancer." Cochrane Database Syst Rev, no. 4 (2007): CD005009; and Calais da Silva, F. E., A. V. Bono, P. Whelan, M. Brausi, A. Marques Queimadelos, J. A. Martin, Z. Kirkali, F. M. Calais da Silva, and C. Robertson. "Intermittent Androgen Deprivation for Locally Advanced and Metastatic Prostate Cancer: Results from a Randomised Phase 3 Study of the South European Uroncological Group." *Eur Rol* 55, no. 6 (2009): 1269–77.

13. Loblaw, D. A., K. S. Virgo, R. Nam, M. R. Somerfield, E. Ben-Josef, D. S. Mendelson, R. Middleton, S. A. Sharp, T. J. Smith, J. Talcott, M. Taplin, N. J. Vogelzang, J. L. Wade, 3rd, C. L. Bennett, and H. I. Scher. "Initial Hormonal Management of Androgen-Sensitive Metastatic, Recurrent, or Progressive Prostate Cancer: 2006 Update of an American Society of Clinical Oncology Practice Guideline." *J Clin Oncol* 25, no. 12 (2007): 1596–605; and Zelefsky, M. J., J. Eastham, O. Sartor, and P. Kantoff. "Cancer of the Prostate." In V. DeVita, T. S. Lawrence, and S. A. Rosenberg, eds., *Cancer: Principles and Practice of Oncology*, pp. 1392–451. Philadelphia: Lippincott Williams & Wilkins, 2008.

14. McLeod, D. G., P. Iversen, W. A. See, T. Morris, J. Armstrong, and M. P. Wirth. "Bicalutamide 150 Mg Plus Standard Care Vs Standard Care Alone for Early Prostate Cancer." *BJU Int* 97, no. 2 (2006): 247–54.

15. Tay, M. H., D. S. Kaufman, M. M. Regan, S. B. Leibowitz, D. J. George, P. G. Febbo, J. Manola, M. R. Smith, I. D. Kaplan, P. W. Kantoff, and W. K. Oh. "Finasteride and Bicalutamide as Primary Hormonal Therapy in Patients with Advanced Adenocarcinoma of the Prostate." *Ann Oncol* 15, no. 6 (2004): 974–78.

16. Shahinian, V. B., Y. F. Kuo, J. L. Freeman, and J. S. Goodwin. "Risk of Fracture After Androgen Deprivation for Prostate Cancer." *N Engl J Med* 352, no. 2 (2005): 154–64.

17. Smith, M. R., B. Egerdie, N. Hernandez Toriz, R. Feldman, T. L. Tammela, F. Saad, J. Heracek, M. Szwedowski, C. Ke, A. Kupic, B. Z. Leder, and C. Goessl. "Denosumab in Men Receiving Androgen-Deprivation Therapy for Prostate Cancer." *N Engl J Med* 361, no. 8 (2009): 745–55; and Smith, M. R., S. B. Malkowicz, F. Chu, J. Forrest, D. Price, P. Sieber, K. G. Barnette, D. Rodriguez, and M. S. Steiner. "Toremifene Increases Bone Mineral Density in Men Receiving Androgen Deprivation Therapy for Prostate Cancer: Interim Analysis of a Multicenter Phase 3 Clinical Study." *J Urol* 179, no. 1 (2008): 152–55; and Michaelson, M. D., D. S. Kaufman, H. Lee, F. J. McGovern, P. W. Kantoff, M. A. Fallon, J. S. Finkelstein, and M. R. Smith. "Randomized Controlled Trial of Annual Zoledronic Acid to Prevent Gonadotropin-Releasing Hormone Agonist-Induced Bone Loss in Men with Prostate Cancer." *J Clin Oncol* 25, no. 9 (2007): 1038–42.

18. Doggrell, S. A. "Clinical Efficacy and Safety of Zoledronic Acid in Prostate and Breast Cancer." *Expert Rev Anticancer Ther* 9, no. 9 (2009): 1211–18.

19. Keating, N. L., A. J. O'Malley, S. J. Freedland, and M. R. Smith. "Diabetes and Cardiovascular Disease During Androgen Deprivation Therapy: Observational Study of Veterans with Prostate Cancer." *J Natl Cancer Inst* 102, no. 1 (2010): 39–46; and Zelefsky, M. J., J. Eastham, O. Sartor, and P. Kantoff. "Cancer of the Prostate." In V. DeVita, T. S. Lawrence, and S. A. Rosenberg, eds., *Cancer: Principles and Practice of Oncology*, pp.1392–451. Philadelphia: Lippincott Williams & Wilkins, 2008.

20. Mohler, J. L. "Castration-Recurrent Prostate Cancer Is Not Androgen-Independent." *Adv Exp Med Biol* 617 (2008): 223–34.

21. Chen, Y., C. L. Sawyers, and H. I. Scher. "Targeting the Androgen Receptor Pathway in Prostate Cancer." *Curr Opin Pharmacol* 8, no. 4 (2008): 440–48.

22. Chen, Y., C. L. Sawyers, and H. I. Scher. "Targeting the Androgen Receptor Pathway in Prostate Cancer." *Curr Opin Pharmacol* 8, no. 4 (2008): 440–48.

23. Tran, C., S. Ouk, N. J. Clegg, Y. Chen, P. A. Watson, V. Arora, J. Wongvipat, P. M. Smith-Jones, D. Yoo, A. Kwon, T. Wasielewska, D. Welsbie, C. D. Chen, C. S. Higano, T. M. Beer, D. T. Hung, H. I. Scher, M. E. Jung, and C. L. Sawyers. "Development of a Second-Generation Antiandrogen for Treatment of Advanced Prostate Cancer." *Science* 324, no. 5928 (2009): 787–90.

24. Attard, G., A. H. Reid, T. A. Yap, F. Raynaud, M. Dowsett, S. Settatree, M. Barrett, C. Parker, V. Martins, E. Folkerd, J. Clark, C. S. Cooper, S. B. Kaye, D. Dearnaley, G. Lee, and J. S. de Bono. "Phase I Clinical Trial of a Selective Inhibitor of Cyp17, Abiraterone Acetate, Confirms That Castration-Resistant Prostate Cancer Commonly Remains Hormone Driven." *J Clin Oncol* 26, no. 28 (2008): 4563–71.

25. Kaasa, S., E. Brenne, J. A. Lund, P. Fayers, U. Falkmer, M. Holmberg, M. Lagerlund, and O. Bruland. "Prospective Randomised Multicenter Trial on Single Fraction Radiotherapy (8 Gy X 1) Versus Multiple Fractions (3 Gy X 10) in the Treatment of Painful Bone Metastases." *Radiother Oncol* 79, no. 3 (2006): 278–84.

26. Zelefsky, M. J., J. Eastham, O. Sartor, and P. Kantoff. "Cancer of the Prostate." In V. DeVita, T. S. Lawrence, and S. A. Rosenberg, eds., *Cancer: Principles and Practice of Oncology*, pp. 1392–451. Philadelphia: Lippincott Williams & Wilkins, 2008.

27. Berry, W., S. Dakhil, M. Modiano, M. Gregurich, and L. Asmar. "Phase III Study of Mitoxantrone plus Low Dose Prednisone versus Low Dose Prednisone Alone in Patients with Asymptomatic Hormone Refractory Prostate Cancer." *J Urol* 168, no. 6 (2002): 2439–43.

28. Petrylak, D. P., C. M. Tangen, M. H. Hussain, P. N. Lara, Jr., J. A. Jones, M. E. Taplin, P. A. Burch, D. Berry, C. Moinpour, M. Kohli, M. C. Benson, E. J. Small, D. Raghavan, and E. D. Crawford. "Docetaxel and Estramustine Compared with Mitoxantrone and Prednisone for Advanced Refractory Prostate Cancer." *N Engl J Med* 351, no. 15 (2004): 1513–20; and Tannock, I. F., R. de Wit, W. R. Berry, J. Horti, A. Pluzanska, K. N. Chi, S. Oudard, C. Theodore, N. D. James, I. Turesson, M. A. Rosenthal, and M. A. Eisenberger. "Docetaxel Plus Prednisone or Mitoxantrone Plus Prednisone for Advanced Prostate Cancer." *N Engl J Med* 351, no. 15 (2004): 1502–12.

29. Sanofi-Aventis. "Rising PSA Study." Sanofi-Aventis USA. http://www.risingpsastudy.net/ (accessed October 30, 2009).

30. Tran, C., S. Ouk, N. J. Clegg, Y. Chen, P. A. Watson, V. Arora, J. Wongvipat, P. M. Smith-Jones, D. Yoo, A. Kwon, T. Wasielewska, D. Welsbie, C. D. Chen, C. S. Higano, T. M. Beer, D. T. Hung, H. I. Scher, M. E. Jung, and C. L. Sawyers. "Development of a Second-Generation Antiandrogen for Treatment of Advanced Prostate Cancer." *Science* 324, no. 5928 (2009): 787–90.

31. Attard, G., A. H. Reid, T. A. Yap, F. Raynaud, M. Dowsett, S. Settatree, M. Barrett, C. Parker, V. Martins, E. Folkerd, J. Clark, C. S. Cooper, S. B. Kaye, D. Dearnaley, G. Lee, and J. S. de Bono. "Phase I Clinical Trial of a Selective Inhibitor of Cyp17, Abiraterone Acetate, Confirms That

Castration-Resistant Prostate Cancer Commonly Remains Hormone Driven." *J Clin Oncol* 26, no. 28 (2008): 4563–71.

32. Knudsen, K. E., and H. I. Scher. "Starving the Addiction: New Opportunities for Durable Suppression of AR Signaling in Prostate Cancer." *Clin Cancer Res* 15, no. 15 (2009): 4792–98.

33. Chi, K. N., A. Zoubeidi, and M. E. Gleave. "Custirsen (Ogx-011): A Second-Generation Antisense Inhibitor of Clusterin for the Treatment of Cancer." *Expert Opin Investig Drugs* 17, no. 12 (2008): 1955–62.

34. Antonarakis, E. S., M. A. Carducci, and M. A. Eisenberger. "Novel Targeted Therapeutics for Metastatic Castration-Resistant Prostate Cancer." *Cancer Lett* (2009); epub.

35. Peggs, K. S., N. H. Segal, and J. P. Allison. "Targeting Immunosupportive Cancer Therapies: Accentuate the Positive, Eliminate the Negative." *Cancer Cell* 12, no. 3 (2007): 192–9.

36. Escorcia, F. E., M. R. McDevitt, C. H. Villa, and D. A. Scheinberg. "Targeted Nanomaterials for Radiotherapy." *Nanomed* 2, no. 6 (2007): 805–15.

37. Feldman, D. R., G. J. Bosl, J. Sheinfeld, and R. J. Motzer. "Medical Treatment of Advanced Testicular Cancer." *JAMA* 299, no. 6 (2008): 672–84.

38. Heiss, G., R. Wallace, G. L. Anderson, A. Aragaki, S. A. Beresford, R. Brzyski, R. T. Chlebowski, M. Gass, A. LaCroix, J. E. Manson, R. L. Prentice, J. Rossouw, and M. L. Stefanick. "Health Risks and Benefits 3 Years After Stopping Randomized Treatment with Estrogen and Progestin." *JAMA* 299, no. 9 (2008): 1036–45.

39. Ornish, D., M. J. Magbanua, G. Weidner, V. Weinberg, C. Kemp, C. Green, M. D. Mattie, R. Marlin, J. Simko, K. Shinohara, C. M. Haqq, and P. R. Carroll. "Changes in Prostate Gene Expression in Men Undergoing an Intensive Nutrition and Lifestyle Intervention." *Proc Natl Acad Sci USA* 105, no. 24 (2008): 8369–74; and Sloan-Kettering. "About Herbs, Botanicals & Other Products." Memorial Sloan-Kettering Cancer Center. http://www.mskcc.org/about-herbs (accessed Oct. 30, 2009).

40. Zelefsky, M. J., J. Eastham, O. Sartor, and P. Kantoff. "Cancer of the Prostate." In V. DeVita, T. S. Lawrence, and S. A. Rosenberg, eds., *Cancer: Principles and Practice of Oncology*, pp. 1392–451. Philadelphia: Lippincott Williams & Wilkins, 2008; and Berger, A. M., et al. *Principles and Practice of Palliative Care and Supportive Oncology*, 3rd ed. Philadelphia: Lippincott Williams & Wilkins, 2007.

GLOSSARY OF TERMS

active surveillance: A strategy for managing disease in which the patient is regularly examined but not treated until the disease shows signs of worsening. Also called *deferred therapy* or *expectant management,* as opposed to traditional **watchful waiting**, which means doing nothing.

acute prostatitis: An inflammation or infection of sudden onset in the prostate.

acute urinary retention: A sudden inability to urinate.

adenocarcinoma: A cancer that begins in epithelial cells of glands and glandlike organs. Almost all prostate cancers are adenocarcinomas.

adrenalectomy: Surgical removal of the adrenal glands, at one time used to treat prostate cancer.

alternative medicine: Approaches outside mainstream medical therapy that are promoted as viable treatment options but are unproven and could be harmful.

androgen: A hormone that stimulates activity of male sex organs or promotes development of male sex characteristics. The principal androgen is testosterone.

androgen deprivation therapy (ADT): A treatment for prostate cancer in which surgery or, more commonly, drugs prevent the body from making or using androgens.

androgen receptor (AR): Molecules that bind to androgens (male hormones) and allow cells to respond to these hormones.

androstenedione (Andro): A steroidal hormone that the body can convert to testosterone. It is naturally produced in testicles, adrenal glands, and ovaries, and has recently been declared a controlled substance by the U.S. government.

antiandrogen withdrawal syndrome: A paradoxical decrease in PSA sometimes associated with shrinkage of a cancer when patients stop taking antiandrogens such as bicalutamide.

antiandrogens: Medications used to block the effects of male hormones. Used as a form of androgen deprivation therapy.

antisense therapy: A form of cancer treatment that involves the administration of synthetic genetic material, usually RNA, that will bind to and turn off a cancer-promoting gene.

apoptosis: Programmed cell death, the natural process by which cells self-destruct to make room for new cells. Cancer cells, resistant to this process, are virtually immortal.

artificial sphincter: A surgically implanted device that replaces the urinary sphincter to treat incontinence.

atypia: Abnormality in cells found on prostate biopsy, often associated with malignancy.

atrophy: A degeneration of cells observed in prostate biopsy samples that can be difficult to distinguish from cancer.

benign: Not malignant, not cancerous; lacking the capacity to spread beyond the organ of origin.

benign prostatic hyperplasia (BPH): Noncancerous overgrowth of cells within the prostate. As the prostate enlarges, it may block the urinary stream.

biochemical recurrence: Return of a prostate cancer after treatment, as measured by a rising PSA.

biopsy: The process of removing tissue from a patient to check for cancer. Also, a sample of tissue removed as part of this process. A "positive" result means cancer has been detected.

bladder: A muscular organ that stores and periodically empties (voids) urine.

bladder neck: The opening of the bladder into the urethra. Contains the internal urinary sphincter.

bladder outlet obstruction: A blockage at the point where the bladder drains into the urethra. BPH is a frequent cause.

bone mineral density: Measure of the strength of a bone, used to determine amount of bone loss after androgen deprivation therapy.

bone scan: A medical test that uses trace amounts of radioisotopes to detect the spread of cancer to bones.

BPH: See **benign prostatic hyperplasia**.

brachytherapy (seed implants): A form of radiation therapy in which the radioactive material is implanted near or in direct contact with the tissue being treated.

cancer: Any disease in which abnormal cells grow in an uncontrolled manner and have the potential to invade nearby tissue and spread to distant sites (metastasize).

cancer-specific mortality rate: The likelihood of dying of prostate cancer at a given time point after diagnosis. Fifteen years is the time point against which most prostate cancer treatments are measured.

capsule: The soft, fibrous outer layer, or "skin," of the prostate.

castration: Blocking the production of testosterone by surgical removal of the testicles (see **orchiectomy**) or with drugs.

castration-resistant prostate cancer: Prostate cancer that recurs after androgen-deprivation therapy.

cavernous (erectile) nerves: The nerves that run along the left and right side of the prostate to the penis and control erections. Surgery or radiation therapy to treat prostate cancer can damage these nerves.

chemotherapeutic drugs: A group of drugs that kill cancer cells and other rapidly dividing cells in the body. These drugs typically have more side effects (e.g., hair loss, nausea, diarrhea, loss of appetite, mouth ulcers) than biologic or immunologic agents.

chemotherapy: Cancer treatment involving one drug or a combination ("cocktail") of drugs.

chronic prostatitis / chronic pelvic pain syndrome (CP/CPPS): The most common type of prostatitis, defined by symptoms that persist for three months or more with no evidence of bacterial infection of the prostate.

chronic prostatitis symptom index (CPSI): A questionnaire used to measure the severity of symptoms in patients with prostatitis.

cold spot: In radiation therapy, an area that has received a lower-than-intended radiation dose, inadequately treating cancer cells.

comorbidity: A disease or medical condition in addition to the condition under consideration. For example, a urologist discussing a man's prostate cancer would consider his heart disease a comorbidity.

complementary medicine: Supportive measures used in addition to conventional medical treatments to alleviate stress, reduce symptoms, and promote a feeling of well-being, e.g., acupuncture, massage.

complete (total) androgen blockade: Hormone therapy that combines an LHRH agonist and an antiandrogen to stop production of male hormones by the testicles and block the effects of the small amount of androgens produced by the adrenal gland.

constricting ring: A ring or band placed at the base of the penis to help maintain an erection.

conventional radiation therapy: A form of external beam therapy in which the radiation is delivered to a box-shaped area around the target organ.

corpora cavernosa (*singular*, corpus cavernosum): Two erectile chambers filled with spongy tissue that run the length of the penis. An influx of blood to these chambers is required for penile erection.

corpus spongiosum: A small erectile chamber near the urethra that runs to the head of the penis.

Cowper's glands: A pair of pea-sized glands that lie beneath the prostate gland and produce part of the seminal fluid.

cryotherapy (cryoablation, cryosurgery): A treatment in which prostate tissue is destroyed by freezing.

cystoscope: A slim, lighted instrument that allows a doctor to visually examine the urethra and the bladder internally.

dehydroepiandrosterone (DHEA): A steroidal hormone alleged to reverse many effects of aging, although its effectiveness and safety are doubtful.

digital rectal exam (DRE): A screening test in which the physician inserts a lubricated, gloved finger into the rectum to detect abnormalities in the prostate.

dihydrotestosterone (DHT): A more powerful male hormone derived from testosterone that is required for development of the prostate and other secondary male characteristics (including male-pattern baldness).

disease state: A distinct stage in the natural history of an illness.

DNA: The molecule that makes up genes and chromosomes and carries all hereditary information.

doubling time: The time required for a tumor to double in size or for the PSA level to double.

dry orgasm: Orgasm without ejaculation.

dysorgasmia: Pain in the penis, scrotum, or perineum during orgasm.

ejaculation: The sudden release of semen through the penis during sexual climax. (The semen is the "ejaculate.")

ejaculatory ducts: Tubes that run from the seminal vesicles and prostate into the urethra near the tip or apex of the prostate.

emission: The discharge of sperm and seminal fluid into the urethra during sexual climax.

endorectal MRI (with spectroscopy): A technique used to visualize the prostate and surrounding tissues using magnetic resonance imaging. A coil placed in the rectum permits greater detail and clarity. Spectroscopy detects chemical signals that distinguish cancer from normal tissue.

epididymis: Long, slender, tightly coiled tube behind the testes in which sperm mature and are stored.

epithelial cells: Cells that line or cover body organs and protect the underlying tissue (e.g., skin). These are the cells that give rise to cancers of the prostate, colon, lung, and breast

erectile dysfunction (ED): A consistent inability to get or maintain an erection satisfactory for sexual intercourse.

erection: A sudden inflow of blood to the penis that causes enlargement and rigidity.

estrogen: A female sex hormone.

expressed prostatic fluid: Liquid expressed from the prostate during a digital rectal exam for diagnostic purposes.

external beam therapy: A treatment for cancer that uses high-energy radiation from an energy source outside the body to kill cancer cells.

external urinary sphincter: The muscular structure that constricts the urethra below the prostate, retaining urine until the sphincter is relaxed. During ejaculation, the external sphincter relaxes while the internal sphincter constricts to allow release of semen through the urethra.

extracapsular extension (ECE): Spread of prostate cancer outside the membranous covering (capsule) of the prostate.

fecal incontinence: The inability to control the passage of feces or gas.

5 alpha-reductase: An enzyme that converts testosterone to dihydrotestosterone (DHT), the male hormone most active in the prostate.

focal therapy: A strategy to reduce the side effects of prostate cancer therapy by treating only the portion of the gland containing cancer.

Foley catheter: A tube inserted through the urethra into the bladder to drain urine.

free PSA: PSA that is not bound to another protein. The ratio of free to total PSA, expressed as a percent (**% free PSA, %fPSA**), helps to distinguish BPH from prostate cancer.

fusion gene: A hybrid gene produced from two separate genes by translocation or other mutation. Often fusion genes are cancer-causing oncogenes.

gene therapy: A process to treat or to prevent disease by inserting genes into cells.

Gleason (sum, score): Used to describe the seriousness of prostate cancer; the sum of the most common Gleason pattern and the second most common Gleason pattern in a given cancer.

Gleason pattern: The degree of disorganization and cellular abnormalities of prostatic glands expressed on a scale from 1 (nearly normal) to 5 (markedly abnormal). Indicates the aggressiveness of a prostate cancer.

grade: A description of a cancer based on how abnormal the cancer cells appear under a microscope, ranked as low (nearly normal), intermediate, or high (markedly abnormal).

Gray (Gy): A unit designating a certain amount of radiation absorbed by the body during radiation therapy (formerly known as a **rad**).

gynecomastia: Breast enlargement, sometimes accompanied by pain or tenderness as a result of hormonal changes.

half-life: The time required for the radioactivity of a given substance to decrease by half. Also, the time required for half the amount of a substance in the body to be eliminated.

hematospermia: Blood in the semen.

hematuria: Blood in the urine.

high-grade prostatic intraepithelial neoplasia (PIN): Premalignant clusters of abnormal cells that have not invaded through the basement membrane of a gland. High-grade PIN is thought to be a precursor of cancer.

high-intensity focused ultrasound (HIFU): A treatment that destroys prostate cells using heat generated by high-frequency sound waves.

hK2 (human kallekrein 2): A protein, closely related to PSA, produced in small amounts by the prostate that can be used as a marker of the presence of or changes in prostate cancer.

hormone: A signaling chemical produced in one organ that regulates the function of another.

hormone-refractory: Referring to prostate cancer that no longer responds to androgen deprivation therapy. See **castration-resistant prostate cancer**.

hormone therapy: See **androgen deprivation therapy.**

hot flash: A sudden, intense feeling of warmth, facial flushing, and perspiration, induced by a reduction in male or female sex hormones.

hot spot: In radiation therapy, an area that receives a higher-than-intended radiation dose, causing damage.

hypophysectomy: Surgical removal or destruction of the pituitary gland. Previously used to treat prostate cancer by eliminating the production of LH.

image-guided radiation therapy (IGRT): Targeted radiation using CT scans.

impotence: See **erectile dysfunction.**

incidental cancer: Small, insignificant cancer found when prostate tissue is removed to treat symptoms of BPH or as part of an operation for bladder cancer.

incontinence: Inability to control the release of urine or feces.

indolent cancer: A tiny cancer that poses no immediate threat to life or health.

infertility: The inability to conceive children.

inflammation: A response of the body to injury or infection.

intensity-modulated radiation therapy (IMRT): A form of external radiation in which the dose is highly targeted to the tumor, increasing effectiveness and decreasing side effects.

internal urinary sphincter: Muscular structure of the bladder neck that retains urine in the bladder until it is voluntarily released.

international prostate symptom score (IPSS): A questionnaire used to assess urinary symptoms.

irritative voiding symptoms: Urinary symptoms (e.g., frequency, urgency, blood in the urine, burning) that result from irritations.

Kegel (pelvic floor) exercises: Repetitive exercises to strengthen the muscles of the pelvic floor to improve urinary control.

laparoscope: A long tubelike instrument used to carry a lens or a camera into the abdominal cavity to view the interior organs for surgery.

laparoscopic prostatectomy: Removal of the entire prostate and seminal vesicles through multiple small incisions, using a laparoscope.

laparoscopic surgery: A surgical technique in which operations are performed through scopes with instruments passed through small incisions in the abdominal wall. Requires a camera and multiple instruments for performing the surgery, and an incision large enough to remove the organ.

laser prostatectomy: The use of laser light to vaporize or excise tissue for the relief of urinary obstruction in men with BPH.

LH (luteinizing hormone): A hormone produced by the pituitary gland that stimulates production of testosterone by the testes.

LHRH agonists: Injectable medications that suppress the body's production of LH (luterinizing hormone, the pituitary hormone that stimulates the testicles to produce androgens). Used as a form of androgen deprivation therapy.

libido: Sexual desire.

lower urinary tract symptoms (LUTS): Urinary problems, including frequent, slow, or painful urination, nocturia, hesitancy, and dribbling.

magnetic resonance imaging (MRI): A diagnostic tool that uses a powerful magnetic field to generate three-dimensional images of internal organs.

malignant: Cancerous; having the capacity to escape an organ of origin and spread to other sites.

meatus: The opening in the head of the penis.

medical informatics: The development of mathematical models designed to improve communication, understanding, and management of medical information.

medical therapy of prostatic symptoms (MTOPs): A clinical trial that compares the control of urinary symptoms with finasteride versus the control of the symptoms with a placebo.

metastasis: The process by which a cancer spreads from the place at which it first arose (primary tumor) to distant locations in the body.

minimal peripheral dose (MPD): In brachytherapy, the least amount of radiation exposure to the edges of the prostate that provides an adequate radiation dose throughout the gland.

monoclonal antibodies: A group of substances produced in the laboratory that track and bind to cancer cells. Monoclonal antibodies have been studied as a means of diagnosing and treating prostate cancer.

morbidity: Any disease condition. Also, the rate of disease; the number of sick people divided by the total population.

mortality: Death. Also, the death rate; the number of deaths from a given cause divided by the total population.

myogenic: Caused by or associated with muscle contractions.

nerve graft: Transfer of a segment of a nerve from one site in the body to another to repair a nerve that has been damaged or removed.

nerve sparing: Radical prostatectomy in which the erectile (cavernous) nerves are preserved.

neurogenic: Caused by or originating in the nervous system.

neuroprotective agents: A group of drugs that protect nerves from damage.

nocturia: Waking at night to urinate.

nocturnal penile tumescence (NPT): Erections that occur during sleep.

nomogram: A mathematical tool for estimating a disease stage or the probability of a medical outcome.

nonsteroidal anti-inflammatory drugs (NSAIDs): A class of substances (e.g., ibuprofen, aspirin) used to relieve pain and suppress inflammation.

obstructive voiding symptoms: Urinary symptoms (e.g., slow stream, hesitancy, intermittency, waking at night to urinate) caused by blockage.

oncogene: A normal gene that, when expressed at high levels, induces a normal cell to become malignant.

open radical prostatectomy: Removal of prostate tissue through an incision in the abdomen.

orchiectomy: Surgical removal of the testes (see **castration**).

organ-confined cancer: A cancer that has not escaped a specific organ, such as the prostate.

osteopenia: A precursor to osteoporosis.

osteoporosis: The thinning of bone and loss of bone density over time that predisposes the bones to fracture. It is seen with greater frequency after androgen deprivation therapy or bone irradiation.

outer urinary sphincter: See **external urinary sphincter.**

overflow incontinence: Urinary incontinence that occurs when there is leakage of urine because the bladder is always full.

Partin tables: Staging tables used to predict what the pathologist will find on examining the prostate after it is surgically removed to treat cancer.

PCPT (Prostate Cancer Prevention Trial): A study to test whether finasteride could prevent prostate cancer.

pelvic lymph node dissection (PLND): A procedure in which lymph nodes near the site of a malignant tumor are removed and examined for cancer.

penile implant (prosthesis): A semi-rigid or inflatable device that is surgically implanted in the penis to enable erections.

penis: The male organ of sexual intercourse and urination.

perineal prostatectomy: Removal of the prostate through an incision between the scrotum and rectum.

perineum: Area between the scrotum and the rectum.

perineural invasion (PNI): The spread of prostate cancer into the sheath surrounding the prostate nerves.

peripheral zone: The part of the prostate beneath the capsule that surrounds the transition zone. Most prostate cancers arise in the peripheral zone.

Peyronie's disease: A condition in which hard areas (fibrous plaques) form in the erectile bodies of the penis, causing it to bend and sometimes feel painful during erections.

photodynamic therapy: An experimental treatment for prostate cancer in which a light source inserted into the prostate activates a therapeutic drug.

placebo: A sham medical intervention that typically involves administering an inert pill to a patient that cannot be distinguished in appearance from the actual medicine being tested.

positive surgical margin: The presence of cancer at the edge of tissue removed during surgery. Suggests that some of the cancer likely remains in the body.

postural hypotension: Lightheadedness or dizziness on standing, an occasional side effect of alpha-blocking drugs.

post-void residual urine: Urine that remains in the bladder after voiding.

priapism: A dangerous condition involving an erection that lasts four hours or more.

proctitis: Inflammation of the mucous membranes that line the rectum; sometimes follows radiation therapy.

progression-free probability: The likelihood at a given time point that a cancer will not return after treatment.

prostadynia: Pain in the prostate.

prostaglandin: Potent hormonelike substance that can trigger inflammation, pain, and various other processes.

ProstaScint: A test for prostate cancer metastases using a monoclonal antibody.

prostate-specific antigen (PSA): A protein, produced in the prostate, normally present in high levels in the semen. Elevated PSA levels in the blood may indicate a problem in the prostate.

prostatectomy: Surgical removal of prostate tissue.

prostatism: Urinary symptoms associated with prostate enlargement.

prostatitis: Inflammation or infection of the prostate.

proton beam radiation: A form of external radiation that uses protons instead of gamma rays.

PSA bounce: A transient rise in the PSA level after radiation.

PSA density (PSAD): The ratio of PSA level to prostate size.

PSA doubling time (PSA velocity): The time required for a man's PSA level to double. PSA velocity is a measure of how quickly the PSA level rises (rate of rise, measured in nanograms per milliliter per year).

PSA nadir: The lowest PSA level after treatment for prostate cancer.

psychogenic: Originating in the mind.

rad: A unit that describes radiation dosage. See **Gray.**

radiation cystitis: Inflammation of the urinary bladder caused by exposure to radiation.

radiation proctitis: Inflammation of the rectum caused by radiation exposure.

radical prostatectomy: Surgery that completely removes the prostate and seminal vesicles.

radiofrequency ablation (RFA): A treatment that uses heat to kill tissue.

rectum: The lowest part of the large intestine, connecting to the anus.

REDEEM trial (Reduction by Dutasteride of Clinical Progression Events in Expectant Management): A study to determine whether dutasteride can retard the growth of prostate cancer.

REDUCE trial (Reduction by Dutasteride of Prostate Cancer Events): A test of dutasteride in chemoprevention of prostate cancer.

retrograde ejaculation: The release of semen into the bladder instead of out through the penis.

robotic surgery: Laparoscopic surgical procedure performed with the assistance of a mechanical robot that translates the surgeon's movements inside the patient's body through surgical instruments.

salvage radiation: Radiation therapy to treat a cancer that has recurred after surgery or other initial treatment.

salvage radical prostatectomy: Removal of the entire prostate, performed to treat prostate cancer that has recurred after radiation or other primary therapy.

seed implants: See **brachytherapy.**

semen: The thick fluid released from the penis during orgasm, containing sperm.

seminal vesicle: One of two glands, connected to the base (top) of the prostate behind the bladder, that secrete a component of seminal fluid.

seminal vesicle invasion (SVI): Spread of prostate cancer into the seminal vesicles.

sex hormone binding globulin (SHBG): A protein in blood that binds testosterone and carries it in the circulation.

simple prostatectomy: A surgical procedure to remove prostate tissue to treat the urinary symptoms of BPH.

sling procedure: A treatment for urinary incontinence in which a piece of synthetic material is attached to the pelvis to compress the urethra.

SPIRIT trial: Test of surgery versus internal radiation (seed implants) in treating patients with Stage II Prostate Cancer.

stage: Describes the size and location of a cancer and how large and extensive it is.

START trial: Trial of surgery versus watchful waiting in early prostate cancer.

stool softeners: Drugs that relieve constipation by causing the stool to contain more moisture, making it easier to pass.

stress incontinence (stress urinary incontinence, SUI): Leakage of urine from an increase in pressure on the abdomen, as from coughing, straining, or sudden movement.

stricture: A narrowing of the urethra caused by scarring.

surgical margin: The outer surface of the tissue that is surgically removed.

telomere: A region of repetitive DNA at the end of a chromosome, which protects the end of the chromosome from destruction.

tenesmus: An urgent desire to empty the bowel, resulting in passage of mucus but little fecal matter.

testis (testicle): One of the two male reproductive glands that produce sperm and testosterone.

testosterone: The principal androgen (male hormone) present in the blood in an active, free form or bound to sex hormone binding globulin (see **sex hormone binding globulin**).

thermal therapy: Use of heat to destroy tissue.

three-dimensional conformal radiation therapy (3D-CRT): A form of external beam radiation therapy in which the tissue exposed to radiation precisely matches the shape of the organ or tumor being targeted.

TNM staging: A system for expressing the size and degree of spread of a cancer by separately describing the extent of tumor as its original location (T), whether and to what extent the cancer has spread to nearby lymph nodes (N), and whether and to what extent the cancer has metastasized to distant sites (M).

total (complete) androgen blockade: Therapy that completely blocks the effects of testosterone.

transition zone: The part of the prostate immediately surrounding the urethra. The transition zone is the site of BPH. Prostate cancers can arise in this zone as well.

transrectal ultrasound (TRUS): Imaging technique in which the prostate is examined through an ultrasound probe inserted in the rectum.

transurethral microwave thermotherapy (TUMT): A nonsurgical treatment for BPH.

transurethral resection of the prostate (TURP): Removal of excess prostate tissue by chipping away with a special instrument. The most common surgical treatment for symptoms of BPH.

tumor suppressor gene: A gene that normally protects a cell from becoming malignant but, when it loses its function, allows cancerous growth to proceed.

ureter: A tube that carries urine from a kidney to the bladder.

urethra: The tube that carries urine from the bladder to the outside of the body.

urethral stricture: See **stricture.**

urge incontinence: A strong, sudden need to urinate immediately.

urinary flow rate: The speed of the stream during urination, measured with a flow meter.

urinary tract: The organs that produce and eliminate urine: the kidneys, ureters, bladder, and urethra.

urodynamic testing: A set of medical tests to measure urinary flow, bladder capacity, and bladder function, used to determine the cause of urinary symptoms.

urology: The field of medicine concerned with the function and disorders of the male genitals and the male and female urinary system.

vaccine: Any preparation designed to prevent or treat disease by stimulating the immune system.

vacuum erection device (VED): Device that induces an erection by creating a vacuum around the penis. A constricting ring maintains the erection.

vas deferens: One of two ducts that carry sperm from the testicles to the prostate.

watchful waiting: An approach to managing prostate cancer. Traditionally, watchful waiting meant to make no attempt to cure or regularly monitor the cancer. Today, the term is often used to mean the deferral of treatment, though patients are actively, regularly monitored and treated when the cancer shows signs of worsening.

GLOSSARY OF MEDICATIONS: INDIVIDUAL DRUGS AND CLASSES OF DRUGS USED TO TREAT PROSTATE DISEASES

Note: Alternative and complementary agents, such as vitamins and nutritional substances, are not included here. They are described in the text and can be located by using the index.

abiraterone: A drug that stops the production of androgens anywhere in the body, including those produced in a cancer.

alfuzosin (Uroxatral): See **alpha blockers.**

alpha blockers: A group of drugs (e.g., doxazosin, terazosin, tamsulosin, and alfuzosin) used to treat urinary symptoms in men. Originally developed to treat high blood pressure, these drugs work by blocking the effects of adrenaline, thus allowing the muscles of the prostate and bladder neck to relax.

alprostadil: A drug used to treat erectile dysfunction, supplied as a suppository (MUSE) or in a syringe for injection (Caverject; also one component of injectable trimix). Alprostadil increases blood flow to the penis, producing an erection.

aminoglutethimide (Cytadren): See **antiandrogens.** The second-line hormonal agent, used for hormone refractory prostate cancer, works by blocking the production of androgens by the adrenal gland. Must be given in combination with steroid hormones (e.g., corticosteroids), which are essential to life but are also blocked by the drug.

ansamycins: A group of experimental drugs being tested as chemotherapeutic agents for prostate cancer.

antiandrogens: A group of drugs (e.g., bicalutamide, flutamide, and nilutamide) used in hormone therapy that block the stimulatory effects of male hormones on prostate cancer cells.

antibiotics: Drugs that kill microorganisms, especially bacteria. Antibiotics can cure both acute and chronic bacterial prostatitis. They are often tried, with limited success, to treat chronic prostatitis/chronic pelvic pain syndrome.

anticholinergics: A group of drugs (e.g., oxybutinin, tolterodine, and banthine) used to relax the bladder and relieve bladder spasms.

anti-CTLA-4: See **ipilimumab.**

Aredia (pamidronate): See **bisphosphonates.**

Avodart (dutasteride): See **dutasteride** and **5 alpha–reductase inhibitors.**

bevasizumab (Avastin): A chemotherapeutic drug that destroys the blood supply required for cancer growth.

bicalutamide (Casodex): See **antiandrogens.** Bicalutamide, taken by mouth, is the most widely prescribed antiandrogen. The dose is lower when bicalutamide is used with LHRH agonists than when it is used alone.

bisphosphonates: A group of drugs (e.g., pamidronate, sodium dodronate, zoledronic acid, and etidronate) used to reduce bone mass loss caused by hormone therapy or by metastases of cancer to bone.

blood thinners. A class of drugs used to hinder the formation of blood clots by preventing the blood from coagulating.

bone protective agent: See **bisphosphonates.**

Bonefos (sodium clodronate): See **bisphosphonates.**

buprenorphine: See **opioids.**

calcium channel blockers: A class of drugs used to treat hypertension.

carboplatin: See **chemotherapeutic drugs.** Carboplatin is an intravenous chemotherapeutic drug with less effect on kidney function than its cousin cisplatinum, but also less effect on cancer.

Cardura (doxazosin): See **alpha blockers.**

Casodex (bicalutamide): See **bicalutamide.**

Caverject (alprostadil): An injectable medication for erectile dysfunction. Caverjet consists of a syringe filled with alprostadil, which can produce an erection by increasing blood flow to the penis.

Celebrex (celecoxib): See **celecoxib.**

celecoxib (Celebrex): See **COX-2 inhibitors.**

Cialis (tadalafil): See **PDE-5 inhibitors.** Tadalafil is sometimes called the "weekend drug" because its effects last longer than those of sildenafil or vardalafil.

Cipro (ciprofloxacin): See **ciprofloxacin.**

ciprofloxacin (Cipro): An antibiotic that is especially effective for urinary tract infections and in preventing infection from prostate biopsies.

codeine: See **opioids.** Codeine, taken by mouth, is an effective medicine for pain after prostate surgery.

Colace (docusate): See **stool softeners.**

Contigen (bovine collagen): A bulking agent that is injected into the urinary sphincter to treat incontinence.

corticosteroids: Hormones (or drugs that have similar hormonal effects) produced by the adrenal gland that reduce inflammation and bleeding from radiation proctitis and prevent nausea and vomiting from chemotherapy.

Coumadin (warfarin): Taken by mouth, this drug prevents clotting of blood by reducing the amount of vitamin K produced by the liver.

COX-2 inhibitors: A group of drugs (e.g., celecoxib and rofecoxib) used to relieve the pain and inflammation of prostatitis and other conditions. Thought to have fewer side effects than aspirin or NSAIDs such as ibuprofen, though the COX-2 inhibitor Vioxx was recently taken off the market when it was found to increase the risk of heart attack and stroke.

custirsen: Experimental antisense inhibitor of clusterin, a gene that retards the death of cancer cells.

Decapeptyl (triptorelin): An LHRH agonist.

denosumab: A monoclonal antibody being studied for the treatment of osteoporosis, which reduces the risk of fracture in prostate cancer patients receiving androgen deprivation therapy.

DES (diethylstilbestrol): A female hormone taken by mouth that stops the production of male hormone by the testicles by blocking the necessary signals from the brain (LHRH).

Detrol (tolterodine): See **anticholinergics.**

Didronel (etidronate): See **bisphosphonates.**

Ditropan (oxybutynin): See **anticholinergics.**

docetaxel (Taxotere): A chemotherapeutic agent used to treat cancer. The combination of docetaxel with other agents has been proven to prolong life in men with hormone-refractory prostate cancer.

doxazosin (Cardura): See **alpha blockers.**

Dulcolax (bisacodyl): A mild laxative, used to relieve constipation; can be taken by mouth or as a rectal suppository.

Durasphere: A bulking agent that is injected into the urinary sphincter as a treatment for incontinence.

dutasteride (Avodart): See **5 alpha-reductase inhibitors**. Dutasteride differs from finasteride in blocking both type I and II reductase enzyme, but it is not clear that this distinction makes any difference in how well it works.

EGFR inhibitor: A substance that stops the action of epidermal growth factor, which promotes cancer.

Eligard (leuprolide): See **LHRH agonists.**

Elmiron (pentosan polysulfate): A drug used to treat bladder pain caused by interstitial cystitis. Elmiron has also been tested as a treatment for chronic prostatitis/chronic pelvic pain syndrome.

erlotinib (Tarceva): A drug used to treat several types of cancer. A tyrosine kinase inhibitor and an EGFR inhibitor.

estradiol: A female hormone in pill form sometimes used to treat prostate cancer.

estramustine: A **chemotherapeutic drug** that combines the effect of an estrogen (female hormone) and a chemotherapeutic agent that kills cancer cells directly, designed especially to treat prostate cancer.

estrogen: Female hormone. Estrogen has been used to treat prostate cancer by inhibiting the production of hormone-stimulating substances (LHRH) in the brain, thus blocking the production of testosterone by the testicles.

etidronate (Didronel): See **bisphosphonates.**

Eulexin (flutamide): See **antiandrogens.**

fentanyl: See **opioids.** Fentanyl provides powerful, quick, but short-lasting pain relief and is often used in epidural anesthesia or as a skin patch for postoperative pain.

finasteride (Proscar, Propecia): See **5 alpha-reductase inhibitors.** Finasteride is approved for use in treating BPH (Proscar) and baldness (Propecia) and may have a role in prostate-cancer prevention.

5 alpha-reductase inhibitors: Drugs (e.g., finasteride, dutasteride) used to treat BPH symptoms by shrinking the prostate. These drugs block the conversion of testosterone to dihydrotestosterone (DHT), the male hormone that stimulates prostate growth.

Flomax (tamsulosin): See **tamsulosin.**

fluoroquinolones: A family of synthetic broad-spectrum antibiotics.

flutamide (Eulexin): See **antiandrogens.**

furosemide (Lasix): A diuretic sometimes used to treat scrotal edema after prostate cancer surgery.

ganciclovir: Antiviral drug used in an experimental gene therapy for prostate cancer.

gefitimib (Iressa): An EGFR inhibitor, used to treat cancers.

gentamicin: See **antibiotics.** Given by injection, gentamicin is one of the most effective antibiotics for urinary infections and prevention of infection after prostate biopsy.

Gleevec (imatinib): The first drug specifically targeted against a mutated gene that causes cancer (chronic myelogenous leukemia). Important as the first drug to prove that targeted cancer therapy works.

goserelin (Zoladex): See **LHRH agonists.**

heparin: See **blood thinners.**

Herceptin (trastuzumab): Monoclonal antibody used to treat prostate cancers that exhibit an excess of the growth-promoting gene HER-2.

histrelin (Vantas): A synthetic male hormone in implant form used to treat symptoms of prostate cancer treatment.

hydrocodone: See **opioids.**

hydrocortisone: See **corticosteroids.**

hydromorphone: See **opioids.**

Hytrin (terazosin): See **alpha blockers.**

imatinib (Gleevec): See **Gleevec.**

Imodium (loperamide): A drug used to treat diarrhea.

ipilimumab (anti-CTLA-4): Human monoclonal antibody, which turns off the natural brakes on the immune system and activates the T-cell response that fights cancer.

ketoconazole (Nizoral): See **antiandrogens.**

ketorolac (Toradol): A powerful anti-inflammatory drug and pain reliever sometimes used to reduce pain after surgery.

Lasix: See **furosemide.**

leuprolide (Lupron, Eligard): See **LHRH agonists.**

Levaquin (levofloxacin): See **antibiotics.**

Levitra (vardenafil): See **PDE-5 inhibitors.**

levofloxacin (Levaquin): See **antibiotics.**

LHRH: Substance that stimulates production of male hormones.

LHRH agonists: A group of drugs used in hormone therapy that shut down testosterone production by the testicles.

lidocaine: A local anesthetic sometimes used before a prostate biopsy.

loperamide (Imodium): A drug used to treat diarrhea.

low-dose estrogens: Small dose of female hormones.

Lupron (leuprolide): See **LHRH agonists**.

MDV3100 (Medivation): An experimental androgen receptor (AR) antagonist, developed for the treatment of hormone-refractory prostate cancer.

Megace (megestrol acetate): Used to treat hot flashes.

megestrol acetate: See **Megace**.

methadone: See **opioids**.

mitoxantrone (Novantrone): See **chemotherapeutic drugs**.

morphine: See **opioids**.

MUSE (medical urethral system for erection): A treatment for erectile dysfunction consisting of a suppository containing alprostadil that is inserted into the urethra. Alprostadil increases blood flow to the penis, which enables an erection.

Nilandron (nilutamide): See **antiandrogens**.

nilutamide (Nilandron): See **antiandrogens**.

nitrates: Drugs used medically to treat chest pain (e.g., nitroglycerin) and recreationally (e.g., "poppers"). Nitrates can interact dangerously with PDE-5 inhibitors.

nitroglycerin: A drug used to treat chest pain (angina).

Nizoral (ketoconazole): See **antiandrogens**.

non-opioid drugs: A group of drugs used to relieve mild to moderate pain (e.g., aspirin, acetaminophen, NSAIDs) that are not addictive.

nonsteroidal anti-inflammatory drugs (NSAIDs): A class of substances (e.g., ibuprofen, aspirin) used to relieve pain and suppress inflammation.

Novantrone (mitoxantrone): See **chemotherapeutic drugs**.

opioids: A group of drugs used to relieve moderate to severe pain. Examples include codeine, tramadol, morphine, methadone, hydrocodone, and buprenorphine.

oxybutynin (Ditropan): See **anticholinergics**.

pamidronate (Aredia): See **bisphosphonates**.

paracetamol (acetaminophen, Tylenol): An analgesic drug (painkiller).

PDE-5 inhibitors: A group of drugs (e.g., sildenafil, vardenafil, tadalafil) used to treat erectile dysfunction by relaxing smooth muscles and increasing blood flow to the penis.

pentosan polysulfate (Elmiron): Prescription drug approved for treating bladder pain caused by interstitial cystitis. Pentosan polysulfate has also been tested as a treatment for chronic prostatitis/chronic pelvic pain syndrome.

Percocet: A combination of the opioid pain reliever hydrocodone and the milder pain reliever acetaminophen. Percocet is often used for relief of pain after surgery.

Percodan: A combination of the opioid pain reliever hydrocodone and the milder pain reliever aspirin. Often used for relief of pain after surgery.

Prednisone: See **corticosteroids**.

progesterone: See **Megace**.

Propecia (finasteride): See **5 alpha-reductase inhibitors**.

Proscar (finasteride): See **5 alpha-reductase inhibitors**.

Provenge (sipuleucel-T): Vaccine used to treat hormone-resistant prostate cancer in its early stages, when PSA is rising.

Rapaflo (silodosin): Alpha blocker that relaxes the prostate, improving urinary flow.

SERMs (selective estrogen-receptor modulators): Drugs (tamoxifen, raloxifene) that act on the estrogen-receptor in ways that vary in different tissues.

sildenafil (Viagra): See **PDE-5 inhibitors**.

silodosin (Rapaflo): See **alpha blockers**.

sipuleucel–T: See **Provenge.**

sodium clodronate (Bonefos): See **bisphosphonates.**

spironolactone (Aldactone): A diuretic used to reduce the swelling and weight gain from fluid retention after surgery.

steroid foam: Medication used to treat rectal irritation, bleeding, and diarrhea.

tadalafil (Cialis): See **PDE–5 inhibitors.**

tamsulosin (Flomax): See **alpha blockers.** Tamsulosin inhibits the specific type of receptor that constricts the bladder neck and the prostate, and may have fewer side effects than doxazosin or terazosin.

Taxotere (docetaxel): See **docetaxel.**

terazosin (Hytrin): See **alpha blockers.**

tobramycin: See **antibiotics.**

tolterodine tartrate (Detrol LA): See **anticholinergics.**

Toradol (ketorolac): See **anti-inflammatory drugs.**

tramadol: See **opioids.**

trastuzumab: See **Herceptin.**

trimethoprim (Trimpex, Proloprim): A drug used for the prevention and treatment of urinary tract infections.

trimix: Injectable mixture of alprostadil, papaverine, and phentolamine used to treat erectile dysfunction by expanding blood vessels and increasing blood flow to the penis. Trimix is not commercially available and must be compounded by a pharmacy.

triptorelin (Decapeptyl): An LHRH agonist.

Uroxatral (alfuzosin): See **alpha blockers.**

Vantas (histrelin): A synthetic male hormone in implant form used to treat symptoms of prostate cancer treatment.

vardenafil (Levitra): See **PDE–5 inhibitors.**

venlafaxine (Effexor): A drug commonly used to treat depression, and also used to reduce the incidence of hot flashes in men on androgen deprivation therapy.

verapamil: See **calcium channel blockers.**

Viagra (sildenafil): See **PDE–5 inhibitors.**

Vicodin: A combination of the opioid pain reliever hydrocodone and the milder pain reliever acetaminophen. Vicodin is often used for relief of pain after surgery.

Vioxx (rofecoxib): See **COX–2 inhibitors.**

warfarin (Coumadin): A blood thinner used to prevent clotting.

Zoladex (goserelin): See **LHRH agonists.**

zoledronic acid (Zometa): See **bisphosphonates.**

Zometa (zoledronic acid): See **bisphosphonates.**

RESOURCES

Countless resources are available to men with prostate diseases and their loved ones. Here is a representative sample of some of the best websites, organizations, and suggested additional readings. Listings are alphabetical by category.

AGING

Rowe, J. W., and R. I. Kan. *Successful Aging.* New York: Dell, 1998.
Based on the findings of the MacArthur Foundation Study of Successful Aging, this book details lifestyle factors that can improve quality of life as we age.

Vaillant, George E. *Aging Well: Surprising Guideposts to a Happier Life from the Landmark Harvard Study of Adult Development.* Boston: Little, Brown, 2002.
This report, based on a fifty-year study of people from highly diverse cultural backgrounds, identifies the apparent keys to successful aging.

ALTERNATIVE AND COMPLEMENTARY MEDICINES

Cassileth, B. R. *The Alternative Medicine Handbook.* New York: W. W. Norton, 1998.
A guide to helpful and harmful alternatives to mainstream medical treatments by a leading expert in the field.

Cassileth, B. R., and C. D. Lucarelli. *Herb-Drug Interactions in Oncology* (CD). Hamilton, Ont.: BC Decker, 2003.
Scientifically based information for cancer patients and physicians on the values and dangers of herbs and remedies.

Moyad, M. A. *ABC's of Nutrition and Supplements for Prostate Cancer.* Chelsea, Mich.: Sleeping Bear Press, 2000.
Practical advice for prostate-cancer patients on nutrients and supplements from a leading expert.

Memorial Sloan-Kettering Cancer Center
www.mskcc.org/mskcc/html/11570.cfm, or go to mskcc.org and search for herbs and botanicals.
1-212-639-2000
Comprehensive information about herbs, botanicals, and other products, as well as a link to the hospital's integrative medicine services and research on alternative healing practices.

National Center for Complementary and Alternative Medicine
www.nccam.nih.gov
1-888-644-6226

An organization of the National Institutes of Health (NIH) that investigates complementary and alternative healing practices in the context of rigorous science. Focuses include research, training, outreach, and integration of proven complementary and alternative practices with conventional medicine.

BENIGN PROSTATIC HYPERPLASIA (BPH)

American Urology Association
www.urologyhealth.org
The patient website of this organization has information on the causes, diagnosis, and treatment of BPH. (The site also offers information on prostate cancer and prostatitis.)

National Guideline Clearinghouse: Guidelines for the Diagnosis and Treatment of BPH
www.guideline.gov/summary/summary.aspx?doc_id=3740&nbr=2966&string=BPH,
or go to www.guideline.gov and type "BPH" in the search bar
info@guideline.gov
Guidelines for the diagnosis and treatment of BPH from the American Urological Association.

National Kidney and Urologic Disease Information Clearinghouse
www.kidney.niddk.nih.gov/kudiseases/pubs/prostateenlargement
1-800-891-5390
Information about BPH, including clinical trials.

CANCER

American Cancer Society
www.cancer.org
1-800-ACS-2345
Information from the leading private cancer organization in the United States.

Información en Español de la NCI
www.nci.nih.gov/espanol
1-800-4-CANCER
Comprehensive information about cancer in Spanish from the National Cancer Institute.

Memorial Sloan-Kettering Cancer Center
www.mskcc.org
1-212-639-2000; 1-800-525-2225
Comprehensive information about all aspects of cancer prevention, diagnosis, and treatment from the world's oldest medical center dedicated to cancer care.

National Cancer Institute (NCI)
www.nci.nih.gov
1-800-4-CANCER
A thorough discussion of cancer screening, diagnosis, and treatment from the government's National Institutes of Health.

NCI List of Designated Cancer Centers
http://www3.cancer.gov/cancercenters/centerslist.html

People Living with Cancer
www.oncology.com/plwc
1-703-797-1914
The patient information website of the American Society of Clinical Oncology (ASCO) provides oncologist-approved information on more than fifty types of cancer and their treatments, clinical trials,

coping, and side effects. Additional resources include a Find an Oncologist database, live chats, message boards, a drug database, and links to patient-support organizations. The site is designed to help people with cancer make informed health-care decisions.

Understanding Cancer
www.cancer.gov/cancertopics
1-800-4-CANCER
Comprehensive information about cancer types, diagnoses, treatments, and clinical trials.

CHEMOTHERAPY

American Cancer Society (ACS)
www.cancer.org/docroot/MBC/MBC_2X_ChemotherapyEffects.asp?sitearea=MBC
1-800-ACS-2345
A comprehensive discussion of chemotherapy, including possible side effects and means to deal with them.

National Cancer Institute (NCI)
www.nci.nih.gov/cancerinfo/chemotherapy-and-you
1-800-4-CANCER
Information about chemotherapy from the National Cancer Institute, including how it works, what to expect during treatment, nutritional needs during therapy, and possible means of financing.

CLINICAL TRIALS

ClinicalTrials.gov
www.clinicaltrials.gov/
1-800-4-CANCER
Information about federally and privately supported clinical trials of new diagnostic tools and treatments for various medical conditions, including all prostate diseases.

Physician Data Query (PDQ)
http://www.cancer.gov/cancertopics/pdq
An NCI database that contains the latest information about cancer treatment, screening, prevention, genetics, supportive care, and complementary and alternative medicine, plus clinical trials.

DRUG INFORMATION

MedlinePlus
www.nlm.nih.gov/medlineplus/druginformation.html
custserv@nlm.nih.gov
Information on prescription and nonprescription drugs.

ERECTILE DYSFUNCTION

Lue, Tom F. *Contemporary Diagnosis and Management of Male Erectile Dysfunction.* Newtown, Pa.: Handbooks in Health Care, 2000.
Written by a prominent urologist, it offers an in-depth look at the causes and treatments for ED.

Mulhall, John P. *Saving Your Sex Life: A Guide for Men with Prostate Cancer.* New York: Hilton, 2008.

Ridwan, Shabsigh, M.D., and Louis Ignarro, Ph.D. *Back to Great Sex: Overcome ED and Reclaim Lost Intimacy.* New York: Kensington, 2002.
Reassuring, scientifically based information on overcoming erectile dysfunction.

National Kidney and Urologic Disease Information Clearinghouse
www.kidney.niddk.nih.gov/kudiseases/pubs/impotence/index.htm
1-800-891-5390

Information about erectile dysfunction from the NIH includes access to a search of the recent medical literature, clinical trials, and resources (*en español también*).

FREE AND SUBSIDIZED SERVICES FOR PATIENTS

Cancer Care
www.cancercare.org
1-800-813-HOPE
One of the oldest private, not-for-profit organizations in the United States. Provides advice and support services free of charge for cancer patients, including counseling, education, information, and referrals, as well as financial assistance.

National Association of Hospital Hospitality Houses, Inc.
www.nahhh.org
1-800-542-9730
Provides lodging and support services to patients and their families who are receiving medical treatment far from their home communities.

National Patient Travel Center
www.patienttravel.org
1-800-296-1217
Provides information and referrals for charitable medical transportation for patients and their families.

Partnership for Prescription Assistance
https://www.pparx.org/
1-888-4PPA-NOW (1-888-477-2669)
This site allows patients and doctors to determine whether the patient is eligible to receive medications free of charge because of financial need.

GENERAL MEDICAL

American Board of Medical Specialties
www.abms.org
1-866-ASK-ABMS
A nonprofit organization of twenty-four specialty societies that list board-certified medical specialists who have completed approved training programs and successfully passed a specialty examination in their fields.

MedlinePlus
www.nlm.nih.gov/medlineplus/healthtopics.html
custserv@nlm.nih.gov
Health information from the National Library of Medicine, including a searchable database of health topics, drug information, a medical encyclopedia and dictionary, health news, and a directory of specialists and hospitals.

NIH SeniorHealth
www.nihseniorhealth.gov
custserv@nlm.nih.gov
Health information from the National Institutes of Health; can be viewed in large type and will read text aloud.

HOSPICE AND OTHER END-OF-LIFE RESOURCES

Hospice services provide comprehensive support services to terminally ill patients and their families.

Hospice Foundation of America
www.hospicefoundation.org
1-305-981-2522

Hospice Net
www.hospicenet.org
Suite 51
401 Bowling Avenue
Nashville, Tenn. 37205-5124

National Hospice and Palliative Care Organization
www.nhpco.org
1-703-837-1500

INCONTINENCE, BOWEL AND URINARY

National Kidney and Urologic Disease Information Clearinghouse
www.kidney.niddk.nih.gov/kudiseases/pubs/uimen/index.htm
1–800–891–5390
A comprehensive source of information about urinary incontinence.

National Digestive Diseases Information Clearinghouse
www.digestive.niddk.nih.gov/ddiseases/pubs/fecalincontinence/index.htm
1-800-891-5389
A comprehensive source of information about fecal incontinence.

INCONTINENCE SUPPLIES

There are many additional online sources for men's incontinence supplies. You can also purchase pads specially designed for men at many drugstores and supermarkets.

At Home Medical
www.athomemedical.com
1-800-526-5895

Direct Medical
directmedicalinc.com/pad.html
1-800-659-8037

UroMed
www.umed.com
1-800-403-9189

PROSTATE CANCER

Campbell, Meredith F., Patrick C. Walsh, and Alan B. Retik. *Campbell's Urology.* 4 vols. Philadelphia: Saunders, 2000.
The definitive textbook of urology, updated every three to five years. Detailed descriptions of the current medical understanding and treatment of BPH, prostatitis, and prostate cancer, with sections on normal anatomy and physiology, and urinary and sexual function and dysfunction.

Ohori, Mak, and P.T. Scardino. "Localized Prostate Cancer" *Current Problems in Surgery* 39 (2002): 833–960.

Vogelzang, N., P.T. Scardino, W. U. Shipley, F. M. J. Debruyne, and W. M. Linehan. *Comprehensive Textbook of Genitourinary Oncology*, 3rd ed. Philadelphia: Lippincott Williams & Wilkins, 2005.
The most comprehensive medical textbook of genitourinary oncology, including prostate cancer, written by international authorities in urology, medical oncology, and radiation therapy. Every aspect of prostate cancer is covered in detail.

Walsh, P. C., and J. F. Worthington. *Dr. Patrick Walsh's Guide to Surviving Prostate Cancer.* New York: Warner Books, 2001.

Department of Defense Congressionally Directed Medical Research Programs
http://cdmrp.army.mil/pcrp
1-301-619-7071
The U.S. Department of Defense is the second largest source of funding for medical research in prostate cancer, after the National Cancer Institute. This site provides information about research grants and research projects.

Memorial Sloan-Kettering Cancer Center
www.mskcc.org/mskcc/html/403.cfm
For information about prostate cancer.

National Cancer Institute: Prostate Cancer
www.cancer.gov/cancerinfo/types/prostate
1-800-4-CANCER
Comprehensive information from the U.S. government's National Institutes of Health about prostate cancer, including support groups and resources, clinical trials, complementary and alternative medicine, statistics, diagnosis and treatment, access to PDQ (a listing of approved clinical trials), and a list of the major research centers for prostate cancer in the United States.

National Comprehensive Cancer Network (NCCN)
www.nccn.org
1-215-690-0300
The NCCN, an alliance of nineteen of the world's leading cancer centers, provides detailed guidelines for the diagnosis and treatment of cancer to help patients and health professionals make informed decisions. For prostate-cancer guidelines, go to www.nccn.org/patient_gls/_english/_prostate/index .htm.

National Guideline Clearinghouse: Guidelines for the Diagnosis and Treatment of Prostate Cancer
http://www.guideline.gov/search/searchresults.aspx?Type=3&txtSearch=prostate+cancer&num=20, or go to www.guideline.gov and type "prostate cancer" in the search bar.
A wide variety of guidelines for screening, diagnosis, and treatment of prostate cancer.

Nomograms: Computer-based tools to predict clinical stage and treatment results.
www.nomograms.org
This URL takes you to a page on the Memorial Sloan-Kettering Cancer Center website that allows you to calculate the probability of success with various treatments for prostate cancer, depending upon the characteristics of your disease (stage, grade, PSA, etc.). Use online or download the software to your computer or PDA.

Phoenix5
www.phoenix5.org
A patient-to-patient site with a particularly good online glossary (www.phoenix5.org/glossary/glossary .html) and abundant links to other patient-oriented resources.

Prostate Cancer Canada Network
www.cpcn.org
1-705-652-9200
The national association of prostate-cancer support groups in Canada.

Prostate Cancer Foundation
www.prostatecancerfoundation.org
1-800-757-CURE
The world's largest source of philanthropic funding for prostate cancer research. Also disseminates information to promote public awareness.

The Prostate Net
www.prostate-online.com/index.html
One man's dedicated effort to provide patient-friendly information about prostate cancer.

Resources in Languages Other Than English
www.cancerindex.org/clinks13.htm
A site with links to cancer resources in many languages.

UrologyHealth.org (See Benign Prostatic Hyperplasia on page 549.)
www.urologyhealth.org
The patient site of the American Urological Association.

Us Too! Prostate Cancer Education and Support
www.ustoo.com
1-630-795-1002; Fax: 1-630-795-1602
Support Hotline: 1-800-80-UsTOO, 1-800-808-7866
The oldest patient support group for men with prostate cancer and their partners, with chapters across the United States and Canada.

PROSTATE CANCER PERSONAL ACCOUNTS

Howe, Desiree Lyon. *His Prostate and Me: A Couple Deals with Prostate Cancer.* Houston: Winedale, 2002.

Korda, Michael. *Man to Man: Surviving Prostate Cancer.* New York: Vintage, 1997.

Martin, W. C. *My Prostate and Me: Dealing with Prostate Cancer.* New York: Cadell & Davies, 1994.

PROSTATITIS

National Guideline Clearinghouse: Guidelines for the Diagnosis and Treatment of Prostatitis
http://www.guideline.gov/search/searchresults.aspx?Type=3&txtSearch=prostatitis&num=20, or go to www.guideline.gov and type "prostatitis" in the search bar.
Prostatitis guidelines from the Association of Genitourinary Medicine in London.

National Kidney and Urologic Disease Information Clearinghouse
www.kidney.niddk.nih.gov/kudiseases/pubs/prostatitis
1-800-891-5390
Information about prostatitis from the NIH; includes access to a search of the recent medical literature.

UrologyHealth.org
(See Benign Prostatic Hyperplasia on page 549.)
www.urologyhealth.org
The patient site of the American Urological Association.

INDEX